Endocrine Imaging

Editor

MARK E. LOCKHART

RADIOLOGIC CLINICS OF NORTH AMERICA

www.radiologic.theclinics.com

Consulting Editor
FRANK H. MILLER

November 2020 • Volume 58 • Number 6

ELSEVIER

1600 John F. Kennedy Boulevard • Suite 1800 • Philadelphia, Pennsylvania, 19103-2899

http://www.theclinics.com

RADIOLOGIC CLINICS OF NORTH AMERICA Volume 58, Number 6
November 2020 ISSN 0033-8389, ISBN 13: 978-0-323-72072-4

Editor: John Vassallo (j.vassallo@elsevier.com)
Developmental Editor: Donald Mumford

Radiologic Clinics of North America (ISSN 0033-8389) is published bimonthly by Elsevier Inc., 360 Park Avenue South, New York, NY 10010-1710. Months of issue are January, March, May, July, September, and November. Periodicals postage paid at New York, NY and additional mailing offices. Subscription prices are USD 513 per year for US individuals, USD 980 per year for US institutions, USD 100 per year for US students and residents, USD 594 per year for Canadian individuals, USD 1253 per year for Canadian institutions, USD 703 per year for international individuals, USD 1253 per year for international institutions, USD 100 per year for Canadian students/residents, and USD 315 per year for international students/residents. To receive student and resident rate, orders must be accompanied by name of affiliated institution, date of term and the signature of program/residency coordinatior on institution letterhead. Orders will be billed at individual rate until proof of status is received. Foreign air speed delivery is included in all *Clinics* subscription prices. All prices are subject to change without notice. **POSTMASTER:** Send address changes to *Radiologic Clinics of North America*, Elsevier Health Sciences Division, Subscription Customer Service, 3251 Riverport Lane, Maryland Heights, MO63043. **Customer Service: Telephone: 1-800-654-2452** (U.S. and Canada); **1-314-447-8871** (outside U.S. and Canada). **Fax: 1-314-447-8029. E-mail: journalscustomerservice-usa@elsevier.com (for print support); journalsonlinesupport-usa@elsevier.com (for online support)**.

Reprints. For copies of 100 or more of articles in this publication, please contact the Commercial Reprints Department, Elsevier Inc., 360 Park Avenue South, New York, New York 10010-1710. Tel.: +1-212-633-3874; Fax: +1-212-633-3820; E-mail: reprints@elsevier.com.

Radiologic Clinics of North America also published in Greek Paschalidis Medical Publications, Athens, Greece.

Radiologic Clinics of North America is covered in *MEDLINE/PubMed (Index Medicus), EMBASE/Excerpta Medica, Current Contents/Life Sciences, Current Contents/Clinical Medicine, RSNA Index to Imaging Literature, BIOSIS, Science Citation Index,* and *ISI/BIOMED.*

Printed in the United States of America.

Contributors

CONSULTING EDITOR

FRANK H. MILLER, MD, FACR
Lee F. Rogers MD Professor of Medical
Education, Chief, Body Imaging Section and
Fellowship Program, Medical Director, MRI,
Department of Radiology, Northwestern
Memorial Hospital, Northwestern University,
Feinberg School of Medicine, Chicago, Illinois

EDITOR

MARK E. LOCKHART, MD, MPH
Professor of Radiology, Chief, Abdominal
Imaging Section, Department of Radiology,
The University of Alabama at Birmingham,
Birmingham, Alabama

AUTHORS

LAUREN F. ALEXANDER, MD
Assistant Professor of Radiology, Mayo Clinic
College of Medicine and Science, Department
of Radiology, Mayo Clinic, Jacksonville, Florida

RONY AVRITSCHER, MD
Professor, Department of Interventional
Radiology, The University of Texas MD
Anderson Cancer Center, Associate Professor,
Department of Interventional Radiology,
Houston, Texas

DEEPTI BAHL, MD
Assistant Professor, The University of Alabama
at Birmingham, Birmingham, Alabama

MELANIE P. CASERTA, MD, FSRU, FSAR
Assistant Professor of Radiology, Mayo Clinic
College of Medicine and Science, Department
of Radiology, Mayo Clinic, Jacksonville, Florida

PHILIP R. CHAPMAN, MD
Associate Professor, Department of Radiology,
School of Medicine, The University of Alabama
at Birmingham, Birmingham, Alabama

NIRVIKAR DAHIYA, MD
Department of Radiology, Mayo Clinic,
Phoenix, Arizona

KHALED M. ELSAYES, MD
Department of Abdominal Imaging, Division
of Diagnostic Imaging, The University of
Texas MD Anderson Cancer Center, Houston,
Texas

LAUREN E. FIORILLO, MD
Assistant Professor, Division of Abdominal
Imaging, Department of Radiology, The Ohio
State University Wexner Medical Center,
Columbus, Ohio

MARY C. FRATES, MD
Professor, Department of Radiology, Brigham
and Women's Hospital, Harvard Medical
School, Boston, Massachusetts

SIDDHARTHA GADDAMANUGU, MD
Assistant Professor, Department of Radiology,
School of Medicine, The University of Alabama
at Birmingham, Birmingham, Alabama

SAMUEL J. GALGANO, MD
Department of Radiology, Sections of
Abdominal Imaging, and Molecular Imaging
and Therapeutics, The University of Alabama at
Birmingham, Birmingham, Alabama

BRANDON A. HOWARD, MD, PhD
Assistant Professor, Division of Nuclear
Medicine, Department of Radiology, Duke
University School of Medicine, Durham, North
Carolina

MALAK ITANI, MD
Assistant Professor, Mallinckrodt Institute of
Radiology, Washington University in St. Louis
School of Medicine, St Louis, Missouri

JOICI JOB, MD
Assistant Professor, Division of
Neuroradiology, Department of Radiology, The
Ohio State University Wexner Medical Center,
Columbus, Ohio

HARMEET KAUR, MD
Professor of Radiology, Department of
Diagnostic Radiology, The University of
Texas MD Anderson Cancer Center,
Houston, Texas

WILLIAM D. MIDDLETON, MD
Professor, Mallinckrodt Institute of Radiology,
Washington University in St. Louis School of
Medicine, St Louis, Missouri

AGATA E. MIGUT, MD
Department of Interventional Radiology, The
University of Texas MD Anderson Cancer
Center, Houston, Texas

AJAYKUMAR C. MORANI, MD
Department of Abdominal Imaging, Division of
Diagnostic Imaging, The University of Texas
MD Anderson Cancer Center, Houston, Texas

DESIREE E. MORGAN, MD
Department of Radiology, Section of
Abdominal Imaging, The University of Alabama
at Birmingham, Birmingham, Alabama

RAJASREE NAMBRON, MD
Clinical Assistant Professor, The University of
Alabama at Birmingham, UAB Multispecialty
Clinic, Montgomery, Alabama

XUAN V. NGUYEN, MD, PhD
Assistant Professor, Division of
Neuroradiology, Department of Radiology, The
Ohio State University Wexner Medical Center,
Columbus, Ohio

MAITRAY D. PATEL, MD
Department of Radiology, Mayo Clinic,
Phoenix, Arizona

NEEMA J. PATEL, MD
Assistant Professor of Radiology, Mayo Clinic
College of Medicine and Science, Department
of Radiology, Mayo Clinic, Jacksonville, Florida

VEERANJANEYULU PRATTIPATI, MD
Assistant Professor, Department of Radiology,
School of Medicine, The University of Alabama
at Birmingham, Birmingham, Alabama

DANIELLE M. RICHMAN, MD, MS
Instructor, Department of Radiology, Brigham
and Women's Hospital, Harvard Medical
School, Boston, Massachusetts

**MICHELLE L. ROBBIN, MD, MS, FACR,
FSRU, FAIUM**
Professor with Tenure, Radiology, UAB School
of Medicine, Department of Radiology, The
University of Alabama at Birmingham,
Birmingham, Alabama

RICHARD ROSENTHAL, MD
Professor, The University of Alabama at
Birmingham, The Kirklin Clinic of UAB Hospital,
Birmingham, Alabama

KEDAR SHARBIDRE, MD
Department of Radiology, Section of
Abdominal Imaging, The University of Alabama
at Birmingham, Birmingham, Alabama

APARNA SINGHAL, MD
Assistant Professor, Department of Radiology,
School of Medicine, The University of Alabama
at Birmingham, Birmingham, Alabama

JENNIFER SIPOS, MD
Professor of Medicine, Director, Benign
Thyroid Disorders Program, Division of
Endocrinology, Diabetes, and Metabolism, The
Ohio State University Wexner Medical Center,
Columbus, Ohio

KATIE SUZANNE TRAYLOR, DO
Neuroradiology Division, Department of
Radiology, Assistant Professor, University of
Pittsburgh Medical Center Presbyterian,
Pittsburgh, Pennsylvania

STEVEN G. WAGUESPACK, MD
Department of Endocrine Neoplasia and
Hormonal Disorders, The University of Texas
MD Anderson Cancer Center, Houston, Texas

CEREN YALNIZ, MD
Department of Abdominal Imaging, Division
of Diagnostic Imaging, The University of
Texas MD Anderson Cancer Center, Houston,
Texas

SCOTT W. YOUNG, MD
Department of Radiology, Mayo Clinic,
Phoenix, Arizona

Contents

Preface: The Breadth and Depth of Imaging of the Endocrine System   xv

Mark E. Lockhart

Diagnosis and Evaluation of Thyroid Nodules-the Clinician's Perspective   1009

Rajasree Nambron, Richard Rosenthal, and Deepti Bahl

> Thyroid nodules are a common clinical problem encountered in an endocrine prac-
> tice. More and more thyroid nodules are now being detected on unrelated imaging
> studies, leading to an increased diagnosis of low-risk thyroid cancers. There is there-
> fore a greater emphasis on risk assessment based on clinical and sonographic fea-
> tures to avoid morbidity secondary to unnecessary therapy. Molecular diagnostics
> are also being widely used to further characterize indeterminate nodules. The Amer-
> ican Thyroid Association and American College of Radiology-Thyroid Imaging Re-
> porting and Data System guidelines are the most commonly used in clinical
> practice for risk assessment.

Thyroid Incidentalomas: Practice Considerations for Radiologists in the Age of Incidental Findings   1019

Xuan V. Nguyen, Joici Job, Lauren E. Fiorillo, and Jennifer Sipos

> Radiologists very frequently encounter incidental findings related to the thyroid
> gland. Given increases in imaging use over the past several decades, thyroid inci-
> dentalomas are increasingly encountered in clinical practice, and it is important
> for radiologists to be aware of recent developments with respect to workup and
> diagnosis of incidental thyroid abnormalities. Recent reporting and management
> guidelines, such as those from the American College of Radiology and American
> Thyroid Association, are reviewed along with applicable evidence in the literature.
> Trending topics, such as artificial intelligence approaches to guide thyroid inciden-
> taloma workup, are also discussed.

Ultrasound of the Normal Thyroid with Technical Pearls and Pitfalls   1033

Danielle M. Richman and Mary C. Frates

> Ultrasound is the best imaging modality for comprehensive evaluation of the thyroid.
> The thyroid is best imaged using a high-frequency linear probe with the patient in a
> supine position with the neck hyperextended. Normal thyroid is homogeneous in
> appearance without defining anatomic landmarks within the gland. A few anatomic
> variants can occur, and it is important for the sonographer and radiologist to be
> aware of these variants, to avoid misidentifying them as a pathology. This article pro-
> vides a comprehensive review of ultrasound of the normal thyroid gland, including
> technique, normal anatomy, anatomic variants, imaging appearance, and technical
> pearls and pitfalls.

Thyroid Ultrasound: Diffuse and Nodular Disease   1041

Lauren F. Alexander, Neema J. Patel, Melanie P. Caserta, and Michelle L. Robbin

> Thyroid ultrasound with gray-scale and color Doppler is the most helpful imaging
> modality to differentiate normal thyroid parenchyma from diffuse or nodular thyroid

disease by evaluating glandular size, echogenicity, echotexture, margins, and vascularity. The various causes of diffuse thyroid disease often have overlapping sonographic imaging features. Thyroid nodules may be hyperplastic or neoplastic, with most due to benign hyperplastic changes in architecture and benign follicular adenomas; only a small percentage are malignant. A systematic approach to nodule morphology that includes evaluation of composition, echogenicity, margin, shape, and any echogenic foci can guide decision to biopsy or follow nodules.

Computed Tomography and MR Imaging of Thyroid Disease   1059

Katie Suzanne Traylor

Over the past several years, there has been an increase in the discovery of thyroid cancers, likely because of the marked increased utilization of computed tomography (CT) and MR imaging. Despite the increase in number of thyroid cancers, the overall mortality remains unchanged because most of these cancers are the differentiated type and have a more indolent behavior. CT and MR imaging are important in the preoperative evaluation of thyroid goiters and thyroid cancer. This article discusses the imaging characteristics of benign and malignant thyroid diseases, and the important information that needs to be relayed to the surgeon.

Parathyroid Imaging   1071

Malak Itani and William D. Middleton

Primary hyperparathyroidism (PHPT) is a common endocrine abnormality, caused in most cases by a single parathyroid adenoma. Surgery remains the first-line curative therapy in PHPT. Imaging plays a vital role in presurgical localization of parathyroid adenomas. Ultrasound provides a safe and quick imaging modality free of ionizing radiation, but is operator dependent. Sestamibi scan offers comparable sensitivity to ultrasound, improved with concurrent tomographic imaging. 4DCT remains a problem-solving technique in challenging cases and after failed neck exploration. We present an overview of various parathyroid imaging modalities, including protocols and findings, in addition to relevant pearls and pitfalls.

Neck Procedures: Thyroid and Parathyroid   1085

Nirvikar Dahiya, Maitray D. Patel, and Scott W. Young

Fine-needle aspiration (FNA) and core biopsy of masses in the neck predominantly include samples from thyroid nodules, parathyroids and lymph nodes. The diagnostic rate of a thyroid nodule FNA improves up to 6 passes and then does not significantly change. Thyroid FNA can be performed on patients who are anticoagulated. Appropriate transducer selection is essential for visualization of the needle. Lymph node biopsies can be additionally sampled for thyroglobulin assay to improve sensitivity for detection of recurrent carcinoma. Parathyroid FNA usually involves additional estimation of parathyroid hormone concentration in needle washouts. Biopsies of the neck are simple procedures with minimal complications.

Imaging of Adrenal-Related Endocrine Disorders   1099

Ceren Yalniz, Ajaykumar C. Morani, Steven G. Waguespack, and Khaled M. Elsayes

Endocrine disorders associated with adrenal pathologies can be caused by insufficient adrenal gland function or excess hormone secretion. Excess hormone secretion may result from adrenal hyperplasia or hormone-secreting (ie, functioning) adrenal masses. Based on the hormone type, functioning adrenal masses can be classified as cortisol-producing tumors, aldosterone producing tumors, and androgen-producing tumors, which originate in the adrenal cortex, as well as catecholamine-producing pheochromocytomas, which originate in the medulla. Nonfunctioning lesions can cause adrenal gland enlargement without causing hormonal imbalance. Evaluation of adrenal-related endocrine disorders requires clinical and biochemical workup associated with imaging evaluation to reach a diagnosis and guide management.

Neuroimaging of the Pituitary Gland: Practical Anatomy and Pathology   1115
Philip R. Chapman, Aparna Singhal, Siddhartha Gaddamanugu, and Veeranjaneyulu Prattipati

The pituitary gland is a small endocrine organ located within the sella turcica. Various pathologic conditions affect the pituitary gland and produce endocrinologic and neurologic abnormalities. The most common lesion of the pituitary gland is the adenoma, a benign neoplasm. Dedicated MR imaging of the pituitary is radiologic study of choice for evaluating pituitary gland and central skull region. Computed tomography is complimentary and allows for identification of calcification and adjacent abnormalities of the osseous skull base. This review emphasizes basic anatomy, current imaging techniques, and highlights the spectrum of pathologic conditions that affect the pituitary gland and sellar region.

Molecular Imaging in the Head and Neck: Diagnosis and Therapy   1135
Brandon A. Howard

This article is a summary of the most up-to-date applications of radiopharmaceuticals to the diagnosis and therapy of benign and malignant diseases involving endocrine or neuroendocrine organs of the head and neck, focusing on radiotracers approved by the US Food and Drug Administration, such as I-123- and I-131-sodium iodide, F-18-fluorodeoxyglucose, Tc99m-sestamibi, as well as the more recently approved tracers Ga-68 DOTATATE and Lu-177 DOTATATE.

Multimodality Imaging of Neuroendocrine Tumors   1147
Samuel J. Galgano, Kedar Sharbidre, and Desiree E. Morgan

Neuroendocrine tumors are rare solid tumors with an estimated 12,000 people in the United States diagnosed each year. Neuroendocrine tumors can occur in any part of the body. There is a wide spectrum of disease, ranging from slow-growing and indolent tumors found incidentally to highly aggressive malignancies with a poor prognosis. Knowledge of neuroendocrine tumor pathology is essential in the diagnostic workup of these patients. This article focuses on the evaluation, detection, and staging of common neuroendocrine tumors with multiple imaging modalities; the information gained with a multimodality approach is often complementary and leads to image-guided treatment decision making.

Neuroendocrine Tumors: Imaging of Treatment and Follow-up   1161
Agata E. Migut, Harmeet Kaur, and Rony Avritscher

Neuroendocrine neoplasms are a heterogeneous group of tumors arising from cells distributed throughout the body. Local and regional disease is managed with surgical resection; however, treatment of higher-grade neuroendocrine tumors (NETs), unresectable or metastatic disease is complex involving a combination of systemic targeted agents, transarterial embolization, and peptide receptor targeted therapies and is discussed in detail. The most important concept in modern NET workup is that an optimal diagnostic strategy requires combination of both anatomic and functional imaging modalities. NETs often present with unknown primary site of disease, and ^{68}Ga-DOTATATE PET can now diagnose these lesions with great sensitivity.

PROGRAM OBJECTIVE

The objective of the *Radiologic Clinics of North America* is to keep practicing radiologists and radiology residents up to date with current clinical practice in radiology by providing timely articles reviewing the state of the art in patient care.

TARGET AUDIENCE

Practicing radiologists, radiology residents, and other healthcare professionals who provide patient care utilizing radiologic findings.

LEARNING OBJECTIVES

Upon completion of this activity, participants will be able to:

1. Describe up-to-date applications of radiopharmaceuticals to the diagnosis and therapy of benign and malignant diseases involving endocrine or neuroendocrine organs of the head and neck.
2. Discuss recent developments with respect to work-up and diagnosis of incidental thyroid abnormalities.
3. Recognize the importance of a multimodality approach in the evaluation, detection, and diagnosis of benign and malignant diseases involving endocrine or neuroendocrine organs of the head and neck.

ACCREDITATION

The Elsevier Office of Continuing Medical Education (EOCME) is accredited by the Accreditation Council for Continuing Medical Education (ACCME) to provide continuing medical education for physicians.

The EOCME designates this journal-based CME activity for a maximum of 12 *AMA PRA Category 1 Credit*(s)™. Physicians should claim only the credit commensurate with the extent of their participation in the activity.

All other healthcare professionals requesting continuing education credit for this enduring material will be issued a certificate of participation.

DISCLOSURE OF CONFLICTS OF INTEREST

The EOCME assesses conflict of interest with its instructors, faculty, planners, and other individuals who are in a position to control the content of CME activities. All relevant conflicts of interest that are identified are thoroughly vetted by EOCME for fair balance, scientific objectivity, and patient care recommendations. EOCME is committed to providing its learners with CME activities that promote improvements or quality in healthcare and not a specific proprietary business or a commercial interest.

The planning committee, staff, authors and editors listed below have identified no financial relationships or relationships to products or devices they or their spouse/life partner have with commercial interest related to the content of this CME activity:

Lauren F. Alexander, MD; Rony Avritscher, MD; Deepti Bahl, MD; Melanie P. Caserta, MD, FSRU, FSAR; Philip R. Chapman, MD; Regina Chavous-Gibson, MSN, RN; Nirvikar Dahiya, MD; Khaled M. Elsayes, MD; Lauren E. Fiorillo, MD; Mary C. Frates, MD; Siddhartha Gaddamanugu, MD; Samuel J. Galgano, MD; Brandon A. Howard, MD, PhD; Malak Itani, MD; Joici Job, MD; Pradeep Kuttysankaran; William D. Middleton, MD; Agata E. Migut, MD; Ajaykumar C. Morani, MD; Desiree E. Morgan, MD; Rajasree Nambron, MD; Xuan V. Nguyen, MD, PhD; Maitray D. Patel, MD; Neema J. Patel, MD; Veeranjaneyulu Prattipati, MD; Danielle M. Richman, MD, MS; Michelle L. Robbin, MD, MS, FACR, FSRU, FAIUM; Richard Rosenthal, MD; Kedar Sharbidre, MD; Aparna Singhal, MD; Jennifer Sipos, MD; Katie Suzanne Traylor, DO; John Vassallo; Steven G. Waguespack, MD; Ceren Yalniz, MD; Scott W. Young, MD.

The planning committee, staff, authors and editors listed below have identified financial relationships or relationships to products or devices they or their spouse/life partner have with commercial interest related to the content of this CME activity:

Harmeet Kaur, MD: owns stock in Nuance Communications, Inc and Twistle, Inc.

UNAPPROVED/OFF-LABEL USE DISCLOSURE

The EOCME requires CME faculty to disclose to the participants:

1. When products or procedures being discussed are off-label, unlabelled, experimental, and/or investigational (not US Food and Drug Administration [FDA] approved); and
2. Any limitations on the information presented, such as data that are preliminary or that represent ongoing research, interim analyses, and/or unsupported opinions. Faculty may discuss information about pharmaceutical agents that is outside of FDA-approved labelling. This information is intended solely for CME and is not intended to promote off-label use of these medications. If you have any questions, contact the medical affairs department of the manufacturer for the most recent prescribing information.

TO ENROLL

To enroll in the *Radiologic Clinics of North America* Continuing Medical Education program, call customer service at 1-800-654-2452 or sign up online at http://www.theclinics.com/home/cme. The CME program is available to subscribers for an additional annual fee of USD 330.00.

METHOD OF PARTICIPATION

In order to claim credit, participants must complete the following:

1. Complete enrolment as indicated above.
2. Read the activity.
3. Complete the CME Test and Evaluation. Participants must achieve a score of 70% on the test. All CME Tests and Evaluations must be completed online.

CME INQUIRIES/SPECIAL NEEDS

For all CME inquiries or special needs, please contact elsevierCME@elsevier.com.

RADIOLOGIC CLINICS OF NORTH AMERICA

FORTHCOMING ISSUES

January 2021
Breast Imaging
Phoebe E. Freer, *Editor*

March 2021
Imaging of the Mediastinum
Brett W. Carter, *Editor*

May 2021
Advanced Neuroimaging in Brain Tumors
Sangam Kanekar, *Editor*

RECENT ISSUES

September 2020
Renal Imaging
Steven C. Eberhardt and Steven S. Raman, *Editors*

July 2020
Vascular Imaging
Christopher J. François, *Editor*

May 2020
Imaging of Disorders Spanning the Spectrum from Childhood into Adulthood
Edward Y. Lee, *Editor*

RELATED SERIES

Advances in Clinical Radiology
www.advancesinclinicalradiology.com
MRI Clinics
www.mri.theclinics.com
Neuroimaging Clinics
www.neuroimaging.theclinics.com
PET Clinics
www.pet.theclinics.com

THE CLINICS ARE AVAILABLE ONLINE!
Access your subscription at:
www.theclinics.com

Preface
The Breadth and Depth of Imaging of the Endocrine System

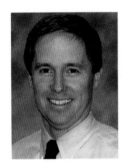

Mark E. Lockhart, MD, MPH
Editor

In 1932, Harvey Cushing made landmark discoveries regarding the details of the neuroendocrine system, but there was a notable absence of imaging at that time. However, imaging now serves as a cornerstone for guidance of both diagnosis and therapy of endocrine disease. The endocrine system plays an important role in human development, and imaging is a key component in the evaluation when the system does not work correctly. Whether there is overproduction, deficiency, or development of malignancy, a variety of techniques can help the physician make the proper diagnosis, and there have been substantial improvements in the imaging armamentarium. For functional and structural changes, molecular imaging, CT, MR imaging, and ultrasound can each provide beneficial information. Detection of vascular flow has greatly improved, especially with contrast-enhanced CT and Doppler ultrasound. Our ability to detect lesions at nearly a cellular level can help with early diagnosis of neuroendocrine cancers. Considering the rapidly changing research in neuroendocrine diseases, it is hoped this update will provide insight for physicians on the myriad of applications for imaging in the field of endocrinology. We hope the readers enjoy the coverage of the topics as much as we enjoyed providing it.

Mark E. Lockhart, MD, MPH
Abdominal Imaging Section
Department of Radiology, JTN 344
University of Alabama at Birmingham
619 19th Street South
Birmingham, AL 35249, USA

E-mail address:
mlockhart@uabmc.edu

Radiol Clin N Am 58 (2020) xv
https://doi.org/10.1016/j.rcl.2020.08.003
0033-8389/20/© 2020 Published by Elsevier Inc.

Diagnosis and Evaluation of Thyroid Nodules-the Clinician's Perspective

Rajasree Nambron, MD[a,1], Richard Rosenthal, MD[b], Deepti Bahl, MD[c,1,*]

KEYWORDS

- Thyroid nodules • Thyroid incidentaloma • Fine needle aspiration • Thyroid cancer
- Thyroid ultrasound • Thyroid imaging

KEY POINTS

- Thyroid nodules are a common clinical problem, and the increased use of imaging techniques has led to increased diagnosis of thyroid incidentalomas and low-risk thyroid cancers.
- Greater emphasis is being placed on risk assessment and sonographic features to avoid unnecessary evaluation and therapy.
- Ultrasound-guided fine need aspiration cytology remains the gold standard test to evaluate thyroid nodules.
- Molecular diagnostics are being widely used for further risk assessment and characterization of indeterminate thyroid nodules.

INTRODUCTION

Epidemiologic studies show that about 5% women and 1% men have palpable nodules in the iodine-sufficient areas of the world.[1] With the advent of high-quality imaging techniques and more patients undergoing radiological imaging for a myriad of clinical problems, thyroid nodules have become a common clinical issue. Most of these nodules are benign; however, the clinical importance lies in the need to exclude cancer.

As per the Surveillance, Epidemiology and End Results (SEER) data, thyroid cancer constitutes 3.0% of all newly diagnosed cancers, and there were an estimated 52,070 new cases diagnosed in 2019. However, the prognosis is excellent, with an overall 5-year survival of 98.2%.[2]

Greater use of thyroid ultrasound has led to an increased diagnosis of low-risk thyroid cancer.[3] Thus, there is a greater emphasis on risk assessment and outcome prediction to minimize morbidity and unnecessary therapy. This strategy led to the changing paradigm in thyroid cancer management from the traditional model of one size fits all to a risk adapted paradigm that involves management based on individualized risk assessment.

THYROID NODULES

A thyroid nodule is a discrete lesion within the thyroid gland that is radiologically and histologically different from the surrounding thyroid parenchyma. Both benign and malignant thyroid disease can cause thyroid nodules. Thyroid cancer occurs in 7% to 15% of any thyroid nodule.[4,5]

PALPABLE AND NONPALPABLE NODULES

The estimated annual incidence rate of thyroid nodules is 0.1% in the United States.[6] The

---

[a] University of Alabama at Birmingham, UAB Multispecialty Clinic, 2119 East South Boulevard, Montgomery, AL 36116, USA; [b] University of Alabama at Birmingham, The Kirklin Clinic of UAB Hospital, 2000 6th Avenue South, Birmingham, AL 35233, USA; [c] University of Alabama at Birmingham, 510 20th Street South, FOT 702, Birmingham, AL 35294-3407, USA
[1] Both of them are first authors.
* Corresponding author. 510, 20th street south, FOT 502, Birmingham, AL 35294.
E-mail address: dbahl@uabmc.edu

Radiol Clin N Am 58 (2020) 1009–1018
https://doi.org/10.1016/j.rcl.2020.07.007

frequency of thyroid nodules, about half of which are solitary on physical examination, increases throughout life.[7] Thyroid nodules are more common in elderly persons, females, people from iodine-deficient geographic areas, and in those with a history of radiation exposure. Single nodules are about 4 times more common in women than in men. Nodules are 10 times more frequent when the gland is examined at autopsy, during surgery, or by ultrasonography. Clinically unrecognized thyroid nodules are common and can be found in up to 50% to 60% of patients at autopsy.[6]

DETECTION

Thyroid nodules can be detected during palpation by the patient or on physical examination by a physician. They are often diagnosed during work-up for hypothyroidism or hyperthyroidism. They are also commonly noted incidentally on imaging studies performed for an unrelated condition. A thyroid nodule discovered during either imaging study or surgery performed because of an unrelated thyroid gland pathology is known as a thyroid incidentaloma. The prevalence rate of a thyroid incidentaloma is 67% with thyroid ultrasound imaging,[8] 16% with computed tomography (CT) or MR imaging,[9] 9.4% by carotid duplex ultrasound,[10] and 2% to 3% with fluorodeoxyglucose (FDG) positron emission tomography (PET).[11] Thyroid incidentalomas, thus, represents a large proportion of patients seen for evaluation of thyroid nodules in an endocrine practice.

INITIAL EVALUATION
History and Physical Examination

The initial evaluation for thyroid nodule(s) is comprised of a thorough history and physical examination. Any personal or family history of benign or malignant thyroid disease should be obtained. The patient should be evaluated for symptoms of hypothyroidism or hyperthyroidism. Pertinent history that increases the risk of malignancy includes a history of head or neck radiation, presentation at extremes of age (less than 14 or more than 70 years), history of rapid growth of the nodule, persistent dysphonia, male gender,[6] and significant family history of differentiated thyroid cancer, medullary thyroid cancer, or multiple endocrine neoplasia (MEN), Type 2.

A complete thyroid examination with palpation of the thyroid gland should be performed. The location, size, and consistency of any palpable nodules should be assessed. Any neck tenderness or cervical adenopathy should also be noted. A complete review of systems for any signs and symptoms of hypothyroidism and hyperthyroidism should also be performed (Table 1).

DIAGNOSIS
Laboratory Studies

The initial laboratory step in the work-up to evaluate a thyroid nodule is obtaining a TSH (thyroid-stimulating hormone) level. A suppressed or low TSH, which signifies a hyperthyroid state, is associated with a decreased probability of malignancy.[12] The management of patients with a low serum TSH is described later in this article. On the other hand, an increased level of serum TSH, even when the level is still within reference limits, is statistically associated with an increased risk of cancer in thyroid nodular disease.[13] Routine measurement of serum thyroglobulin and serum calcitonin is not recommended in the initial evaluation of thyroid nodules.[14]

Imaging
Thyroid ultrasound

All patients with a suspected thyroid nodule, a known nodular goiter, or a thyroid nodule incidentally diagnosed on any other imaging study should undergo a diagnostic thyroid ultrasound. High-resolution ultrasound is the most sensitive imaging technique to detect thyroid nodules, and it is well-suited to evaluate the gland architecture.[15] Thyroid ultrasound should be used to determine the size and number of nodules and provide a description of any abnormal lymphadenopathy in the neck. The size and sonographic features of the nodules (eg, composition, echogenicity, shape, margins, and echogenic foci) are taken into consideration while deciding the need for fine needle aspiration (FNA) as described later in this article.[16,17]

Table 1 Shows the symptoms associated with a hypothyroid and hyperthyroid state	
Hyperthyroidism	**Hypothyroidism**
Palpitations	Dry skin and hair
Heat intolerance	Cold intolerance
Weight loss	Weight gain
Frequent bowel movements	Constipation
Anxiety	Fatigue
Oligomenorrhea	Menorrhagia
Increased appetite	Decreased appetite

Thyroid ultrasound is not indicated in patients with medical thyroid disease if the gland is normal in size without evidence of a palpable nodule on physical examination. It is also not indicated as a screening test except in patients with high genetic risk or possibly in those with history of radiation to the head or neck region.

Ultrasound elastography, which uses both sonography and a computational module to measure tissue stiffness, has been used in some institutions to assess cancer risk. Recently, larger clinical trials show that ultrasound elastography has been inferior to gray scale sonography, especially with partially cystic or cystic nodules.[18] Patients with multinodular goiter, coalescence of nodules, obese patients, or those with nodules that are inferior or posterior are not candidates for ultrasound elastography.[19]

Other imaging modalities

A chest radiograph is not useful and therefore not recommended for evaluation of the thyroid gland, although it may indicate a substernal goiter, which typically presents as a mass associated with tracheal narrowing, tracheal stenosis, and mediastinal widening causing shortness of breath.

Cross-sectional imaging with CT scan is recommended to evaluate and confirm substernal extension and tracheal compression. It is also recommended in suspected advanced thyroid cancer to assess for nodal disease and widespread metastases.[14] Iodinated contrast administration should be avoided in patients with suspected thyroid cancer, as it will delay therapy with radioactive iodine (RAI).

FDG-PET imaging is not recommended for the evaluation of patients with newly detected thyroid nodules or thyroid disease. Incidental FDG-PET uptake in the thyroid gland is seen in 2% to 3% patients and can be either focal or diffuse.[11] Focal FDG-PET uptake in the thyroid is associated with an approximately 35% risk of being cancerous.[20] For PET-positive nodules greater than 1 cm diameter, a dedicated ultrasound and FNA are recommended. However, diffuse FDG uptake in conjunction with sonographic and clinical evidence of chronic lymphocytic thyroiditis does not require further imaging or FNA.

MULTINODULAR GOITER AND TOXIC NODULES

A radioactive iodine uptake and scan should be obtained if the TSH is low to assess whether the nodule is hyperfunctioning.[21] The pattern of uptake in a patient with a single hyperfunctioning nodule generally shows focal uptake in the adenoma with suppressed uptake in the surrounding and contralateral thyroid tissue (**Fig. 1**).

No further cytology evaluation is generally recommended for a hyperfunctioning nodule, as these nodules rarely harbor malignancy. However, the prevalence of thyroid cancer in hyperfunctioning nodules is approximately 3%.[22] Therefore, in clinical practice, FNA of a hyperfunctioning nodule should be considered in patients with risk factors for thyroid cancer, any nodules with suspicious sonographic features, and those that show growth on surveillance.

Patients with a suppressed TSH who are noted to have one or more hyperfunctioning nodules on uptake and scan should also undergo thyroid ultrasound to evaluate the presence of nodules concordant with the hyperfunctioning areas on the scan and other nonfunctioning nodules that might be present (**Fig. 2**).

A multicenter study looked at association of thyroid cancer in patients with nodular Graves' disease and found the rate of carcinoma in a cold nodule was 15% (n = 140 patients). In patients with nodular Graves' disease, ultrasound-guided FNA is useful before radioiodine therapy or surgery.[23]

The risk of thyroid cancer in patients with a multinodular goiter is the same as in those with a solitary nodule.[24,25] Therefore, all nodules within a multinodular goiter that meet sonographic and size criteria concerning for malignancy should undergo biopsy.[14]

Fine Needle Aspiration

FNA is the procedure of choice in the histologic evaluation of thyroid nodules. The nodule size at initial ultrasound, the ultrasound characteristics, and definite increase in size during follow-up are generally considered as reasonable criteria for deciding whether to proceed with FNA. FNA should be performed under ultrasound guidance to ensure optimal placement of the needle tip for nodule sampling.

In the United States, the two commonly used guidelines to estimate risk of malignancy, and thus assess a need for FNA, are the ATA (American Thyroid Association) guidelines[14] and the ACR TI-RADS (American College of Radiology Thyroid Imaging Reporting and Data System).[16,26]

Table 2 shows the ATA ultrasound features and criteria for biopsy as per the guidelines.[14] In comparison, **Fig. 3** shows thyroid nodule imaging features and guidelines for biopsy as recommended by the ACR TI-RADS reporting system.[16]

Both guidelines recommend biopsy if size of the thyroid nodule is over 1 cm and there are high-suspicion sonographic features. For intermediate-

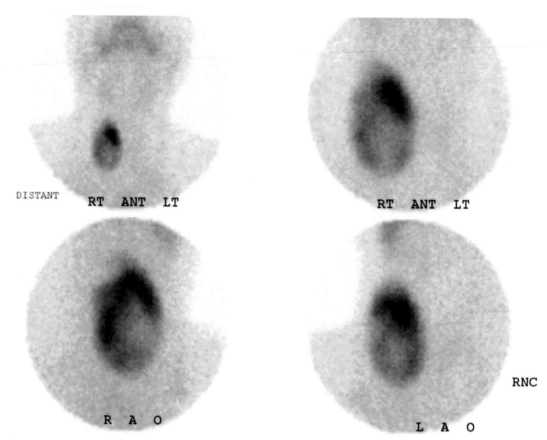

Fig. 1. Thyroid scan with I-131 of a solitary functioning nodule in the right thyroid lobe in a 22-year-old woman noted to have a suppressed TSH. A functioning nodule is nearly always benign, whereas, a nonfunctioning nodule (approximately 90% of nodules) has a 5% to 15% risk of being malignant.

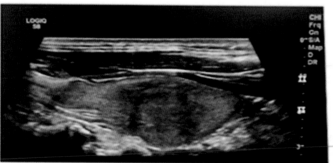
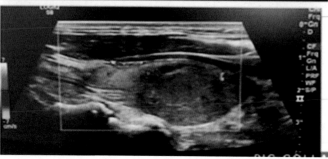

Fig. 2. A 62-year-old man presented with thyrotoxicosis from Graves' disease. Thyroid ultrasound showed a left thyroid lobe solid nodule 2.3 × 1.9 cm (ACR TI-RADS 4). A nuclear uptake scan reported this nodule to be cold, and biopsy proved to be medullary thyroid cancer.

Table 2
Ultrasound features and criteria for fine need aspiration

High Risk of Malignancy (70%–90%)	Intermediate Risk of Malignancy (10%–20%)	Low Risk of Malignancy (5%–10%)	Very Low Risk of Malignancy (<3%)	Benign(<1%)
Hypoechoic nodule with • Microcalcifications • Taller than wide • Irregular margins • Evidence of extrathyroidal extension	Hypoechoic nodule with regular margins	Hyperechoic nodule Isoechoic nodule Partially cystic nodule with eccentric solid component	Spongiform nodule Partially cystic nodule with no concerning features	Purely cystic nodule
FNA at greater than equal to 1 cm	FNA at greater than equal to 1 cm	FNA at greater than equal to 1.5 cm	FNA at greater than equal to 2 cm or observation without FNA	No biopsy

and low- suspicion nodules, there is some variability in the size criteria when the 2 guidelines are compared. FNA can be performed based on patient and clinician preference, availability of high-resolution ultrasound, and a high-volume skilled radiologist. There is currently an ongoing international effort to harmonize recommendations on the management of thyroid nodules based on ultrasound.

CYTOLOGY
Bethesda Classification

Recent efforts to standardize the reporting of thyroid nodule cytology have improved the consistency of this aspect of thyroid disease diagnosis. The Bethesda classification was developed to maintain consistency in reporting and classification of cytology of thyroid nodules.[27,28] The categories can be described as

Composition	Echogenic	Margins	Shape	Foci
Cystic - 0 Spongiform - 0 Mixed cystic/solid -1 Completely solid - 2	Anechoic - 0 Hyperechoic/isoechoic - 1 Hypoechoic - 2 Very hypoechoic - 3	Wider than tall - 0 Taller than wide - 3	Smooth - 0 Ill-defined - 0 Lobulated/irregular - 2 Extra-thyroidal extension - 3	None/comet tail - 0 Macro-calcifications - 1 Peripheral (rim) calcifications - 2 Punctate echogenic foci - 3

Add points from all above categories

0 points	2 points	3 points	4–6 points	>7 points
TR1	**TR2**	**TR3**	**TR4**	**TR5**
Benign	Not suspicious	Mildly suspicious	Moderately suspicious	Highly suspicious
No FNA	No FNA	FNA >2.5 cm Follow if >1.5 cm	FNA >1.5 cm Follow >1 cm	FNA >1 cm Follow >0.5 cm

Fig. 3. Imaging features of thyroid nodules based on ACR TI-RADS reporting system. The total score is determined by adding the number of points assigned to each feature including composition, echogenicity, margins, shape, and the presence of calcifications in the nodule.

Category 1 - nondiagnostic; the estimated risk of malignancy is 1% to 4%

Category 2 - benign cytology implies a less than 3% likelihood of cancer

Category 3 – follicular lesion of undetermined significance (FLUS) or atypia of undetermined significance (AUS); the risk for malignancy is 5% to 15%

Category 4 – follicular neoplasm/suspicious for follicular neoplasm (FN/SFN), Hurthle cell neoplasm or suspicious for Hurthle cell neoplasm; risk for malignancy is 15% to 30%

Category 5 – suspicious for malignancy; there is a 60% to 75% chance of papillary thyroid cancer

Category 6 – malignant

Table 3
The common mutations seen in papillary and follicular thyroid cancer

Papillary	Follicular
BRAF (40%–50%)	RAS (40%–50%)
RAS (7%–20%)	PAX8/PPAR(30%–35%)
RET/PTC(10%–20%)	TP53(21%)
EGFR (5%)	PTEN(8%)
TRK(<5%)	PIK3CA(7%)
PIK3CA(2%)	BRAF(2%)

Data from Roth MY, Witt RL, Steward DL. Molecular testing for thyroid nodules: Review and current state. Cancer. 2018;124(5):888-98.

Role of Molecular Markers

FNA cytology is the reference standard test to distinguish benign versus malignant thyroid nodule, but it is not without limitations. Cibas and colleagues evaluated 635 patients with 776 surgically resected nodules and found substantial inter- and intraobserver variability in the cytopathologic and histopathologic evaluation of thyroid nodules. This variability was higher for AUS and FLUS (atypia and follicular lesions) using the Bethesda criteria.[29]

These nodules are indeterminate on FNA cytology and need to be further characterized to help clinicians decide the best course of action and avoid unnecessary diagnostic thyroid surgeries. Therein arises the application of molecular markers in the management of thyroid nodules. The two commonly used molecular tests to better characterize indeterminate nodules are the Gene Expression Classifier (GEC) and Next Generation Sequencing[30]

GEC was developed to rule out malignancy and thereby decrease the rate of surgeries for indeterminate cytology. GEC was proposed as a rule-out test because of its relatively high sensitivity (92%) and negative predictive value (93%). GEC tests for a panel of mRNAs that assigns a low risk of malignancy similar to a benign FNA.[31]

Mutational testing was proposed for use as a rule-in test because of relatively high reported specificity (86%–100%) and positive predictive value (84%–100%). **Table 3** shows a panel of common mutations in differentiated thyroid cancer.

The Cancer Genome Atlas project mapped mutations to various forms of differentiated thyroid cancer. This subsequently led to development of Next Generation Sequencing (ThyroSeq) to improve the sensitivity and negative predictive

value with mild reduction in specificity and thereby identify benign versus malignant cytology.[32] Both these tests are being optimized for Hurthle cell and follicular tumors. Another approach to molecular testing with high sensitivity and specificity is microRNA testing. Patients should be counseled regarding the potential benefits and limitations of the testing, and about the possible uncertainties in the therapeutic and long-term clinical implications of the results.

Medical Management

Historically, TSH suppression with levothyroxine has been practiced in an effort to decrease the size and prevent growth of existing or new thyroid nodules. The data regarding this practice, however, show modest clinical efficacy while increasing the risk of adverse effects from iatrogenic thyrotoxicosis, which include atrial fibrillation and reduced bone density.[33,34] Therefore, routine TSH suppression for benign thyroid nodules is not recommended.[14] An adequate dietary iodine intake (150 μg daily) has shown some benefit in reducing nodule size.[35] However, it has not been shown whether dietary modification can affect risk of thyroid malignancy.

Surgical Management

Surgery should be considered for benign nodules (Bethseda Category 2) that are large (>4 cm), continue to grow and/or are causing compressive symptoms including dysphonia, dysphagia, or dyspnea.[36,37] (**Fig. 4**).

A single-center study evaluated the FNA results and ultrasound features in patients with nodules over 4 cm. Of the subset of 125 nodules that were identified as benign in preoperative FNA, 10.4% were malignant on postoperative pathology.[38] Another retrospective study confirmed

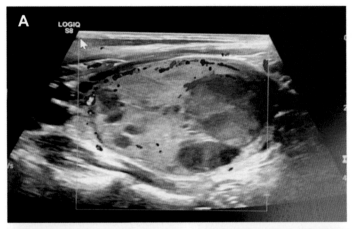

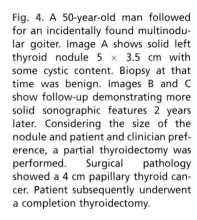

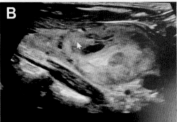

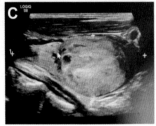

Fig. 4. A 50-year-old man followed for an incidentally found multinodular goiter. Image A shows solid left thyroid nodule 5 × 3.5 cm with some cystic content. Biopsy at that time was benign. Images B and C show follow-up demonstrating more solid sonographic features 2 years later. Considering the size of the nodule and patient and clinician preference, a partial thyroidectomy was performed. Surgical pathology showed a 4 cm papillary thyroid cancer. Patient subsequently underwent a completion thyroidectomy.

that patients with initially benign FNA had a low mortality risk during long-term follow-up even though they had a low, but real risk of false negatives.[39]

Surgical excision of indeterminate thyroid nodules (AUS/FLUS-Bethesda Category 3) should be considered if repeat biopsy or molecular testing or both is either not performed or is conclusive or suspicious.

Surgical excision is also recommended for follicular neoplasms (FN/SFN-Bethesda Category 4). In these patients, thyroid lobectomy is the initial procedure of choice. Total thyroidectomy, however, should be considered in patients with high clinical suspicion, presence of high-risk sonographic features, suspicious molecular diagnostics, presence of risk factors, presence of multiple nodules, and patient preference.

Surgical management is similar to that of a malignant nodule for lesions classified Suspicious for Malignancy (Bethesda Category 5). Historically, total thyroidectomy has been the recommended approach to a patient with biopsy-proven malignant disease (Bethesda Category 6). However, recent data have suggested similar outcomes in patients with unilateral or bilateral thyroid surgery in appropriately chosen patients with low-risk disease.[40,41] Total thyroidectomy is recommended for patients with large tumors (>4 cm), gross extrathyroidal extension, and either regional nodal or distant metastasis. For patients with tumors greater than 1 cm but less than 4 cm with no evidence of extrathyroidal spread or metastatic disease, the initial procedure of choice can be a lobectomy versus total thyroidectomy based on clinical concern and patient preference. Thyroid lobectomy is the procedure of choice for patients with tumors less than 1 cm and no evidence of extrathyroidal extension, nodal, or distant metastatic disease.[42]

For patients with a nondiagnostic cytology (Bethesda Category 1), FNA should be repeated, preferably with onsite cytologic evaluation.[43] Surgery should be considered in nondiagnostic nodules with high-suspicion sonographic features, growth during surveillance, or presence of clinical risk factors for malignancy.

Toxic Nodules

Radioactive iodine therapy and surgery are the recommended treatment modalities for patients with toxic multinodular goiter and toxic adenomas. The size and number of nodules, sonographic features, other comorbidities, and patient preference should be taken into consideration when deciding on the treatment. For patients with hyperfunction, surgery is usually recommended for patients with large multiple nodules, presence of compressive symptoms, substernal or retrosternal extension, concern for thyroid cancer, or need for rapid correction of hyperthyroid state. RAI therapy should be considered for patients with contraindications to surgery, advanced age, and prior surgery or other comorbidities. FNA biopsy should be performed for any nodules with suspicious sonographic features before radioactive iodine therapy, if chosen. Antithyroid drugs may be considered for patients with small nodules and mild hyperthyroidism, in those with advanced age, and patients with contraindications to both surgery and radioactive iodine therapy.

Nodules in Pregnancy

Clinically relevant nodules in a pregnant patient are evaluated the same as in nonpregnant adults. However, radioactive diagnostic scanning is contraindicated in pregnancy. Patients with nodules diagnosed as differentiated thyroid cancer during the course of pregnancy should be monitored sonographically; delaying surgery until after delivery has not been shown to affect outcome.[44] Surgery should be considered in the second trimester if there is evidence of growth of the nodule, cervical lymphadenopathy, or distant metastasis.

FOLLOW-UP

Thyroid ultrasound is used for follow-up over time to assess for changes in nodule size and characteristics. A significant increase in nodule size, defined as increase in size of nodule by 20% in 2 dimensions or a 50% increase in volume is an indication for repeat sampling/FNA.[14] As described elsewhere, the possibility of malignancy is best judged by the ultrasound characteristics, rather than growth. As per the ATA 2015 guidelines, any thyroid nodule with high-suspicion sonographic features and benign FNA cytology should be followed with a repeat ultrasound or FNA in 12 months. For the nodules with intermediate suspicion, the recommended interval of follow-up is typically 12 to 24 months. For a low-suspicion nodule, ultrasound can be repeated in more than 24 months. During the course of surveillance, if the nodule shows any growth or change in characteristic or development of high-risk sonographic features, a repeat FNA should be performed.

The ACR TI-RADS system guidelines have similar recommendations as the ATA 2015 with regards to long-term follow-up of benign thyroid nodules. ACR TI-RADS recommends following nodules up to 5 years and discontinuing surveillance if stable. However, repeat imaging or continued surveillance should be done if there is increase in ACR TI-RADS score or increase in nodule size.

SUMMARY

Thyroid nodules are a common clinical problem encountered in an endocrine practice. Increasingly, thyroid nodules are being detected incidentally, leading to an increased diagnosis of low-risk thyroid cancers. There is, therefore, a greater emphasis on risk assessment based on clinical and sonographic features to avoid morbidity secondary to unnecessary therapy. Molecular diagnostics are also being widely used to further characterize indeterminate nodules. The ATA and ACR TI-RADS guidelines are the most used in clinical practice for risk assessment. Ultimately, it is important to take into consideration a patient's risk factors, clinical findings, comorbidities, life expectancy, and preference prior to making management decisions.

DISCLOSURE

The authors have nothing to disclose.

REFERENCES

1. Vander JB, Gaston EA, Dawber TR. The significance of nontoxic thyroid nodules. Final report of a 15-year study of the incidence of thyroid malignancy. Ann Intern Med 1968;69(3):537–40.
2. SEER-Database. 2019. Available at: https://seer.cancer.gov/statfacts/html/thyro.html. Accessed February 2, 2020.
3. Haymart MR, Banerjee M, Reyes-Gastelum D, et al. Thyroid ultrasound and the increase in diagnosis of low-risk thyroid cancer. J Clin Endocrinol Metab 2019;104(3):785–92.
4. Hegedüs L. The thyroid nodule. N Engl J Med 2004;351(17):1764–71.
5. Mandel SJ. A 64-year-old woman with a thyroid nodule. JAMA 2004;292(21):2632–42.
6. Dean DS, Gharib H. Epidemiology of thyroid nodules. Best Pract Res Clin Endocrinol Metab 2008;22(6):901–11.
7. Mazzaferri EL. Management of a solitary thyroid nodule. N Engl J Med 1993;328(8):553–9.
8. Ezzat S, Sarti DA, Cain DR, et al. Thyroid incidentalomas: prevalence by palpation and ultrasonography. Arch Intern Med 1994;154(16):1838–40.
9. Youserm D, Huang T, Loevner LA, et al. Clinical and economic impact of incidental thyroid lesions found with CT and MR. AJNR Am J Neuroradiol 1997;18(8):1423–8.
10. Steele SR, Martin MJ, Mullenix PS, et al. The significance of incidental thyroid abnormalities identified during carotid duplex ultrasonography. Arch Surg 2005;140(10):981–5.
11. Cohen MS, Arslan N, Dehdashti F, et al. Risk of malignancy in thyroid incidentalomas identified by

fluorodeoxyglucose-positron emission tomography. Surgery 2001;130(6):941–6.

12. Boelaert K, Horacek J, Holder RL, et al. Serum thyrotropin concentration as a novel predictor of malignancy in thyroid nodules investigated by fine-needle aspiration. J Clin Endocrinol Metab 2006;91(11):4295–301.

13. Gerschpacher M, Göbl C, Anderwald C, et al. Thyrotropin serum concentrations in patients with papillary thyroid microcancers. Thyroid 2010;20(4):389–92.

14. Haugen BR, Alexander EK, Bible KC, et al. 2015 American Thyroid Association Management guidelines for adult patients with thyroid nodules and differentiated thyroid cancer: The American Thyroid Association Guidelines Task Force on Thyroid Nodules and Differentiated Thyroid Cancer. Thyroid 2016;26(1):1–133.

15. Radecki PD, Arger PH, Arenson RL, et al. Thyroid imaging: comparison of high-resolution real-time ultrasound and computed tomography. Radiology 1984;153(1):145–7.

16. Tessler FN, Middleton WD, Grant EG, et al. ACR Thyroid Imaging, Reporting and Data System (TIRADS): white paper of the ACR TI-RADS committee. J Am Coll Radiol 2017;14(5):587–95.

17. Fish SA, Langer JE, Mandel SJ. Sonographic imaging of thyroid nodules and cervical lymph nodes. Endocrinol Metab Clin North Am 2008;37(2):401–17.

18. Moon HJ, Sung JM, Kim E-K, et al. Diagnostic performance of gray-scale US and elastography in solid thyroid nodules. Radiology 2012;262(3):1002–13.

19. Azizi G, Keller J, Lewis M, et al. Performance of elastography for the evaluation of thyroid nodules: a prospective study. Thyroid 2013;23(6):734–40.

20. Soelberg KK, Bonnema SJ, Brix TH, et al. Risk of malignancy in thyroid incidentalomas detected by 18f-fluorodeoxyglucose positron emission tomography: a systematic review. Thyroid 2012;22(9):918–25.

21. Ross DS, Burch HB, Cooper DS, et al. 2016 American Thyroid Association guidelines for diagnosis and management of hyperthyroidism and other causes of thyrotoxicosis. Thyroid 2016;26(10):1343–421.

22. Mirfakhraee S, Mathews D, Peng L, et al. A solitary hyperfunctioning thyroid nodule harboring thyroid carcinoma: review of the literature. Thyroid Res 2013;6(1):7.

23. Kraimps JL, Bouin-Pineau MH, Mathonnet M, et al. Multicentre study of thyroid nodules in patients with Graves' disease. Br J Surg 2000;87(8):1111–3.

24. Marqusee E, Benson CB, Frates MC, et al. Usefulness of ultrasonography in the management of nodular thyroid disease. Ann Intern Med 2000;133(9):696–700.

25. Papini E, Guglielmi R, Bianchini A, et al. Risk of malignancy in nonpalpable thyroid nodules: predictive value of ultrasound and color-doppler features. J Clin Endocrinol Metab 2002;87(5):1941–6.

26. Grant EG, Tessler FN, Hoang JK, et al. Thyroid ultrasound reporting lexicon: white paper of the ACR thyroid imaging, reporting and data system (TIRADS) Committee. J Am Coll Radiol 2015;12(12 Pt A):1272–9.

27. Baloch ZW, LiVolsi VA, Asa SL, et al. Diagnostic terminology and morphologic criteria for cytologic diagnosis of thyroid lesions: a synopsis of the national cancer institute thyroid fine-needle aspiration state of the science conference. Diagn Cytopathol 2008;36(6):425–37.

28. Cibas ES, Ali SZ. The 2017 Bethesda system for reporting thyroid cytopathology. Thyroid 2017;27(11):1341–6.

29. Cibas ES, Baloch ZW, Fellegara G, et al. A prospective assessment defining the limitations of thyroid nodule pathologic evaluation. Ann Intern Med 2013;159(5):325–32.

30. Roth MY, Witt RL, Steward DL. Molecular testing for thyroid nodules: Review and current state. Cancer 2018;124(5):888–98.

31. Patel KN, Angell TE, Babiarz J, et al. Performance of a genomic sequencing classifier for the preoperative diagnosis of cytologically indeterminate thyroid nodules. JAMA Surg 2018;153(9):817–24.

32. Nikiforova MN, Mercurio S, Wald AI, et al. Analytical performance of the ThyroSeq v3 genomic classifier for cancer diagnosis in thyroid nodules. Cancer 2018;124(8):1682–90.

33. Sdano MT, Falciglia M, Welge JA, et al. Efficacy of thyroid hormone suppression for benign thyroid nodules: meta-analysis of randomized trials. Otolaryngol Head Neck Surg 2005;133(3):391–6.

34. Yousef A, Clark J, Doi SAR. Thyroxine suppression therapy for benign, non-functioning solitary thyroid nodules: a quality-effects meta-analysis. Clin Med Res 2010;8(3–4):150–8.

35. Grussendorf M, Reiners C, Paschke R, et al. Reduction of thyroid nodule volume by levothyroxine and iodine alone and in combination: a randomized, placebo-controlled trial. J Clin Endocrinol Metab 2011;96(9):2786–95.

36. Shin JJ, Caragacianu D, Randolph GW. Impact of thyroid nodule size on prevalence and post-test probability of malignancy: a systematic review. Laryngoscope 2015;125(1):263–72.

37. Aydoğan Bİ, Şahin M, Ceyhan K, et al. The influence of thyroid nodule size on the diagnostic efficacy and accuracy of ultrasound guided fine-needle aspiration cytology. Diagn Cytopathol 2019;47(7):682–7.

38. Wharry LI, McCoy KL, Stang MT, et al. Thyroid nodules (≥4 cm): can ultrasound and cytology reliably exclude cancer? World J Surg 2014;38(3):614–21.

39. Nou E, Kwong N, Alexander LK, et al. Determination of the optimal time interval for repeat evaluation after

a benign thyroid nodule aspiration. J Clin Endocrinol Metab 2014;99(2):510–6.

40. Matsuzu K, Sugino K, Masudo K, et al. Thyroid lobectomy for papillary thyroid cancer: long-term follow-up study of 1,088 cases. World J Surg 2014; 38(1):68–79.

41. Barney B, Hitchcock Y, Sharma P, et al. Overall and cause-specific survival for patients undergoing lobectomy, near-total, or total thyroidectomy for differentiated thyroid cancer. Head Neck 2011;33: 645–9.

42. Nixon IJ, Ganly I, Patel SG, et al. Thyroid lobectomy for treatment of well differentiated intrathyroid malignancy. Surgery 2012;151(4):571–9.

43. Lin DM, Tracht J, Rosenblum F, et al. Rapid on-site evaluation with telecytology significantly reduced unsatisfactory rates of thyroid fine-needle aspiration: a case-control study. Am J Clin Pathol 2020;153(3): 342–5.

44. Moosa M, Mazzaferri EL. Outcome of differentiated thyroid cancer diagnosed in pregnant women. J Clin Endocrinol Metab 1997;82(9):2862–6.

Thyroid Incidentalomas
Practice Considerations for Radiologists in the Age of Incidental Findings

Xuan V. Nguyen, MD, PhD[a],*, Joici Job, MD[a], Lauren E. Fiorillo, MD[b],
Jennifer Sipos, MD[c]

KEYWORDS

• Thyroid • Incidentaloma • Nodule • ACR TI-RADS • Thyroid cancer

KEY POINTS

• Thyroid incidentalomas are very common and can be initially detected on computed tomography, MR, ultrasound, PET, or other modalities.
• Most thyroid nodules are benign, and most malignant nodules are papillary carcinomas with a favorable prognosis.
• Appropriateness of dedicated sonographic evaluation of incidental thyroid nodules depends on nodule size, presence of aggressive imaging features, patient age, and absence of comorbidities that limit life expectancy.
• Thyroid ultrasound permits stratification of malignancy risk of thyroid incidentalomas and can guide decisions for biopsy or follow-up with imaging.

INTRODUCTION

In routine clinical practice, radiologists are very likely to encounter incidental thyroid abnormalities during interpretation of imaging studies of the neck, chest, or spine. Occasionally, a diffuse thyroid abnormality, such as goiter, may be incidentally encountered (**Fig. 1**), particularly in areas with iodine deficiency, but this article will primarily discuss recent literature relevant to the thyroid incidentaloma or incidental thyroid nodule (ITN), a term that refers to an asymptomatic thyroid nodule identified on imaging studies not specifically intended for assessment of thyroid pathologic conditions. Although incidental detection of an ITN often leads to further evaluation to exclude or diagnose malignancy, fortunately, most ITNs are benign,[1] and most thyroid cancers are papillary thyroid carcinomas, which generally have an excellent prognosis.[2] Familiarity with existing guidelines and evidence-based recommendations regarding ITNs will enable radiologists to more effectively and appropriately communicate the significance of incidentally detected abnormalities to patients and referring providers.

PREVALENCE OF THYROID INCIDENTALOMAS

A familiarity with ITNs is crucial because they are exceedingly common in clinical and radiology practice, with reported prevalence varying by the examined population and assessment

[a] Division of Neuroradiology, Department of Radiology, The Ohio State University Wexner Medical Center, 395 West 12th Avenue, Columbus, OH 43210, USA; [b] Division of Abdominal Imaging, Department of Radiology, The Ohio State University Wexner Medical Center, 395 West 12th Avenue, Columbus, OH 43210, USA; [c] Division of Endocrinology, Diabetes, and Metabolism, The Ohio State University Wexner Medical Center, 1581 Dodd Drive, McCampbell Hall, Columbus, OH 43210, USA
* Corresponding author.
E-mail address: Xuan.Nguyen@osumc.edu

Radiol Clin N Am 58 (2020) 1019–1031
https://doi.org/10.1016/j.rcl.2020.06.005
0033-8389/20/© 2020 Elsevier Inc. All rights reserved.

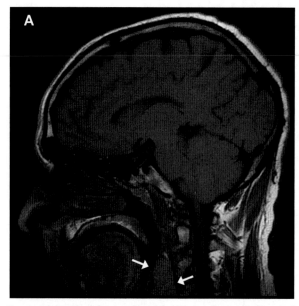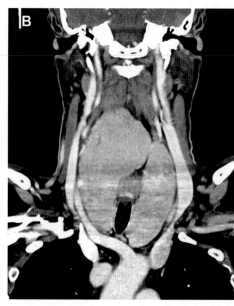

Fig. 1. An incidental retropharyngeal mass (*arrows*) detected on an emergent brain MR performed for headache (*A*) was confirmed to represent goiter on a subsequent neck CT (*B*). This case illustrates the extent to which thyroid abnormalities can be detected on imaging unrelated to thyroid pathologic conditions.

technique. Based on postmortem examinations of thyroid glands of asymptomatic subjects, thyroid nodules are present in approximately half the population.[3] In contrast, thyroid palpation detects nodules in roughly a fifth of asymptomatic subjects.[4] In general, thyroid nodule prevalence varies somewhat linearly with age and shows a strong female predominance.[4,5] Incidentalomas on imaging are reported at frequencies between that of autopsy and palpation, although one should keep in mind that imaging utilization, which varies with age and gender,[6] can have confounding effects on the prevalence and malignancy risk of ITNs.

On neck computed tomography (CT) examinations, ITNs have a prevalence of 16% to 18% based on retrospective investigations,[7,8] but they are described in clinical radiology reports at a lower rate of 6%.[7] About 1 in 4 contrast-enhanced chest CT examinations have an ITN,[9] and lung cancer screening chest CTs can potentially contribute to incidental detection of thyroid abnormalities.[10] CT represents a very common modality on which ITNs or incidental thyroid cancers are initially detected.[11–14] Prevalence of ITNs on MR imaging (**Fig. 2**A, B) is similar to that of CT.[7] However, MR imaging represents a much smaller contribution to incidentaloma detection than CT.[11,12,14]

Ultrasound (US) is generally the modality of choice for characterizing ITNs, but US studies performed for unrelated indications, such as assessing neck vasculature or in a screening context, can result in incidental detection of nodules. US-detected thyroid nodules represent a sizable component of ITNs.[11,12,14] Sonography in randomly selected individuals in a Finnish study detected ITNs in 21% and diffuse abnormalities in 6%.[15] An Italian study examining US examinations in individuals without thyroid disease reported an ITN prevalence of 33%,[16] similar to findings from a large Korean study showing prevalence of thyroid nodules or cysts to be 34% among subjects undergoing thyroid US during routine health evaluations.[17] Prevalence of ITNs as high as 67% on US has been reported.[4]

Focal thyroid gland uptake on fluorodeoxyglucose (FDG)-PET (**Fig. 3**) is detected in only 2% to 3% of oncologic PET studies.[18,19] Nonetheless, PET-detected ITNs comprise a substantial portion of imaging-detected incidentalomas[12,14] and account for a quarter of thyroid cancers initially detected on imaging.[12] Other modalities may detect incidental thyroid cancers and nodules, such as other nuclear medicine studies (octreotide scans), chest radiography, and echocardiography,[11,12] but incidentalomas detected on these modalities are much less common.

AN ERA OF INCIDENTAL FINDINGS?

According to the Surveillance, Epidemiology, and End Results (SEER) Program, thyroid cancer incidence is 15.8/100,000 per year, with a mortality

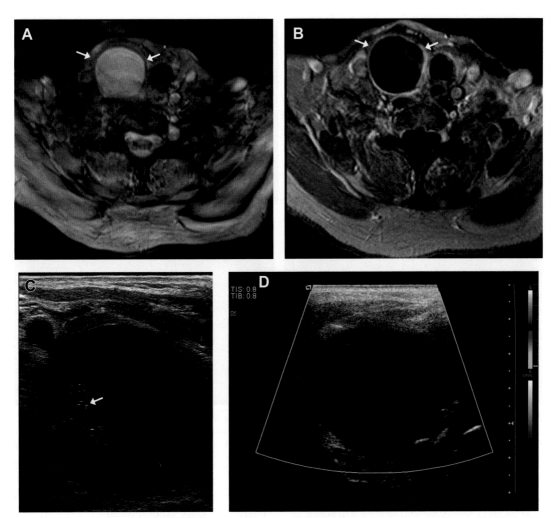

Fig. 2. Axial T2-weighted (A) and postcontrast T1-weighted (B) MR images show a rounded nonenhancing T2-hyperintense lesion (arrows) in the right thyroid lobe. Grayscale (C) and color Doppler (D) US images show an anechoic cyst lacking vascular flow and containing echogenic foci that have comet-tail artifacts (arrow) and likely represent colloid inclusions. This is considered benign by both ATA and ACR TI-RADS criteria.

of 0.5/100,000 per year[2] Much has been written about the seemingly alarming increase in thyroid cancer incidence of approximately 3-fold over the past 4 decades.[20,21] Most of the increased incidence is attributable to more frequent detection of subcentimeter papillary thyroid carcinomas.[20] However, because overall mortality from thyroid cancer has remained relatively stable,[21] several investigators have described this phenomenon as a problem of overdiagnosis.[21–23] One mechanistic explanation underlying the observed increase in thyroid cancer incidence is the presence of a large reservoir of asymptomatic, indolent thyroid cancers that may never reach clinical attention. The near-ubiquity of clinically occult thyroid cancers is demonstrated in 1 study that found foci of papillary carcinoma, most of which

were less than 1 cm, in 36% of consecutive autopsies,[24] indicating a high prevalence of small foci meeting histologic criteria for carcinoma that may never manifest as a clinically apparent cancer.

There are other factors that may contribute to increased detection of incidental findings. Increasing utilization of cross-sectional imaging modalities, including a 10% per year growth in CT imaging use over a similar time period[25] and increased use of point-of-care sonography,[26] because of higher quality and lower cost of US equipment, is thought to contribute to a large portion of the observed increase in thyroid cancer diagnoses. In addition, incidental cancers may also be detected at a greater rate because of rising rates of fine-needle aspiration (FNA) and thyroid

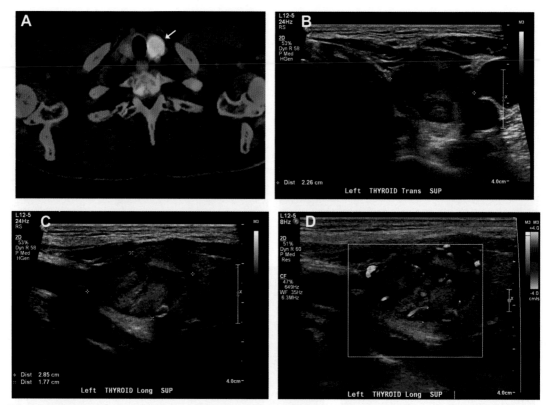

Fig. 3. Staging PET-CT (*A*) for lung cancer shows a hypermetabolic thyroid nodule (*arrow*). Grayscale US (*B, C*) shows a 2.9-cm solid isoechoic-to-hypoechoic nodule (*calipers*) with a smooth regular margin, wider-than-tall shape, and absence of echogenic foci. Doppler US (*D*) demonstrates vascular flow within the nodule. FNA results were suspicious for a follicular neoplasm.

surgeries. One study of claims databases from 2006 to 2011 demonstrated annual increases of 16% for thyroid FNAs and 12% for total thyroidectomies in the United States.[27] Therefore, increased imaging detection or increased diagnostic scrutiny could potentially result in higher thyroid cancer incidences over time.

However, some investigators have reported a small yearly change in incidence-based thyroid cancer mortality on the order of 1% per year,[28] raising the possibility of a relatively small superimposed increase in true cancer risk in addition to effects of increased detection. Incidence of clinically symptomatic or palpable cancers has also increased,[29] suggesting that there may be other factors contributing to these thyroid cancer incidence trends. Regardless of the cause of the observed growth in thyroid cancer diagnoses, the relatively indolent course of most incidental thyroid malignancies has led to a growing interest in the radiology community to refine and standardize radiology reporting and management recommendations for this very common incidental finding.

CANCER RISK IN THYROID INCIDENTALOMAS
Thyroid Nodule Epidemiology

Most ITNs are benign. Malignancy risks among ITNs have been reported at approximately 12% in patients undergoing US-guided FNA.[30] Estimates of malignancy risk among CT-detected ITNs are similar at 11%.[31] FNA and surgical series tend to overestimate malignancy risk for ITNs because of ascertainment bias, because many low-risk nodules will not undergo FNA or surgery, and therefore, would be underrepresented in the cytopathologic or histopathologic data. A population-based study estimating cancer risk among thousands of patients who underwent US evaluation of ITNs found a malignancy risk of 1.6% for thyroid nodules at least 5 mm.[1] Although this malignancy risk estimate is lower than that obtained in FNA or surgical series, the linking of a cohort of more than 8000 patients with cancer registry data allowed that study to capture cancers detected as late as 6 years after the US evaluation. Therefore, it likely yields a more reliable and unbiased estimate of malignancy risk for incidentalomas, irrespective of decisions to perform FNA at the time of imaging.

What Patient Factors Affect Malignancy Risk and/or Prognosis?

One of the early studies examining ITNs in both CT and US detected an increased malignancy risk for thyroid incidentalomas in patients less than 35 years of age.[31] One later study showed better prediction of malignancy when dichotomizing at an age threshold of 52 years.[32] From age 20 to 60, relative risk of malignancy decreases 2.2% per year.[33] However, the effects of age are complicated by the observation that despite the lower risk of malignancy among elderly patients, thyroid cancers identified in older patients are more likely to demonstrate higher-risk histologies.[33] Nonetheless, existing literature offers some justification for a less aggressive management approach for elderly patients. In 1 study of patients at least 70 years of age who had undergone US and FNA for thyroid nodules, the likelihood of death from thyroid cancer, as assessed during follow-up intervals averaging 4 years, was very low (<1%),[34] and 94% of deaths in this cohort were due to causes unrelated to thyroid disease. Of those who did die from thyroid cancer, all had significant-risk thyroid cancers that were not subtle on imaging and/or cytology and were easily discerned at the time of thyroid nodule evaluation. Other potential factors that may increase risk of malignancy in ITNs include male gender,[32,35] radiation exposure in childhood,[36,37] and family history of thyroid cancer.[38]

What Nodule Imaging Characteristics Affect Malignancy Risk and/or Prognosis?

Imaging findings for most ITNs on CT or MR imaging do not permit reliable determination of benignity or malignancy,[31] but the presence of some highly suspicious findings, such as aggressive local invasion, suspicious lymphadenopathy, or systemic metastatic disease, can be used to assign higher risk to nodules seen on CT or MR imaging[8] (Fig. 4). Most of the literature quantifying malignancy risk in ITNs is based on ultrasonographic features, but size is 1 property that can be assessed on different modalities. The relationship between nodule size and malignancy risk in the literature is variable, ranging from absent[35] to a modest positive correlation.[32,39] A study using population-based SEER data to predict thyroid cancer outcomes as a function of tumor and patient variables using a proportional hazards model found that tumor size only increased mortality when size exceeded 2.5 cm.[40] Another

population-based study following all patients who had thyroid nodules examined under US found size greater than 2 cm to be one of 3 sonographic findings significantly associated with cancer risk.[1]

The other 2 sonographic determinants of cancer risk in the above population-based study were microcalcifications and an entirely solid composition.[1] Microcalcifications in a solitary solid thyroid nodule confer a 48% chance of malignancy based on regression analysis of FNA data in 1 study.[35] In a separate multi-institutional series, thyroid nodules with solid composition had a malignancy risk of 13% compared with 4% for mixed solid and cystic nodules.[41] In addition to nodule composition and calcifications, other imaging features in the sonographic literature that affect risk of malignancy in thyroid nodules include echogenicity, shape, and margins.[35,42–44] Sonographic determinants of malignancy have been reviewed in further detail in recent publications.[45,46]

PUBLISHED GUIDELINES FOR REPORTING AND EVALUATING INCIDENTAL THYROID LESIONS
Overview of Existing Guidelines

Before efforts by the American College of Radiology (ACR) to adopt a standardized reporting system, there had been high variability among radiologists regarding the reporting of ITNs[47,48] and subsequent workup of reported incidentalomas.[49] Reduction in ITN workup can be achieved with minimal risk of missing aggressive cancers by applying varying size thresholds for different levels of estimated malignancy risk.[8,11,14,50,51] Several approaches to stratifying malignancy risk on sonography have been proposed, including pattern-based categorization systems proposed by the American Thyroid Association (ATA)[52] and other organizations.[53,54] In 2017, the ACR finalized a feature-based grading system, designated ACR Thyroid Imaging Reporting and Data System (ACR TI-RADS), loosely modeled after the Breast Imaging Reporting and Data System for mammography reporting.[46] Most of the discussion in the following subsections focuses primarily on recommendations from the ACR and ATA.

Decision to Pursue Dedicated Thyroid Ultrasonography

ITNs are frequently detected on CT, MR imaging, or PET as nonspecific nodular findings. In general, ultrasonography allows more definitive characterization of these nodules, but the need to detect potential thyroid malignancy must be weighed against the potential harms of pursuing definitive

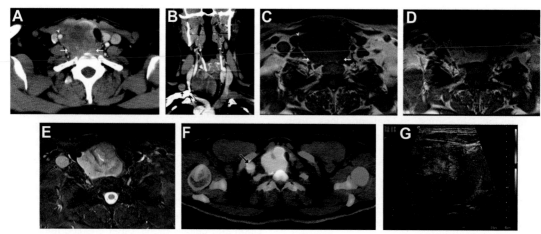

Fig. 4. Axial (*A*) and coronal (*B*) contrast-enhanced CT images and axial precontrast T1-weighted (*C*), postcontrast T1-weighted (*D*), and short tau inversion recovery (*E*) MR images show a large abnormality in the right thyroid lobe with highly suspicious findings, including extrathyroidal extension with loss of adjacent fat planes (*white arrows*) and encasement of the right common carotid artery (*arrowhead*). There is an enlarged, rounded right supraclavicular lymph node (*black arrow* in *B*, *C*, and *E*). PET-CT (*F*) shows FDG avidity in both the thyroid lesion and the right supraclavicular lymph node (*black arrow*). US (*G*) shows a solid hypoechoic mass. Histopathology was anaplastic carcinoma.

evaluation and treatment of a predominantly indolent and asymptomatic incidental finding.[23] A radionuclide thyroid scan is unnecessary in most patients and is only helpful in the setting of low serum thyroid-stimulating hormone.[52] Often, before pursuing further evaluation, review of prior available imaging may be helpful to determine the presence or absence of the nodule on a prior imaging study, even if not explicitly mentioned in the imaging report, and interval change can provide critical information regarding the malignancy risk of the nodule. For instance, a nodule with long-term stability is unlikely to represent a malignancy, whereas a nodule not present on a scan a year ago or having doubled in size over a short time interval raises concern.

A diagnostic thyroid US examination typically involves a high-resolution sonographic evaluation of the neck in hyperextension with imaging performed in longitudinal and transverse planes and includes assessment of the thyroid gland and cervical lymph nodes.[55] Sonographic findings determine the need for FNA or sonographic follow-up or may reassure against the need for further nodule evaluation, but not all ITNs require dedicated evaluation with sonography. The 2015 ATA guidelines[52] state that dedicated thyroid sonography "should be performed in all patients with a suspected thyroid nodule, nodular goiter, or radiographic abnormality suggesting a thyroid nodule incidentally detected on another imaging study," but also include a general statement that evaluation with FNA should only be performed in nodules

greater than 1 cm along with an acknowledgment that subcentimeter nodules may occasionally warrant workup because of symptoms or lymphadenopathy. The general practice of avoiding workup of most subcentimeter nodules is supported by data showing subcentimeter thyroid carcinomas have a favorable prognosis amenable to nonsurgical management using imaging surveillance.[56]

An ACR white paper published in 2015 provides evidence-based recommendations for communicating workup recommendations for ITNs incidentally detected on radiologic imaging.[57] According to these recommendations, dedicated ultrasonography should be performed on all ITNs that are accompanied by suspicious imaging features, such as evidence of local invasion or lymphadenopathy, regardless of nodule size or patient age. For this purpose, focal radiotracer uptake on a nuclear medicine study is considered a suspicious imaging feature, because focal ITN uptake on PET confers a relatively high risk of malignancy (as high as 50%–60%).[18,19,58,59]

In otherwise healthy patients without suspicious imaging features, the ACR recommends US for nodules meeting a minimum size threshold of 1 cm in patients younger than 35 years and 1.5 cm in patients 35 years and older.[57] Pursuing sonographic evaluation may not necessarily be warranted in patients with comorbidities that limit life expectancy or increase treatment risks. For patients with such comorbidities, the ACR white paper recommends against further evaluation in the absence of suspicious imaging features, even if nodules exceed the aforementioned size thresholds. For example, in most patients with stage IV lung cancer incidentally noted to have an ITN on staging scans, further workup of the ITN is generally not indicated. Treatment of the more aggressive malignancy is preferable to interrupting therapy to investigate a much less concerning thyroid neoplasm. In an elderly cohort of patients with ITNs undergoing US and FNA described above, close to half had a comorbidity, such as coronary artery disease, or another primary malignancy at the time of nodule evaluation that more than doubles the risk of all-cause mortality,[34] suggesting that even if workup yields a malignant cytologic diagnosis, there may be relatively little benefit on overall survival.

Decision to Perform Fine-Needle Aspiration or Surveillance

High-resolution thyroid ultrasonography is the test of choice for determining the need for tissue sampling or imaging surveillance. Nodule size can be reliably assessed on US and has been incorporated into both the ATA guidelines and the ACR TI-RADS management recommendations in the form of size thresholds for FNA or surveillance that vary depending on the risk categorization for a given nodule[52,60,61] (Table 1). In ACR TI-RADS, points are assigned based on sonographic determination of composition (cystic/solid characteristics), dominant echogenicity pattern, shape, margins, and echogenic foci,[45,46,60,62] with sonographic features associated with higher malignancy risk, such as taller-than-wide shape or microcalcifications (Fig. 5), awarded more points. These points are summed for the nodule of interest to determine placement in one of 5 risk categories (Table 2). Validation of the ACR TI-RADS criteria has been performed in a multi-institutional study of more than 3000 nodules that found that the vast majority (86%) of nodules showed empiric malignancy risks within 1% of the specified ACR TI-RADS risk thresholds.[41] One of the main differences between ACR TI-RADS and other systems is that it uses a set of imaging characteristics that can be independently assessed, whereas the ATA and several other systems use a pattern-based approach.[52] Both the ATA and ACR TI-RADS systems recommend against FNA for nodules falling under their most benign risk category (Fig. 2C, D). At the highest-risk category, both use a 1-cm threshold for recommending FNA. Between these extremes, ACR TI-RADS and ATA differ slightly in the size threshold used, with ACR TI-RADS using higher size thresholds for FNA. In addition, ACR TI-RADS does not recommend FNA of spongiform nodules (Fig. 6), whereas ATA recommends FNA for spongiform nodules above 2 cm.

Compared with ATA, the ACR TI-RADS system results in a greater biopsy yield of malignancy (14% vs 10%) and a lower estimated frequency of biopsy rate among benign nodules (47% vs 78%).[63] Under the ACR TI-RADS system, nodules classified as at least mildly suspicious but not

Table 1
Thyroid nodule management options under American College of Radiology Thyroid Imaging Reporting and Data System and American Thyroid Association

Management Options	ACR TI-RADS Risk Categories	ATA Risk Categories
FNA	TR5: Highly suspicious (if ≥1.0 cm) TR4: Moderately suspicious (if ≥1.5 cm) TR3: Mildly suspicious (if ≥2.5 cm)	High suspicion (if ≥1 cm) Intermediate suspicion (if ≥1 cm) Low suspicion (if ≥1.5 cm) Very low suspicion (if ≥2 cm)
Surveillance if benign cytology on FNA[a]	TR5: Highly suspicious (if ≥0.5 cm) TR4: Moderately suspicious (if ≥1.0 cm) TR3: Mildly suspicious (if ≥1.5 cm)	High suspicion[b] Intermediate suspicion Low suspicion Very low suspicion
No further workup	TR2: Not suspicious TR1: Benign TR3, TR4, and TR5 (if not meeting surveillance size threshold)	Benign

[a] Or, under ACR TI-RADS, if FNA is not indicated, but the nodule meets listed size thresholds for surveillance. Timing of surveillance varies for each risk category and differs between ACR TI-RADS and ATA.
[b] In addition to repeat FNA.
Data from Refs.[46,52]

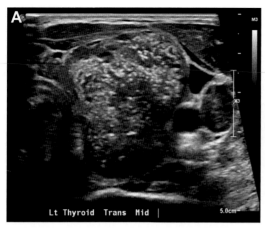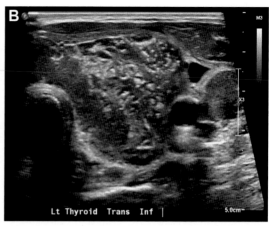

Fig. 5. Axial US images of the left thyroid lobe (*A, B*) illustrate microcalcifications and taller-than-wide shape, which are 2 sonographic findings that are assigned the maximum number of points in their respective feature categories in ACR TI-RADS and are also considered high-risk features in ATA.

Table 2
Risk category assignment under American College of Radiology Thyroid Imaging Reporting and Data System and American Thyroid Association

ACR TI-RADS		ATA	
Risk Category	Description	Risk Category	Description
TR5: Highly suspicious	Composition[a] + Echogenicity[b] + Shape[c] + Margin[d] + Echogenic foci[e] = Total score $\geq$7	High suspicion	Solid hypoechoic nodule or nodular component & $\geq$1 high-risk feature [f]
TR4: Moderately suspicious	Total score = 4, 5, or 6	Intermediate suspicion	Solid hypoechoic nodule with smooth margins & no high-risk features
TR3: Mildly suspicious	Total score = 3	Low suspicion	Solid hyperechoic or isoechoic nodule OR partially cystic nodule with an eccentric solid component & no high-risk features
TR2: Not suspicious	Total score = 2	Very low suspicion	Spongiform or partially cystic nodules without any of the above sonographic patterns
TR1: Benign	Total score = 0	Benign	Simple cysts

[a] Composition score = {cystic or spongiform = 0; mixed = 1; solid or cannot be determined due to calcification = 2}. If the nodule is spongiform, the scores for all the remaining feature categories are 0. If mixed, scores for the remaining categories are assigned based on the predominant solid component.
[b] Echogenicity score = {anechoic = 0; hyperechoic or isoechoic or cannot be determined = 1; hypoechoic = 2; very hypoechoic = 3}. Echogenicity is assessed relative to adjacent parenchyma.
[c] Shape score = {wider-than-tall = 0; taller-than-wide = 3}.
[d] Margin score = {smooth or ill-defined or cannot be determined = 0; lobulated or irregular = 2; extrathyroidal extension = 3}.
[e] Echogenic foci score = {none or large comet-tail = 0; macrocalcifications = 1; rim calcifications = 2; punctate = 3}.
[f] ATA high-risk features: irregular margins, microcalcifications, taller-than-wide shape, interrupted rim calcifications, extrathyroidal extension.
Data from Refs.[46,52]

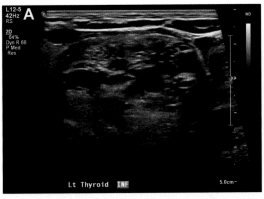 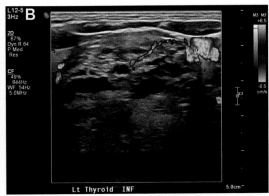

Fig. 6. Grayscale (*A*) US image shows a benign spongiform pattern, considered Very Low Suspicion under ATA and TR1 Benign under ACR TI-RADS. On color Doppler (*B*), there is no abnormal vascularity within the nodule.

meeting size criteria for FNA are followed by US for 5 years in lieu of FNA if they meet size criteria for surveillance. A definitive recommendation against further workup can potentially be made in 32% of nodules under ACR TI-RADS, compared with 1.5% under the ATA guidelines.[63] One advantage of the point-based system used in ACR TI-RADS is that it allows all nodules to be characterized, whereas 3% to 14% of nodules, such as nonhypoechoic nodules with microcalcifications, do not match one of the defined patterns in the ATA system[63,64] (see **Table 2**). Moreover, these unclassifiable nodules have malignancy risks slightly higher than those classified as intermediate risk.[64] The ACR TI-RADS system also has some limitations. Some definitively benign but relatively uncommon sonographic appearances, such as the "giraffe" pattern and "white knight" pattern associated with Hashimoto thyroiditis,[65] would not be categorized as benign under the ACR TI-RADS points system.[46] Another limitation of a points-based system is that the alteration in risk associated with a given finding in 1 feature category theoretically could vary depending on findings in other categories; in other words, simple addition of points from each category may not lead to an accurate risk estimate if the feature categories do not independently and linearly contribute to malignancy risk.

The ATA pattern-based approach may be more efficient among experienced sonographers, whereas the ACR TI-RADS points-based system may be more user-friendly and somewhat easier to implement in clinical practice. Some may find the follow-up guidelines in ACR TI-RADS to be clearer. Until data are available demonstrating superiority of any 1 system in terms of reliability or cost-effectiveness, the risk stratification system used will likely depend on an individual provider's familiarity, comfort, and experience.

FUTURE DIRECTIONS FOR IMPROVING INCIDENTALOMA MANAGEMENT

With better standardization of diagnostic reporting and increasing availability of large-scale clinical and outcomes data, prediction models can be developed to allow more personalized risk assessment and management for individual patients. For instance, 1 group using regression analysis to identify variables predicting malignancy risk made their prediction model accessible in the form of an online calculator (http://thyroidcancerrisk.brighamandwomens.org) that computes risk of malignancy for a thyroid nodule for any combination of selection choices for 5 demographic and US input variables.[32] Although this model requires validation, cancer risk models will continue to evolve in the era of Big Data, and more robust predictions of individualized risk may enable more customized tailoring of management to match each patient's risk tolerance.

Machine learning and other artificial intelligence approaches represent a growing area of interest in the medical arena that could potentially improve prediction of malignancy risk in ITNs. One 2016 study using various machine learning classifier models to predict malignancy risk from a combination of clinical variables and US features performed better than an inexperienced radiologist but not as well as an experienced radiologist.[66] Recently, a machine learning approach was used to tweak point assignments for sonographic features in ACR TI-RADS, producing a simpler set of point assignments with improved specificity.[67] It is likely that new data made available through adoption of standardized reporting practices and ongoing collection of relevant outcomes data will help guide any future adjustments to the various risk stratification systems.

Deep-learning approaches can also be applied to more rapidly assess sonographic images in the context of computer vision. Many studies have applied texture analysis to obtain imaging features from a nodule's sonographic appearance for computer-aided prediction of malignancy.[68] Some studies applied semiautomated or automated techniques to extract texture or morphologic features from US images to serve as input to train machine learning models to predict a nodule's final benign or malignant classification.[69,70] Computer-aided diagnosis (CAD) was recently incorporated into a US workflow in which manual selection of a region of interest yielded an automated real-time prediction of benign or malignant status for a given nodule.[71] In that study, the performance of the CAD system alone was comparable to that of a radiologist, but a radiologist assisted by the CAD showed improved diagnostic sensitivity. Another study reported a detection system for automated thyroid nodule localization on US, feature extraction, and real-time prediction of a nodule's malignant status that performs comparably to experienced radiologists by most metrics, including overall accuracy of 90%, and even shows higher specificity for thyroid malignancy than experienced radiologists.[72] In addition, risk stratification can be extended further to assist in identifying nodules with high-risk genetic profiles; 1 study found that a deep-learning model applied to sonographic images of thyroid nodules can differentiate between high-risk and low-risk genetic mutations with an overall accuracy of 77%.[73] Although many of these artificial intelligence approaches are not currently in widespread clinical use, they likely represent additional future adjunctive mechanisms to facilitate risk stratification of incidentalomas and allow providers to more efficiently prioritize treatment of higher-risk incidentalomas.

WHAT THE REFERRING PHYSICIAN WANTS TO KNOW

- What is the approximate malignancy risk?
- If incidentally detected on a study other than a dedicated thyroid sonogram, is dedicated sonographic evaluation warranted?
- Does the nodule require FNA?
- What is the recommended interval for follow-up imaging?

PEARLS

- ITNs are very common, but most nodules are benign, and most malignant nodules have favorable prognosis.

- Avoid recommending unnecessary tests and review prior imaging studies if available.
- US is the test of choice for stratifying a thyroid nodule's malignancy risk and to guide decisions of whether to biopsy and/or follow-up with imaging.

SUMMARY

Because of their high prevalence, ITNs are likely to be encountered in everyday radiology practice on various modalities, including CT, MR, US, and PET. Increased utilization of cross-sectional imaging modalities over the past several decades likely contributes to rising numbers of ITNs detected. Based on ACR recommendations and the predominantly benign prognosis of thyroid nodules, not all ITNs require further evaluation with US, but when indicated, dedicated thyroid sonography is the best imaging test for estimation of a nodule's malignancy risk and can guide decisions for biopsy and/or surveillance. Standardized reporting practices, appropriate application of evidence-based guidelines, and future efforts to improve predictive accuracy for malignancy risk will likely help curtail the number of ITNs subjected to unnecessary biopsies.

DISCLOSURE

The authors have nothing to disclose.

REFERENCES

1. Smith-Bindman R, Lebda P, Feldstein VA, et al. Risk of thyroid cancer based on thyroid ultrasound imaging characteristics: results of a population-based study. JAMA Intern Med 2013;173(19):1788–96.
2. Howlader N, Noone AM, Krapcho M, et al. SEER Cancer Statistics Review, 1975-2016, based on November 2018 SEER data submission. Available at: https://seer.cancer.gov/csr/1975_2016/. Accessed January 31, 2020.
3. Mortensen JD, Woolner LB, Bennett WA. Gross and microscopic findings in clinically normal thyroid glands. J Clin Endocrinol Metab 1955;15(10):1270–80.
4. Ezzat S, Sarti DA, Cain DR, et al. Thyroid incidentalomas. Prevalence by palpation and ultrasonography. Arch Intern Med 1994;154(16):1838–40.
5. Mazzaferri EL. Management of a solitary thyroid nodule. N Engl J Med 1993;328(8):553–9.
6. Lang K, Huang H, Lee DW, et al. National trends in advanced outpatient diagnostic imaging utilization: an analysis of the medical expenditure panel survey, 2000-2009. BMC Med Imaging 2013;13:40.
7. Yousem DM, Huang T, Loevner LA, et al. Clinical and economic impact of incidental thyroid lesions found

with CT and MR. AJNR Am J Neuroradiol 1997;18(8): 1423–8.

8. Nguyen XV, Choudhury KR, Eastwood JD, et al. Incidental thyroid nodules on CT: evaluation of 2 risk-categorization methods for work-up of nodules. AJNR Am J Neuroradiol 2013;34(9):1812–7.

9. Ahmed S, Horton KM, JR B Jr, et al. Incidental thyroid nodules on chest CT: review of the literature and management suggestions. AJR Am J Roentgenol 2010;195(5):1066–71.

10. Nguyen XV, Davies L, Eastwood JD, et al. Extrapulmonary findings and malignancies in participants screened with chest CT in the national lung screening trial. J Am Coll Radiol 2017;14(3):324–30.

11. Bahl M, Sosa JA, Eastwood JD, et al. Using the 3-tiered system for categorizing workup of incidental thyroid nodules detected on CT, MRI, or PET/CT: how many cancers would be missed? Thyroid 2014;24(12):1772–8.

12. Bahl M, Sosa JA, Nelson RC, et al. Imaging-detected incidental thyroid nodules that undergo surgery: a single-center experience over 1 year. AJNR Am J Neuroradiol 2014;35(11):2176–80.

13. Chaikhoutdinov I, Mitzner R, Goldenberg D. Incidental thyroid nodules: incidence, evaluation, and outcome. Otolaryngol Head Neck Surg 2014; 150(6):939–42.

14. Hobbs HA, Bahl M, Nelson RC, et al. Journal Club: incidental thyroid nodules detected at imaging: can diagnostic workup be reduced by use of the Society of Radiologists in Ultrasound recommendations and the three-tiered system? AJR Am J Roentgenol 2014;202(1):18–24.

15. Brander A, Viikinkoski P, Nickels J, et al. Thyroid gland: US screening in a random adult population. Radiology 1991;181(3):683–7.

16. Bartolotta TV, Midiri M, Runza G, et al. Incidentally discovered thyroid nodules: incidence, and grey-scale and colour Doppler pattern in an adult population screened by real-time compound spatial sonography. Radiol Med 2006;111(7):989–98.

17. Moon JH, Hyun MK, Lee JY, et al. Prevalence of thyroid nodules and their associated clinical parameters: a large-scale, multicenter-based health checkup study. Korean J Intern Med 2018;33(4):753–62.

18. Chen W, Parsons M, Torigian DA, et al. Evaluation of thyroid FDG uptake incidentally identified on FDG-PET/CT imaging. Nucl Med Commun 2009;30(3): 240–4.

19. Nishimori H, Tabah R, Hickeson M, et al. Incidental thyroid "PETomas": clinical significance and novel description of the self-resolving variant of focal FDG-PET thyroid uptake. Can J Surg 2011;54(2): 83–8.

20. Davies L, Welch HG. Increasing incidence of thyroid cancer in the United States, 1973-2002. JAMA 2006; 295(18):2164–7.

21. Davies L, Welch HG. Current thyroid cancer trends in the United States. JAMA Otolaryngol Head Neck Surg 2014;140(4):317–22.

22. Hoang JK, Nguyen XV, Davies L. Overdiagnosis of thyroid cancer: answers to five key questions. Acad Radiol 2015;22(8):1024–9.

23. Hoang JK, Nguyen XV. Understanding the risks and harms of management of incidental thyroid nodules: a review. JAMA Otolaryngol Head Neck Surg 2017; 143(7):718–24.

24. Harach HR, Franssila KO, Wasenius VM. Occult papillary carcinoma of the thyroid. A "normal" finding in Finland. A systematic autopsy study. Cancer 1985;56(3):531–8.

25. Hoang JK, Roy Choudhury K, Eastwood JD, et al. An exponential growth in incidence of thyroid cancer: trends and impact of CT imaging. AJNR Am J Neuroradiol 2013. https://doi.org/10.3174/ajnr.A3743.

26. Moore CL, Copel JA. Point-of-care ultrasonography. N Engl J Med 2011;364(8):749–57.

27. Sosa JA, Hanna JW, Robinson KA, et al. Increases in thyroid nodule fine-needle aspirations, operations, and diagnoses of thyroid cancer in the United States. Surgery 2013;154(6):1420–6 [discussion: 1426–7].

28. Lim H, Devesa SS, Sosa JA, et al. Trends in thyroid cancer incidence and mortality in the United States, 1974-2013. JAMA 2017;317(13):1338–48.

29. Bahl M, Sosa JA, Nelson RC, et al. Trends in incidentally identified thyroid cancers over a decade: a retrospective analysis of 2,090 surgical patients. World J Surg 2014;38(6):1312–7.

30. Nam-Goong IS, Kim HY, Gong G, et al. Ultrasonography-guided fine-needle aspiration of thyroid incidentaloma: correlation with pathological findings. Clin Endocrinol (Oxf) 2004;60(1):21–8.

31. Shetty SK, Maher MM, Hahn PF, et al. Significance of incidental thyroid lesions detected on CT: correlation among CT, sonography, and pathology. AJR Am J Roentgenol 2006;187(5):1349–56.

32. Angell TE, Maurer R, Wang Z, et al. A cohort analysis of clinical and ultrasound variables predicting cancer risk in 20,001 consecutive thyroid nodules. J Clin Endocrinol Metab 2019;104(11): 5665–72.

33. Kwong N, Medici M, Angell TE, et al. The influence of patient age on thyroid nodule formation, multinodularity, and thyroid cancer risk. J Clin Endocrinol Metab 2015;100(12):4434–40.

34. Wang Z, Vyas CM, Van Benschoten O, et al. Quantitative analysis of the benefits and risk of thyroid nodule evaluation in patients ≥70 years old. Thyroid 2018;28(4):465–71.

35. Frates MC, Benson CB, Doubilet PM, et al. Prevalence and distribution of carcinoma in patients with solitary and multiple thyroid nodules on sonography. J Clin Endocrinol Metab 2006;91(9):3411–7.

36. Sklar C, Whitton J, Mertens A, et al. Abnormalities of the thyroid in survivors of Hodgkin's disease: data from the Childhood Cancer Survivor Study. J Clin Endocrinol Metab 2000;85(9):3227–32.

37. Schneider AB, Ron E, Lubin J, et al. Dose-response relationships for radiation-induced thyroid cancer and thyroid nodules: evidence for the prolonged effects of radiation on the thyroid. J Clin Endocrinol Metab 1993;77(2):362–9.

38. Charkes ND. On the prevalence of familial nonmedullary thyroid cancer in multiply affected kindreds. Thyroid 2006;16(2):181–6.

39. Shin JJ, Caragacianu D, Randolph GW. Impact of thyroid nodule size on prevalence and post-test probability of malignancy: a systematic review. Laryngoscope 2015;125(1):263–72.

40. Nguyen XV, Roy Choudhury K, Tessler FN, et al. Effect of tumor size on risk of metastatic disease and survival for thyroid cancer: implications for biopsy guidelines. Thyroid 2018;28(3):295–300.

41. Middleton WD, Teefey SA, Reading CC, et al. Multi-institutional analysis of thyroid nodule risk stratification using the American College of Radiology thyroid imaging reporting and data system. AJR Am J Roentgenol 2017;208(6):1331–41.

42. Chen SP, Hu YP, Chen B. Taller-than-wide sign for predicting thyroid microcarcinoma: comparison and combination of two ultrasonographic planes. Ultrasound Med Biol 2014;40(9):2004–11.

43. Moon HJ, Kwak JY, Kim EK, et al. A taller-than-wide shape in thyroid nodules in transverse and longitudinal ultrasonographic planes and the prediction of malignancy. Thyroid 2011;21(11):1249–53.

44. Kim EK, Park CS, Chung WY, et al. New sonographic criteria for recommending fine-needle aspiration biopsy of nonpalpable solid nodules of the thyroid. AJR Am J Roentgenol 2002;178(3):687–91.

45. Grant EG, Tessler FN, Hoang JK, et al. Thyroid ultrasound reporting lexicon: white paper of the ACR Thyroid Imaging, Reporting and Data System (TI-RADS) Committee. J Am Coll Radiol 2015;12(12 Pt A):1272–9.

46. Tessler FN, Middleton WD, Grant EG, et al. ACR Thyroid Imaging, Reporting and Data System (TI-RADS): white paper of the ACR TI-RADS Committee. J Am Coll Radiol 2017;14(5):587–95.

47. Grady AT, Sosa JA, Tanpitukpongse TP, et al. Radiology reports for incidental thyroid nodules on CT and MRI: high variability across subspecialties. AJNR Am J Neuroradiol 2015;36(2):397–402.

48. Hoang JK, Riofrio A, Bashir MR, et al. High variability in radiologists' reporting practices for incidental thyroid nodules detected on CT and MRI. AJNR Am J Neuroradiol 2014. https://doi.org/10.3174/ajnr.A3834.

49. Tanpitukpongse TP, Grady AT, Sosa JA, et al. Incidental thyroid nodules on CT or MRI: discordance between what we report and what receives workup. AJR Am J Roentgenol 2015;205(6):1281–7.

50. Bahl M, Sosa JA, Nelson RC, et al. Thyroid cancers incidentally detected at imaging in a 10-year period: how many cancers would be missed with use of the recommendations from the Society of Radiologists in ultrasound? Radiology 2014;271(3):888–94.

51. Hobbs HA, Bahl M, Nelson RC, et al. Applying the Society of Radiologists in Ultrasound recommendations for fine-needle aspiration of thyroid nodules: effect on workup and malignancy detection. AJR Am J Roentgenol 2014;202(3):602–7.

52. Haugen BR, Alexander EK, Bible KC, et al. 2015 American Thyroid Association Management Guidelines for Adult Patients with Thyroid Nodules and Differentiated Thyroid Cancer: the American Thyroid Association Guidelines Task Force on Thyroid Nodules and Differentiated Thyroid Cancer. Thyroid 2016;26(1):1–133.

53. Gharib H, Papini E, Valcavi R, et al. American Association of Clinical Endocrinologists and Associazione Medici Endocrinologi Medical Guidelines for clinical practice for the diagnosis and management of thyroid nodules. Endocr Pract 2006;12(1):63–102.

54. Shin JH, Baek JH, Chung J, et al. Ultrasonography diagnosis and imaging-based management of thyroid nodules: revised Korean Society of Thyroid Radiology consensus statement and recommendations. Korean J Radiol 2016;17(3):370–95.

55. American Institute of Ultrasound in Medicine. American College of Radiology, Society for Pediatric Radiology, Society of Radiologists in Ultrasound. AIUM practice guideline for the performance of a thyroid and parathyroid ultrasound examination. J Ultrasound Med 2013;32(7):1319–29.

56. Ito Y, Miyauchi A, Inoue H, et al. An observational trial for papillary thyroid microcarcinoma in Japanese patients. World J Surg 2010;34(1):28–35.

57. Hoang JK, Langer JE, Middleton WD, et al. Managing incidental thyroid nodules detected on imaging: white paper of the ACR Incidental Thyroid Findings Committee. J Am Coll Radiol 2015;12(2):143–50.

58. Soelberg KK, Bonnema SJ, Brix TH, et al. Risk of malignancy in thyroid incidentalomas detected by 18F-fluorodeoxyglucose positron emission tomography: a systematic review. Thyroid 2012;22(9):918–25.

59. Salvatori M, Melis L, Castaldi P, et al. Clinical significance of focal and diffuse thyroid diseases identified by (18)F-fluorodeoxyglucose positron emission tomography. Biomed Pharmacother 2007;61(8):488–93.

60. Tessler FN, Middleton WD, Grant EG. Thyroid imaging reporting and data system (TI-RADS): a user's guide. Radiology 2018;287(1):29–36.

61. Maxwell C, Sipos JA. Clinical diagnostic evaluation of thyroid nodules. Endocrinol Metab Clin North Am 2019;48(1):61–84.

62. Horvath E, Majlis S, Rossi R, et al. An ultrasonogram reporting system for thyroid nodules stratifying cancer risk for clinical management. J Clin Endocrinol Metab 2009;94(5):1748–51.

63. Middleton WD, Teefey SA, Reading CC, et al. Comparison of performance characteristics of American College of Radiology TI-RADS, Korean Society of Thyroid Radiology TIRADS, and American Thyroid Association Guidelines. AJR Am J Roentgenol 2018;210(5):1148–54.

64. Yoon JH, Lee HS, Kim EK, et al. Malignancy risk stratification of thyroid nodules: comparison between the thyroid imaging reporting and data system and the 2014 American Thyroid Association Management Guidelines. Radiology 2016;278(3):917–24.

65. Virmani V, Hammond I. Sonographic patterns of benign thyroid nodules: verification at our institution. AJR Am J Roentgenol 2011;196(4):891–5.

66. Wu H, Deng Z, Zhang B, et al. Classifier model based on machine learning algorithms: application to differential diagnosis of suspicious thyroid nodules via sonography. AJR Am J Roentgenol 2016;207(4):859–64.

67. Wildman-Tobriner B, Buda M, Hoang JK, et al. Using artificial intelligence to revise ACR TI-RADS risk stratification of thyroid nodules: diagnostic accuracy and utility. Radiology 2019;292(1):112–9.

68. Sollini M, Cozzi L, Chiti A, et al. Texture analysis and machine learning to characterize suspected thyroid nodules and differentiated thyroid cancer: where do we stand? Eur J Radiol 2018;99:1–8.

69. Chi J, Walia E, Babyn P, et al. Thyroid nodule classification in ultrasound images by fine-tuning deep convolutional neural network. J Digit Imaging 2017; 30(4):477–86.

70. Yu Q, Jiang T, Zhou A, et al. Computer-aided diagnosis of malignant or benign thyroid nodes based on ultrasound images. Eur Arch Otorhinolaryngol 2017;274(7):2891–7.

71. Yoo YJ, Ha EJ, Cho YJ, et al. Computer-aided diagnosis of thyroid nodules via ultrasonography: initial clinical experience. Korean J Radiol 2018;19(4):665–72.

72. Wang L, Yang S, Yang S, et al. Automatic thyroid nodule recognition and diagnosis in ultrasound imaging with the YOLOv2 neural network. World J Surg Oncol 2019;17(1):12.

73. Daniels K, Gummadi S, Zhu Z, et al. Machine learning by ultrasonography for genetic risk stratification of thyroid nodules. JAMA Otolaryngol Head Neck Surg 2019;1–6. https://doi.org/10.1001/jamaoto.2019.3073.

Ultrasound of the Normal Thyroid with Technical Pearls and Pitfalls

Danielle M. Richman, MD, MS*, Mary C. Frates, MD

KEYWORDS

- Thyroid • Thyroid anatomy • Normal anatomic variants of the thyroid • Ultrasound
- Technical pitfalls • Technical pearls

KEY POINTS

- Ultrasound is the best screening and diagnostic test for evaluation of the thyroid gland.
- Thyroid ultrasound is best performed with the patient in a supine position with the neck hyperextended.
- The normal thyroid gland is homogeneous in appearance.
- There are a few anatomic variants to consider when imaging the thyroid gland as to not mistake normal anatomy for pathology.

INTRODUCTION

The thyroid is a superficial structure in the anterior neck. Because of this superficial location, ultrasound is the imaging modality of choice for evaluation of the thyroid gland. It is safe, inexpensive, and an effective diagnostic test. Furthermore, the components of ultrasound of the thyroid gland are well established, including the appearance of the normal thyroid gland and thyroid pathology.

IMAGING PROTOCOLS

The thyroid is imaged using a high-frequency linear transducer (7–15 MHz) with the patient lying supine with the neck in hyperextension. Placing a rolled towel beneath the upper shoulders can help extend the neck in larger patients or in patients with a low-lying gland. Ideally, the highest frequency available should be used to evaluate the thyroid gland; however, in certain clinical circumstances the frequency should be decreased to optimize tissue penetration. Both lobes should be imaged in transverse and longitudinal planes, and the isthmus should be imaged in the transverse plane. Measurements should be obtained for each lobe including the anteroposterior, transverse, and sagittal dimensions. The anteroposterior dimension of the isthmus should be measured in the transverse plane. Color Doppler images are obtained to supplement gray scale images in the appropriate clinical setting (ie, suspected thyroiditis) and to help characterize a focal abnormality or nodule. Imaging should also extend superiorly in the midline to detect a pyramidal lobe or thyroglossal duct cyst.

A complete evaluation of the thyroid also includes imaging of the internal jugular lymph node chain bilaterally to assess for the presence of enlarged or abnormal-appearing lymph nodes.[1] The bilateral internal jugular chains are imaged in the transverse plane from the clavicle to the level of the hyoid (levels III, IV, and VI). Any enlarged benign-appearing lymph nodes or

Department of Radiology, Brigham and Women's Hospital, Harvard Medical School, 75 Francis Street, Boston, MA 02115, USA
* Corresponding author.
E-mail address: DMRichman@partners.org

Radiol Clin N Am 58 (2020) 1033–1039
https://doi.org/10.1016/j.rcl.2020.06.006

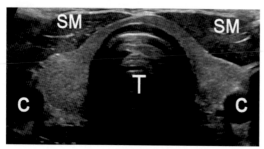

Fig. 1. Normal transverse thyroid on grayscale ultrasound. C = carotid artery; SM = strap muscles; T = trachea. Note the homogenous echotexture and symmetric morphology without enlargement.

abnormal-appearing lymph nodes of any size are measured in three planes (anteroposterior, transverse, sagittal). Because enlarged benign-appearing lymph nodes are commonly identified in levels IA and IB and are almost universally related to the mouth and not the thyroid, these levels are not included in the standard thyroid protocol.

IMAGING FINDINGS

The thyroid is a bilobed structure in the neck that is located anterior to the trachea, with the lobes extending vertically along the right and left sides of the trachea (Fig. 1). The isthmus is the portion of the thyroid gland that connects the two lobes anteriorly. The trachea lies immediately posterior to the isthmus and is air-filled. Posterolateral to the thyroid lobe on each side is the carotid sheath, containing the common carotid artery medially and internal jugular vein laterally. Immediately anterior (superficial) to the thyroid are the strap muscles. The strap muscles include the sternohyoid and sternothyroid

anterior to the thyroid, the sternocleidomastoid muscles anterolateral to the thyroid, and the longus colli muscles posteriorly. The esophagus is most commonly located posterior to the left lobe of the thyroid and can contain air (Fig. 2). When evaluating the thyroid in the context of pathology that the thyroid lacks a true capsule, it does typically have a well-defined peripheral margin.

Sonographically, the normal thyroid gland is homogeneously echogenic with increased echogenicity as compared with the adjacent strap muscles. There are no specific anatomic landmarks within the thyroid. The size of the normal thyroid gland is variable, but in adults, each lobe measures approximately 5 × 2 × 2 cm (sagittal × anteroposterior × transverse) with the isthmus measuring up to 0.3 cm in anteroposterior dimension.[2–6] A thyroid gland that is larger than these measurements is typically considered enlarged. An additional imaging finding that can further suggest that the thyroid is enlarged is bulging of the anterior surface of each lobe because this surface is typically symmetric and flat appearing (Fig. 3A). Extension of the gland over the anterior surface of the common carotid artery on a transverse image is evidence of gland enlargement (Fig. 3B). The normal thyroid gland can also extend over the surface of the carotid, but the anterior contour is typically flat. In children, gland shape and contour are used to indicate gland enlargement rather than size.

Sonographic evaluation of lymph nodes in the mid and low neck (levels III, IV, and VI) should be part of every thyroid ultrasound. Size and sonographic characteristics of the nodes should be assessed. Although size criteria are varied, at our institution a lymph node is considered enlarged if it measures greater than or equal to 7 mm in transverse diameter.[2] Size and location

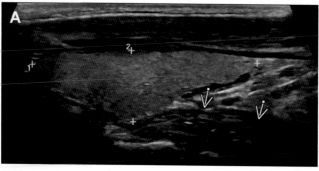
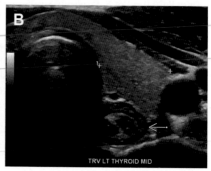

Fig. 2. (A) Sagittal left lobe of the thyroid on grayscale ultrasound (calipers). The esophagus is seen posteriorly (arrows). (B) Transverse image of the left lobe of the thyroid (calipers) with the esophagus located more posterior (arrow).

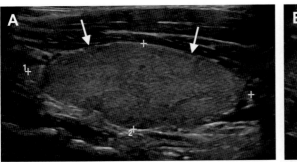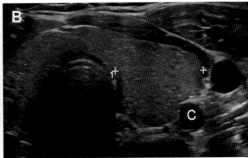

Fig. 3. (A) Sagittal grayscale ultrasound image of the thyroid (*calipers*) with bulging of the anterior potion (*arrows*), which suggests an enlarged gland. (B) Transverse grayscale ultrasound image of an enlarged left lobe of the thyroid (*calipers*) extending over the carotid artery (C).

of benign nodes meeting the criteria for enlargement are included in the report. Sonographic characteristics that are highly correlated with benign etiologies include an elongated shape, tapered or pointed ends, and a thin echogenic hilum. Color Doppler is used to visualize a single vessel entering the node at the hilum and branching toward each end of the node.[7]

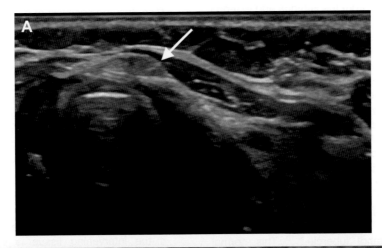

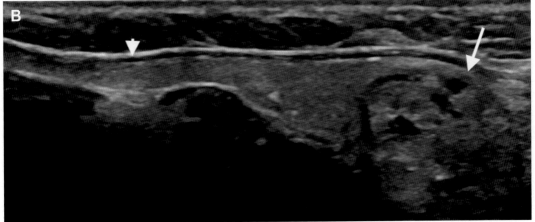

Fig. 4. (A) Transverse grayscale image of a pyramidal lobe (*arrow*) in a patient with surgical absence of the left lobe. (B) Sagittal grayscale image of the pyramidal lobe (*arrowhead*). The imaged portion of the right lobe contains a nodule (*arrow*).

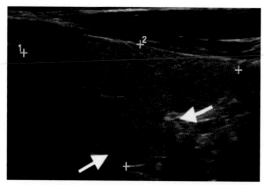

Fig. 5. Sagittal grayscale image of the right lobe with normal thyroid tissue arising from the posterior margin of the gland (*arrows*), also known as the tubercle of Zuckerkandl. Note the similar echotexture as the rest of the gland.

ANATOMIC VARIANTS

- *Pyramidal lobe*: Appears as normal thyroid tissue that arises from the isthmus and extends superiorly, anterior to the trachea. It may lay slightly to the right or left of true midline (**Fig. 4**). It is important to recognize and report this normal variant, because nodules can occur in this lobe, and it could potentially be overlooked by the surgeon during a thyroidectomy.
- *Zuckerkandl tubercle*: A protuberance of the normal thyroid tissue that arises from the posterior margin of the gland and extends posterior to the tracheoesophageal groove, most commonly on the right (**Fig. 5**). It is an important anatomic landmark for surgeons because of its relationship with the recurrent laryngeal nerve, which is typically located medial to the Zuckerkandl tubercle.[8–10] This normal

protuberance of tissue can mimic a thyroid nodule in the transverse plane (pseudonodule); however scanning in the sagittal plane confirms that the area is contiguous with normal thyroid tissue and is not a discrete nodule.

- *Thyroglossal duct remnant:* During normal embryonal development, the thyroid descends from the foramen cecum at the base of the tongue to its normal anatomic location in the low anterior neck. A remnant thyroglossal duct can remain along the path of descent, and residual thyroid tissue is seen in this area, manifested as a pyramidal lobe if connected to the gland, and as ectopic thyroid tissue if separate. If descent of the gland continues below the normal anatomic location, thyroid tissue is seen inferiorly within the mediastinum.
- *Partial or complete congenital absence of the thyroid:* Rarely, the thyroid gland is partially or completely absent at birth. In partial agenesis there may be agenesis of one lobe with resultant compensatory hypertrophy of the remaining lobe (**Fig. 6**).[11] There could also be sonographically normal thyroid tissue located ectopically, including laterally (**Fig. 7**), at the base of the tongue (lingual gland), in the superior mediastinum/thymus, or along the remnant thyroglossal duct (**Fig. 8**).[12,13] Newborn infants are routinely screened for the presence of thyroid hormone to exclude complete agenesis of the thyroid, because thyroid hormone is critical for normal development.

IMAGING PITFALLS

- In some patients with a Zuckerkandl tubercle, if the intervening tissue is very thin, the appearance can mimic a nodule on transverse

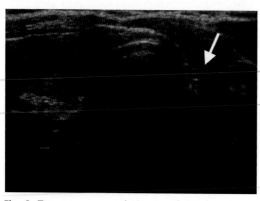

Fig. 6. Transverse grayscale image of the thyroid in a patient with congenital absence of the left lobe (*arrow*). The right lobe contains a partially cystic nodule.

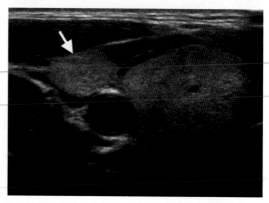

Fig. 7. Transverse grayscale image of the right lobe of the thyroid with ectopic thyroid tissue more lateral to the thyroid bed (*arrow*).

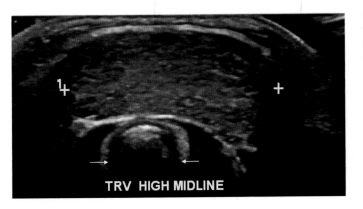

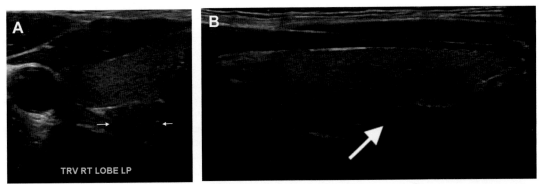

Fig. 9. (*A*) Transverse grayscale image of the right lobe with a thin echogenic interface and additional tissue noted posteriorly in the lower pole, mimicking the appearance of a posterior nodule (*arrows*). (*B*) Sagittal grayscale image of the right lobe demonstrates that this posterior lower pole thyroid tissue (*arrow*) is contiguous with adjacent thyroid tissue, consistent with a pseudonodule.

imaging. However, on sagittal images this thyroid tissue is contiguous with the more superior thyroid tissue, and the finding is actually a pseudonodule (**Fig. 9**).

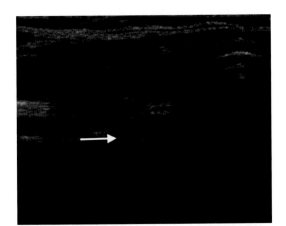

Fig. 10. Transverse grayscale image of the right lobe with the esophagus posterior to the thyroid (*arrow*). The esophagus may occasionally be seen to the right of the trachea.

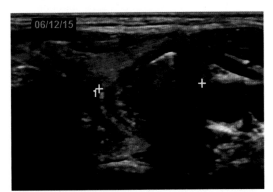

Fig. 11. Transverse grayscale image of the left lobe. Posterolateral to the left lobe is an esophageal duplication cyst containing gas within the lumen (*calipers*) that displaces the normal gland anteriorly.

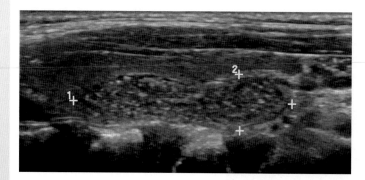

Fig. 12. Sagittal grayscale image of the right lobe with thymus posterior to the thyroid gland (*calipers*).

- Occasionally, the esophagus can appear posteriorly to the right lobe and should not be mistaken for pathology (**Fig. 10**). Esophageal pathology on either side can mimic thyroid pathology (**Fig. 11**).
- In young children, the thymus is almost always visible immediately inferior to the lower poles of the thyroid in the superior mediastinum, and it should not be mistaken for pathology. The normal thymus appears heterogeneous and hypoechoic relative to normal thyroid tissue, with multiple prominent linear echogenic foci.[14] Normal thymic tissue can extend into the thyroid bed, typically posterior to the gland (**Fig. 12**).[15] Occasionally, thymic tissue is located within the gland and mimics a nodule.[16]

TECHNICAL PEARLS

- Place a towel roll or pad behind the shoulders to improve neck hyperextension, particularly in larger patients or those with a short neck.
- In obese patients or patients with a thyroid that extends into the superior mediastinum, a lower frequency probe is used for increased penetration.
- Consider imaging the soft tissue superior to the thyroid isthmus to look for normal anatomic variants, such as a pyramidal lobe, or pathology, such as a thyroglossal duct cyst.

SUMMARY

Ultrasound is the best imaging modality for a comprehensive evaluation of the thyroid. The thyroid is best imaged using a high-frequency linear probe with the patient in a supine position with the neck hyperextended. Normal thyroid is homogeneous in appearance without defining anatomic landmarks within the gland. A few anatomic variants can occur, and it is important for the sonographer and radiologist to be aware of these variants, to avoid misidentifying them as a pathology.

DISCLOSURE

No disclosures.

REFERENCES

1. AIUM–ACR–SPR–SRU Practice Parameter for the Performance and Interpretation of a Diagnostic Ultrasound Examination of the Extracranial Head and Neck. J Ultrasound Med 2018;37:E6–12.
2. Frates MC. Thyroid and parathyroid and other glands. In: McGahan JP, Goldberg BB, editors. Diagnostic ultrasound: a logical approach. New York: Informa Healthcare USA, Inc; 2008. p. 211–34.
3. Solbiati L, Livraghi T, Ballarati E, et al. Thyroid gland. In: Solbiati L, Rizzatto G, editors. Ultrasound of superficial structures: high frequencies, Doppler and interventional procedures. New York: Churchill Livingstone; 1995. p. 49–85.
4. Nachiappan AC, Metwalli ZA, Hailey BS, et al. The thyroid: review of imaging features and biopsy techniques with radiologic-pathologic correlation. Radiographics 2014;34(2):276–93.
5. Loevner LA. Imaging of the thyroid gland. Semin Ultrasound CT MR 1996;17(6):539–62.
6. Yalcin B, Tatar I, Ozan H. The Zuckerkandl tubercle and the recurrent laryngeal nerve. Am J Surg 2008; 196:311–2.
7. Prativadi R, Dahiya N, Kamaya A, et al. Ultrasound characteristics of benign vs malignant cervical lymph nodes. Semin Ultrasound CT MR 2017;38: 506–15.
8. Won HJ, Won HS, Kwak DS, et al. Zuckerkandl tubercle of the thyroid gland: correlations between findings of anatomic dissections and CT imaging. AJNR Am J Neuroradiol 2017;38(7):1416–20.
9. Lee TC, Selvarajan SK, Curtin H, et al. Zuckerkandl tubercle of the thyroid: a common imaging finding that may mimic pathology. AJNR Am J Neuroradiol 2012;33(6):1134–48.
10. Mirilas P, Skandalakis JE. Zuckerkandl's tubercle: Hannibal ad Portas. J Am Coll Surg 2003;196(5): 796–801.

11. Chang J, Gerscovich EO, Dublin AB, et al. Thyroid hemiagenesis: a rare finding. J Ultrasound Med 2011;30:1309–10.

12. Muir A, Daneman D, Daneman A, et al. Thyroid scanning, ultrasound and serum thyroglobulin in determining the origin of congenital hypothyroidism. Am J Dis Child 1988;142:214–8.

13. Ueda D, Mitamura R, Suzuki N, et al. Sonographic imaging of the thyroid gland in congenital hypothyroidism. Pediatr Radiol 1992;22:102–5.

14. Nasseri F, Eftekhari F. Clinical and radiologic review of the normal and abnormal thymus: pearls and pitfalls. Radiographics 2010;30(2):413–28.

15. Costa NS, Laor T, Donnelly LF. Superior cervical extension of the thymus: a normal finding that should not be mistaken for a mass. Radiology 2010;256:238–42.

16. Frates MC, Benson CB, Dorfman DM, et al. Ectopic intrathyroidal thymic tissue mimicking thyroid nodules in children: case series and review. J Ultrasound Med 2018;37:783–91.

Thyroid Ultrasound
Diffuse and Nodular Disease

Lauren F. Alexander, MD[a],*, Neema J. Patel, MD[a], Melanie P. Caserta, MD, FSRU, FSAR[a], Michelle L. Robbin, MD, MS, FSRU[b]

KEYWORDS

- Thyroiditis • Thyroid nodules • Thyroid cancer • Diffuse thyroid disease
- Thyroid imaging reporting and data system • Ultrasound

KEY POINTS

- Thyroid ultrasound can diagnose diffuse thyroid disease by evaluating glandular size, echogenicity, echotexture, margins, and vascularity.
- Ultrasound of chronic lymphocytic thyroiditis shows a diffusely heterogeneous gland with patchy, nodular hypoechoic areas intermixed with echogenic parenchymal bands, giving the gland a micronodular appearance.
- The classic sonographic appearance of Graves disease is an enlarged gland with increased parenchymal vascularity and arteriovenous shunting creating a "thyroid inferno" appearance with a smooth or scalloped glandular contour.
- Ultrasound assessment of thyroid nodules should include description of internal composition, echogenicity, margins, shape, and presence of any echogenic foci.
- Thyroid nodule morphologic features suspicious for malignancy include hypoechoic and very hypoechoic echogenicity, taller-than-wide shape, irregular margins, echogenic foci in solid nodules, and focal increased [18]FDG activity on PET imaging.

INTRODUCTION

The normal thyroid gland lies in the anterior neck, superficial to the trachea, deep to the strap muscles, and medial to the carotid arteries and jugular veins. The superficial location of the thyroid makes high-resolution ultrasound the imaging modality of choice for evaluation of diffuse and focal processes. Patients may be referred for imaging because of laboratory or palpable abnormalities. The anatomy and sonographic technique to evaluate the thyroid gland is discussed in detail in the Danielle M. Richman and Mary C. Frates' article, "Ultrasound of the Normal Thyroid with Technical Pearls and Pitfalls," elsewhere in this issue. This article focuses on diffuse and focal abnormalities of the thyroid parenchyma, and an approach to thyroid nodules for an understanding of how ultrasound can guide management of thyroid pathology.

DIFFUSE THYROID DISEASE

Thyroid ultrasound with gray-scale and color Doppler is the most helpful imaging modality to differentiate normal thyroid parenchyma from diffuse or nodular thyroid disease by evaluating glandular size, echogenicity, echotexture, margins, and vascularity. The various causes of diffuse thyroid disease often have overlapping sonographic imaging features.[1]

The adult thyroid can vary in size with patient body habitus, ranging from 4 to 6 cm cranial to caudal length, 2 to 3 cm transverse width, and 1.5 to 2.0 cm anteroposterior depth.[1] The anteroposterior diameter of the thyroid can also be divided into categories that consist of normal range (1–2 cm), decreased size (<1 cm), and enlarged size (>2 cm).[2] With diffuse thyroid diseases, the thyroid is often enlarged. The term "goiter" is defined as generalized enlargement of

[a] Department of Radiology, Mayo Clinic, 4500 San Pablo Road, Jacksonville, FL 32224, USA; [b] Department of Radiology, University of Alabama – Birmingham, JTN 358; 619 S 19th Street South, Birmingham, AL 35294, USA
* Corresponding author.
E-mail address: alexander.lauren1@mayo.edu

Radiol Clin N Am 58 (2020) 1041–1057
https://doi.org/10.1016/j.rcl.2020.07.003
0033-8389/20/© 2020 Elsevier Inc. All rights reserved.

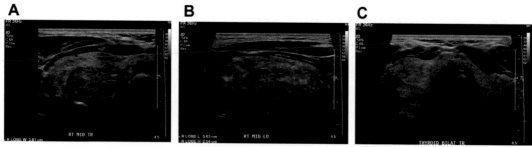

Fig. 1. A 66-year-old woman with multinodular goiter. (*A, B*) Gray-scale images demonstrate enlarged nodular goiter with coalescent nodules virtually replacing the gland without discrete suspicious-appearing nodule in the right lobe transverse (*A*) and longitudinal planes (*B*). (*C*) Transverse image of both enlarged, lobular thyroid lobes. Cursors on (*A*), (*B*) represent thyroid lobe measurements in the transverse and longitudinal planes.

the thyroid, and refers to both normal parenchyma and diffuse or nodular disease. Patients with a diffuse multinodular goiter have an enlarged gland with multiple hyperplastic or adenomatous nodules of variable size, usually all similar in appearance, with or without normal-appearing tissue between the nodules[3,4](**Fig. 1**).

Thyroid parenchymal echogenicity is described as isoechoic, hypoechoic, markedly hypoechoic, or hyperechoic using the strap musculature as an internal reference.[2] The normal thyroid is usually homogeneous and slightly hyperechoic due to its follicular composition, with a thin echogenic border and smooth margins.[4] The term border is preferred over capsule,[5] as the thin connective tissue along the outer surface of the thyroid has heterogeneous thickness and composition, and discontinuous distribution, consistent with a pseudocapsule rather than a true fibrous capsule.[6] Thyroid echotexture is described as fine, coarse, or micronodular pattern.[2] In diffuse thyroid disease, the thyroid can have increased or decreased parenchymal echogenicity and coarsened echotexture with nodular (micro- or macrolobulated) margins.[2,7]

Glandular vascularity with color Doppler sonography is categorized as normal, mildly increased, markedly increased, or decreased. Normal thyroid color Doppler flow should be fairly symmetric and evenly distributed. Diffuse thyroid disease presents with variable vascularity that can be normal, increased, or decreased.[1,2,4,7]

A combination of 2 or more abnormal features had 82% sensitivity and 84% specificity for diffuse thyroid disease in one multicenter study.[7] Kim and colleagues[2] demonstrated that a combination of 3 or more ultrasound characteristics of diffuse thyroid disease had a high sensitivity and specificity (88% and 92%, respectively) for the identification of diffuse thyroid disease over 2 sonographic features. No single feature provided both high specificity and sensitivity, but the absence of any sonographic features of diffuse thyroid disease essentially excluded asymptomatic diffuse thyroid disease.[2,7] The most specific features of diffuse thyroid disease include anteroposterior diameter greater than 2 cm, marked hypoechogenicity, coarse echotexture, markedly increased (or decreased) vascularity, and macrolobulated margins.[2]

THYROIDITIS

Thyroiditis encompasses a wide group of disorders that cause inflammation of the thyroid gland and diffuse thyroid disease (**Box 1**). These

---

Box 1
Types of thyroiditis

Autoimmune

    Chronic autoimmune lymphocytic (Hashimoto disease)

    Subacute granulomatous (DeQuervain disease)

    Graves disease

Medication induced

    Amiodarone

    Interleukins (IL-2)

    Interferon-alpha

    Tyrosine kinase inhibitors

    Immunomodulating cancer therapies

Infectious

    Acute suppurative

Uncertain etiology

    Riedel thyroiditis

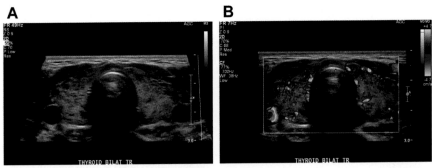

Fig. 2. A 39-year-old woman with Hashimoto thyroiditis. (*A*) On gray-scale, mall patchy hypoechoic nodules scattered diffusely throughout the gland in the transverse plane. (*B*) Color Doppler can be increased in the acute phase, as in this patient, shown in the transverse plane.

conditions have various etiologies, clinical symptomatology, imaging findings, and treatment.

Chronic Lymphocytic (Hashimoto) Thyroiditis

Chronic lymphocytic thyroiditis, or Hashimoto thyroiditis, is the most common autoimmune disorder of the thyroid and the most common cause of hypothyroidism in iodine-sufficient areas, affecting up to 10% of individuals in the United States with an overall female predominance of 8 to 9:1. Patients develop antibodies targeting thyroglobulin, thyroid peroxidase (TPO), an enzyme for thyroid hormonogenesis, and the thyroid-stimulating hormone (TSH) receptor. The thyroid becomes infiltrated with lymphocytes, which incite progressive replacement of follicular cells with eventual fibrosis and atrophy.[1,3,7,8]

The typical sonographic appearance of chronic lymphocytic thyroiditis is a diffusely heterogeneous gland with patchy, nodular hypoechoic

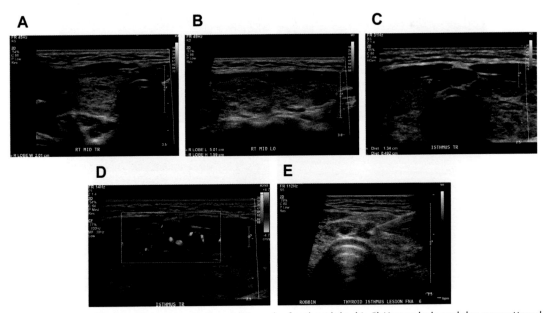

Fig. 3. A 17-year-old girl with Hashimoto thyroiditis and a focal nodule. (*A, B*) Hypoechoic nodules are scattered throughout the gland with increased echogenic bands in-between the nodules, the "giraffe skin" appearance, in the right lobe transverse (*A*) and longitudinal planes (*B*) on gray-scale imaging. (*C, D*) Focal 2.1-cm hypoechoic nodule in the isthmus, on gray-scale (*C*) with internal color Doppler flow (*D*), classified as ACR TI-RADS TR-4. (*E*) FNA is shown with needle in the nodule; sampling revealed focal lymphocytic infiltrate consistent with Hashimoto thyroiditis, without features of a focal nodule. Cursors on (*A, B*) represent thyroid lobe measurements in the transverse and longitudinal planes; (*D*) Isthmus nodule measurement is shown in the transverse plane. Longitudinal measurement of the nodule was 2.1 cm, not shown.

areas of lymphocytic infiltration intermixed with echogenic parenchymal bands between the nodules, giving the gland a micronodular or "giraffe skin" appearance[4,9] (**Figs. 2** and **3**). In the acute phase, this thyroiditis can present with a painless, lobular goiter; normal size gland; or small gland, sometimes with increased vascularity.[4] As inflammation and fibrosis progresses, hyperechoic linear and curvilinear bands can occur with heterogeneous appearance while the surface contour becomes more nodular and the gland more atrophic at end stage, sometimes with the appearance of "pseudonodules" (see **Fig. 3**; **Fig. 4**).[1] Ultrasound often identifies an increased number of benign, hyperplastic lymph nodes in cervical levels II, III, and IV compared with patients without thyroid disease.[10,11]

Patients with chronic lymphocytic thyroiditis are at risk for developing primary thyroid lymphoma, which is usually a B-cell lymphoma and represents less than 5% of all thyroid malignancies.[12] This diagnosis should be suspected if an atrophic gland quickly enlarges or develops hypoechoic masses

with increased through transmission, particularly in the setting of systemic symptoms[1,12] (**Fig. 5**).

Subacute Granulomatous (DeQuervain) Thyroiditis

DeQuervain or subacute thyroiditis is a rare, often self-limiting condition likely due to an immune response following a viral or upper respiratory tract infection (**Box 2**) and represents approximately 3% to 6% of all thyroid diseases.[1,3] The classic presentation is an acutely painful neck with tender glandular swelling, jaw and ear pain, and occasional systemic symptoms, such as fever, fatigue, weight loss, elevated erythrocyte sedimentation rate or C-reactive protein, suppressed TSH level, and dysphagia.[1,3,4,13] In the acute phase, patients may be hyperthyroid but often later become hypothyroid until returning to a euthyroid state after approximately 6 to 18 months.[1,3]

The typical ultrasound appearance of the gland includes patchy, ill-defined hypoechoic regions in one or both lobes with significantly decreased vascularity within the thyroid parenchyma

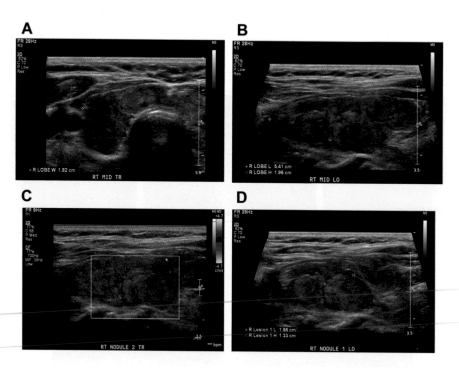

Fig. 4. A 67-year-old woman with Hashimoto thyroiditis and discrete possible nodule. (*A*, *B*) Heterogeneous gland with hypoechoic nodules diffusely in the right lobe on gray-scale in the transverse (*A*) and longitudinal planes (*B*). (*C*) On color Doppler, there is little flow in the nodule and thyroid in this chronic phase. (*D*) Discrete 1.9-cm ACR TI-RADS TR-3 nodule was biopsied (before TI-RADS implementation); pathology was benign lymphocytic infiltration. Note that nodule measurement was made before ACR TI-RADS implementation in the longitudinal plane; note that TI-RADS nodule measurement requires only cranial-caudal measurement in the longitudinal plane, and both AP and transverse measurements should be obtained in the transverse plane, as in **Fig. 3**. Cursors on (*A*, *B*) represent thyroid lobe measurements in the transverse and longitudinal planes.

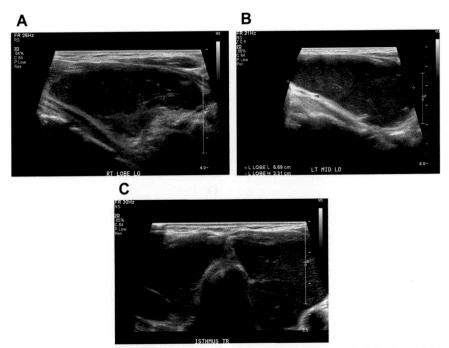

Fig. 5. An 84-year-old woman with large B-cell lymphoma on gray-scale ultrasound of the thyroid. (*A–C*) Thyroid gland is enlarged with near-complete replacement of gland with hypoechoic infiltrate in the right longitudinal (*A*), left longitudinal (*B*), and bilateral lobe transverse view (*C*). Biopsy showed large B-cell lymphoma. Cursors on (*B*) represent thyroid lobe measurement in the longitudinal plane.

(**Fig. 6**). Often, these hypoechoic areas elongate and do not result in discrete nodules but have a "pseudonodule" appearance.[3] Sometimes the appearance is described as "lava flow," with diffuse and confluent hypoechoic areas.[13,14] The acute phase may demonstrate hypervascularity, whereas the subacute phase may reflect diffuse hypovascularity. Imaging features may take weeks to months to resolve.[1]

Box 2
Viruses associated with subacute granulomatous thyroiditis

Hepatitis B

Hepatitis C

Mumps

Cytomegalovirus

Coxsackie virus (A and B)

Enterovirus

Data from Dighe M, Barr R, Bojunga J, et al. Thyroid Ultrasound: State of the Art Part 1 - Thyroid Ultrasound reporting and Diffuse Thyroid Diseases. *Med Ultrason.* 2017;19(1):79-93.

Graves Disease

Graves disease is an autoimmune disorder with female predominance, in which antibodies stimulate the TSH and cause epithelial hyperplasia, glandular enlargement, bowing of the anterior margin, parenchymal coarsening, and hyperthyroidism, occasionally with the presence of a pyramidal lobe due to gland hypertrophy.[1,3] The classic sonographic appearance of Graves disease is an enlarged gland with increased parenchymal vascularity and arteriovenous shunting creating a "thyroid inferno" appearance with a smooth or scalloped glandular contour[1,4] (**Fig. 7**). The gland may demonstrate decreased echogenicity due to increased blood flow, increased cellularity, and decreased colloid.[3,4]

Medication-Induced Thyroiditis

Various medications result in thyroid dysfunction (see **Box 1**), with sonographic features that overlap with other causes. Amiodarone is an iodine-rich medication used in the treatment of cardiac arrhythmia with side effects of both hyperthyroidism and hypothyroidism. Thyrotoxicosis can occur in up to 15% of patients on this therapy independent of dose or duration of therapy. Despite stopping amiodarone when possible, patients often require additional medical treatment for the

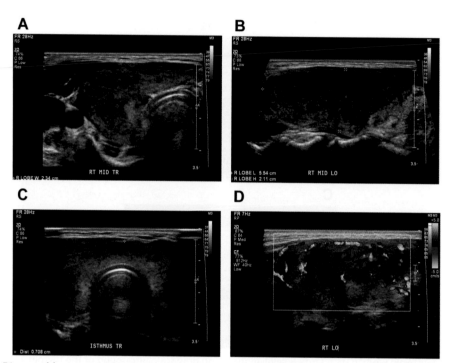

Fig. 6. A 51-year-old woman with subacute thyroiditis, likely post viral. (*A–C*) Gray-scale images in transverse (*A, C*) and longitudinal (*B*) planes show diffuse small hypoechoic areas throughout an enlarged thyroid, with focal areas of overall decreased echogenicity, so-called "lava flow" pattern. (*D*) In the acute phase, increased color Doppler flow is present in the right lobe between the hypoechoic areas. Cursors on (*A, B*) represent thyroid lobe measurements in the transverse and longitudinal planes; cursors on (*C*) show the measurement of isthmus thickness, which is enlarged at greater than 3 mm.

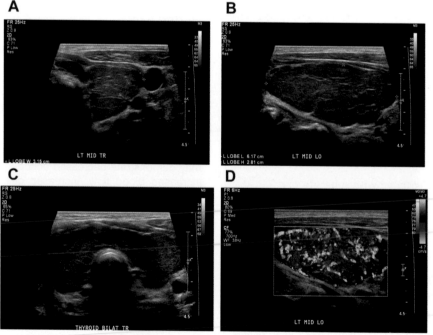

Fig. 7. A 42-year-old woman with Graves disease. (*A–C*) Enlarged, mildly heterogeneous gland with decreased echotexture, and a scalloped, nodular contour without focal nodules on gray-scale. (*D*) Increased color Doppler flow due to hyperemia is shown in the left lobe, longitudinal plane. Cursors on (*A, B*) represent thyroid lobe measurements in the transverse and longitudinal planes.

hyperthyroidism.[15–17] Interferon medication can induce thyroid disease with sonographic features detectable even before abnormal thyroid function or antibody status could be measured, occurring with increased incidence in female individuals and patients with a preexisting thyroglobulin or TPO antibodies and viral load. It presents as a destructive process on ultrasound with no specific imaging features.[3]

Immunotherapy-related thyroiditis may be increasing in prevalence given the wider use of immunotherapy for various malignancies. These agents can induce autoimmune responses beyond the malignant target, known as immune-related adverse events (IRAEs), usually occurring within 3 to 6 months of initiation of therapy. Approximately 5% to 10% of patients experience endocrine IRAEs, most commonly reported to affect thyroid and pituitary hormones, with typical thyroid disorder presenting as thyrotoxicosis and eventual hypothyroidism if the IRAE causes inflammatory damage to the gland.[18,19] The imaging features can overlap with other types of thyroiditis, including heterogeneous glandular tissue with increased or decreased vascularity and hypoechoic nodular areas.[20,21]

Riedel Thyroiditis

Riedel thyroiditis is a rare, local form of fibrosclerosis of the thyroid that presents in patients 30 to 50 years of age with uncertain etiology, thought to be due to an autoimmune process.[3] It results in very firm neck swelling due to thyroid fibrosis and invasion of adjacent neck soft tissue structures with inflammatory cell infiltrates.[3,22] This condition is most common in women and can be associated with mediastinal or retroperitoneal fibrosis like immunoglobulin G4–mediated diseases.[3] The gland is enlarged, hypoechoic, hypovascular, and coarsened with a pseudonodular appearance that has fibrotic bands and perithyroid extension.[3]

Acute Suppurative Thyroiditis

This is a rare disease that occurs in immunosuppressed patients or children and young adults with branchial anomalies. It presents with inflammation including fever, sore throat, painful swelling, skin erythema, and lymphadenopathy in a euthyroid state. On ultrasound, the thyroid gland has nonspecific hypoechoic and anechoic areas with normal or increased vascularity. Occasionally, an abscess can occur and can be cured with antibiotic therapy or drainage.[3]

FOCAL THYROID ABNORMALITIES

The American Thyroid Association (ATA) defines a nodule as "a discrete lesion within the thyroid gland that is radiographically distinct from the surrounding thyroid parenchyma."[23] The incidence and prevalence of thyroid nodules can be difficult to pin down due to the overall increase in imaging studies and the goal of the imaging study, as nodules may be identified incidentally on chest computed tomography imaging or carotid ultrasound, or as part of a dedicated thyroid study for abnormal laboratory values or physical examination. Detection of nonpalpable nodules by imaging studies may be as high as 70%[24] and can vary by imaging modality. Thyroid nodules may be hyperplastic or neoplastic, with most due to benign hyperplastic changes in architecture and benign follicular adenomas; only a small percentage are malignant. Occasionally, focal thyroiditis can mimic a nodule.

Thyroid malignancies are listed in **Box 3**. In 2016, there were an estimated 822,242 people living with thyroid cancer in the United States. The American Cancer Society estimates approximately 52,070 new cases in 2019, which has tripled over the past 3 decades. Death rates remain low, with estimated 2170 deaths in 2019, and overall 5-year survival of 98%.[25,26]

Box 3
Thyroid malignancies

Follicular epithelial cell origin
  Papillary
  Follicular
  Hurthle cell
  Poorly differentiated
  Anaplastic
Neuroendocrine C-cell origin
  Medullary
Metastases (from)
  Lung
  Renal cell
  Breast
  Melanoma
Lymphoma

Data from Refs.[4,28]

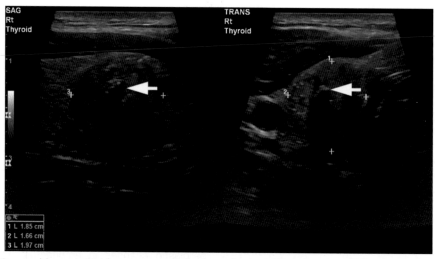

Fig. 8. A 40-year-old man with biopsy-proven follicular variant papillary thyroid cancer. Transverse and longitudinal gray-scale ultrasound images show a hypoechoic nodule with ill-defined margins, PEF, and shadowing calcifications (*arrow*), and taller-than-wide shape, as measured by the calipers. Taller-than-wide shape is a highly specific indicator of malignancy.

Differentiated thyroid cancers arise from the follicular epithelial cells, and include papillary, follicular, and Hurthle cell subtypes.

Papillary thyroid cancer is the most common subtype in the United States, accounting for up to 90% of all thyroid cancers. This cancer occurs more frequently in women, with peak incidences in the third and seventh decades. The tumors are hypoechoic due to closely packed cells, and up to 35% have calcified psammomatous bodies, which are not found in follicular or medullary carcinoma[27] (Figs. 8 and 9). Metastases occur most commonly by lymphatic spread to cervical lymph nodes, which should be carefully assessed for cystic change and echogenic foci indicative of metastases even in the setting of normal nodal size.[27,28] Papillary microcarcinoma presents as small tumors of less than 10 mm, often with metastatic adenopathy. With high-resolution scanning, these small tumors can be identified by their suspicious features[4] (Fig. 10).

Follicular carcinoma accounts for 5% to 15% of cancers and also occurs more frequently in women. Tumors are often homogeneous and well-encapsulated, making them difficult to differentiate from hyperplastic nodules by imaging. The Bethesda System for Reporting Thyroid Cytopathology is a category-based reporting system for specimens obtained with fine-needle aspiration (FNA) to allow for clear communication between pathologists and referring clinicians that samples fall into 1 of 6 diagnostic categories: (I) nondiagnostic or unsatisfactory; (II) benign; (III) atypia of undetermined significance (AUS) or follicular lesion of undetermined significance (FLUS); (IV) follicular neoplasm or suspicious for a follicular neoplasm; (V) suspicious for malignancy; and (VI) malignant. Because follicular tumors cannot be

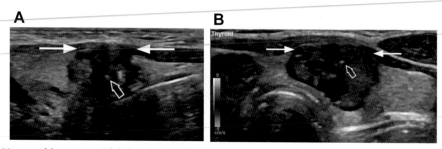

Fig. 9. A 41-year-old woman with bilateral papillary thyroid cancer. (*A*) Longitudinal (*A*) and transverse (*B*) grayscale image demonstrates a right hypoechoic nodule with calcifications (*open arrow*) and extrathyroidal extension into the adjacent sternothyroid muscle (*arrows*).

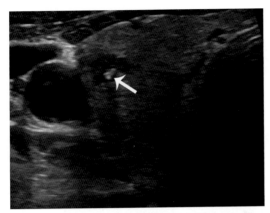

Fig. 10. A 66-year-old woman with a 4-mm papillary thyroid carcinoma in the mid-right thyroid on gray-scale image. Although small, the nodule is hypoechoic with irregular margins and contains a shadowing macrocalcification (*arrow*).

reliably categorized by FNA alone, they may be characterized as a Bethesda III or Bethesda IV.[29] Molecular testing can be used for additional risk stratification at the time of initial FNA to reduce the number of surgeries for benign nodules.[30] Follicular carcinoma is more likely to metastasize by hematogenous spread.[4,28]

Medullary thyroid cancer arises from the neuroendocrine C-cells and represents approximately 2% to 5% of cancers. Up to 20% of these cancers occur in patients with multiple endocrine neoplasia type 2. Metastatic lymph nodes can be found in up to 70% of patients at presentation.[28]

Anaplastic thyroid cancer is an aggressive malignancy that presents with widespread involvement rather than as a focal nodule and carries a poor prognosis. Patients often present with a rapidly enlarging neck mass, and often have metastatic disease to the lungs, bone, or brain at presentation.[28]

Metastases to the thyroid are more commonly found in autopsy specimens than with a clinical presentation. Tumors that most commonly spread to the thyroid include renal cell carcinoma, lung, breast, and gastrointestinal tract malignancies. These lesions tend to present similarly to other thyroid nodules, as either a palpable finding or incidentally on a diagnostic imaging study.[31]

APPROACH TO THYROID NODULES

Because thyroid malignancies most commonly present as focal nodules, multiple endocrinology and radiology societies have developed morphologic and size criteria to identify nodules most suspicious for underlying malignancy, guide follow-up examinations, and reduce unnecessary

biopsies.[5,32–40] The development of these risk-stratification systems over the past 2 decades, from qualitative and pattern approaches to quantitative scoring systems, is nicely reviewed by Ha and colleagues.[41]

Although a detailed review of all the thyroid nodule scoring systems is beyond the scope of this article, a common theme among the scoring systems is the description of morphologic features that determine suspicion of malignancy, to guide further assessment with FNA and imaging follow-up. Because the morphologic features that are suspicious for malignancy overlap between scoring systems, we focus on the features of the American College of Radiology Thyroid Imaging, Reporting and Data System (ACR TI-RADS) released in 2017,[5] which defines 5 morphologic categories to assess at ultrasound (**Box 4**). For each nodule, the categories are evaluated and scored, and the final score corresponds to a suspicion for malignancy, guiding the decision of whether to perform FNA based on nodule size and features (**Fig. 11**).[5]

Composition

Nodule composition describes the internal material in the nodule as 1 of the following: (1) cystic or almost completely cystic, (2) spongiform, (3) mixed cystic and solid, or (4) solid or almost completely solid.[5] A cystic nodule is well circumscribed and anechoic with increased through transmission (**Fig. 12**). Spongiform nodules are composed of small cystic spaces that account for greater than 50% of the nodule; the cystic spaces are relatively similar in size and distributed throughout the nodule[35] (**Fig. 13**). Larger cystic spaces can be a part of spongiform nodules, but if large solid components are present, the nodule is mixed cystic and solid, not spongiform.[42] Both cystic and spongiform nodules are nearly always benign.[43,44] The solid component of mixed cystic and solid nodules should be carefully analyzed for suspicious features such as nodularity or calcification. Color Doppler flow of these areas can

---

Box 4
Sonographic features to assess risk of malignancy in thyroid nodules

Composition

Echogenicity

Margin

Shape

Echogenic foci

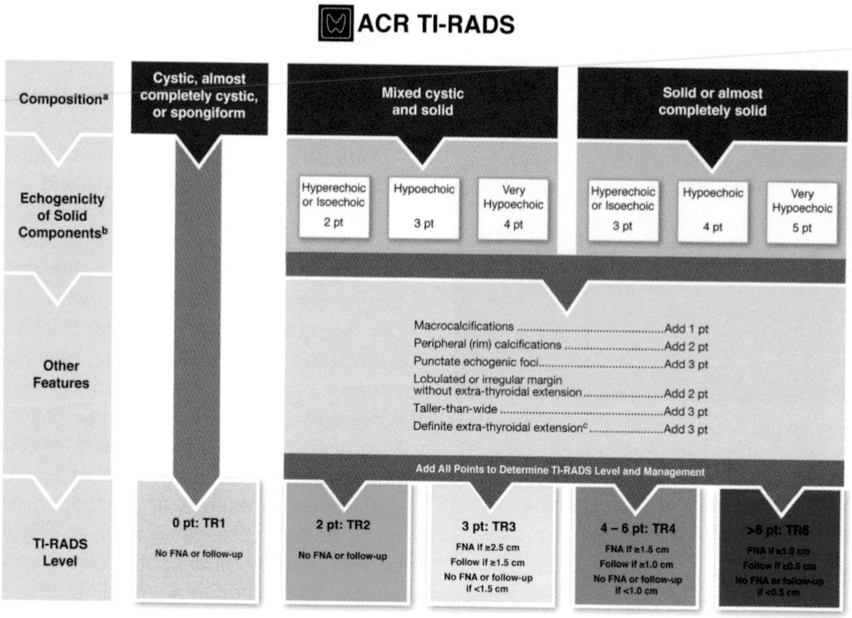

Fig. 11. ACR TI-RADS scoring system flow chart. [a] Classify nodule as solid if composition cannot be determined. [b] Classify nodule as isoechoic if echogenicity cannot be determined. [c] Nodules with definite extrathyroidal extension should be considered malignant until proven otherwise. (From https://www.acr.org/-/media/ACR/Files/RADS/TI-RADS/TI-RADS-Alternative-chart.pdf from ACR Thyroid Imaging, Reporting and Data System (TI-RADS™); with permission.)

help differentiate solid tissue from blood products or layering debris. Solid nodules may have a small cystic component, usually 5% or less, when the nodule is viewed in its entirety.[45]

Echogenicity

The echogenicity of solid nodules is determined by comparison with adjacent thyroid tissue, and nodules may be hyperechoic, isoechoic, or hypoechoic based on the appearance of most of the nodule (Fig. 14). The "very hypoechoic" descriptor refers to hypoechoic nodules that are more hypoechoic than the adjacent neck strap musculature.[35] Anechoic is included in the lexicon for description of cystic nodules.[5] Color Doppler flow can differentiate solid, very hypoechoic nodules from avascular cysts.

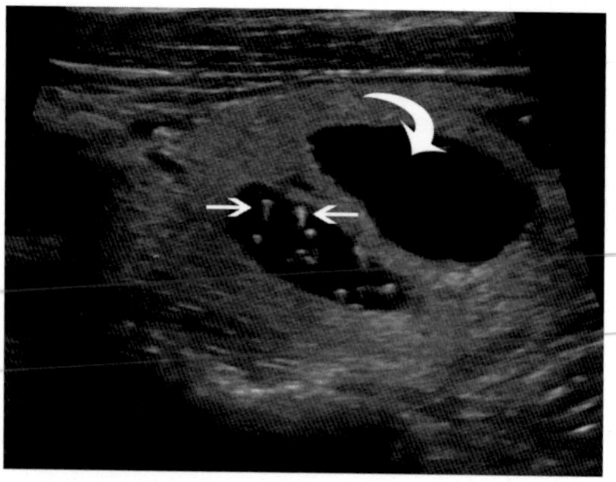

Fig. 12. A 76-year-old woman with a history of amiodarone thyrotoxicosis. Longitudinal gray-scale image of the left upper thyroid demonstrates a colloid cyst with multiple echogenic foci demonstrating large comet-tail artifact (arrows). There is an adjacent anechoic cyst (curved arrow).

Shape

The shape of the nodule should be assessed in the transverse plane with measurement of the transverse and anterior-posterior (AP) dimensions. "Taller-than-wide" nodule shape has longer AP length compared with transverse (Fig. 15), with low sensitivity but high specificity for malignancy,[34,35,46,47] as many malignant nodules have round or oval shape that is longer in the AP direction compared with the transverse. Although this appearance can be assessed visually, a recent study suggests than an AP-to-transverse ratio greater than 1.2 can improve specificity.[48] Three-dimensional measurement is completed by a cranial-caudal measurement of the nodule in the longitudinal plane. The largest of these 3 measurements is used to determine subsequent management.

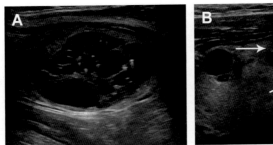
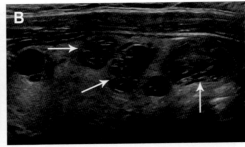

Fig. 13. Spongiform nodules. (A) 66-year-old woman with a multinodular goiter. Longitudinal gray-scale image shows a spongiform nodule characterized by multiple small cystic spaces. Spongiform architecture is strongly associated with benign cytology. (B) A 66-year-old man with metastatic papillary thyroid cancer (not shown) also has multiple spongiform nodules (arrows) in the right thyroid on longitudinal gray-scale ultrasound. Note the nodules contain PEF indicating the backwalls of small simple cysts.

Margin

The nodule margin, or its border with the adjacent parenchyma, can be categorized as (1) smooth, with well-defined and uninterrupted curvilinear edge; (2) ill-defined, or unable to distinguish from neighboring tissue; or (3) irregular (spiculated, jagged, or angulated margins) or lobular (focal rounded protrusions) (Fig. 16). Of note, for partially cystic nodules, the margin of the solid component should be assessed, not the entire nodule margin.[49] If the nodule has an interface with the borders of the thyroid, this margin should be assessed for extrathyroidal extension.[5,35] Minimal extrathyroidal extension can be suspected if the nodule abuts the thyroid border, bulges the thyroid contour, or there is loss of the echogenic thyroid border at the nodule-thyroid border interface[50]

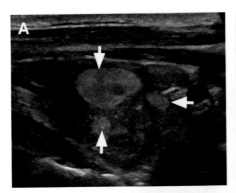
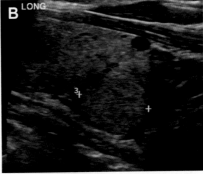
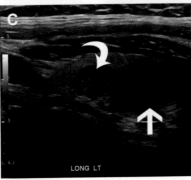

Fig. 14. Nodule echogenicity on gray-scale ultrasound. (A) An 88-year-old man with hyperechoic nodules (arrows) and Hashimoto thyroiditis. (B) A 65-year-old woman with an isoechoic nodule (calipers). (C) A 51-year-old woman with nodules that are hypoechoic (curved arrow) and very hypoechoic (arrow).

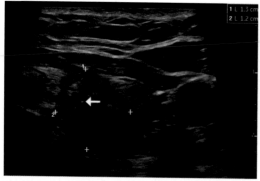

Fig. 15. A 58-year-old woman with well-differentiated papillary thyroid cancer in the left thyroid. Transverse gray-scale image demonstrates a taller-than-wide shape (*calipers*) and PEF (*arrow*).

(**Fig. 17**). Clear invasion of soft tissues beyond the thyroid is characterized as extensive extrathyroidal extension, which is highly associated with malignancy, and a poor prognostic factor[51] (**Fig. 18**).

Echogenic Foci

Nodules can contain echogenic foci, defined as focal areas with markedly increased echogenicity within or along the margins of the nodule, and these foci may represent calcification, colloid, or microcyst wall interfaces. Macrocalcifications are coarse, echogenic foci that produce posterior acoustic shadowing and may be within the nodule or around the periphery (see **Figs. 8** and **10**). The

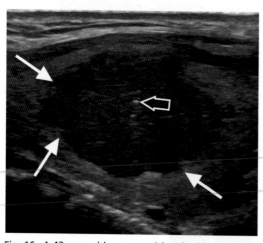

Fig. 16. A 42-year-old woman with palpable right thyroid nodule detected on annual physical exam. Longitudinal gray-scale ultrasound shows a hypoechoic solid nodule with irregular margins (*arrows*) and PEF without shadowing or comet-tail artifact (*open arrow*). Final pathology was medullary thyroid carcinoma.

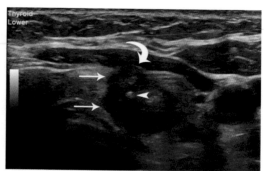

Fig. 17. A 58-year-old woman with well-differentiated papillary thyroid cancer. Transverse gray-scale ultrasound image shows a hypoechoic solid nodule with irregular margins (*arrows*), extension to the thyroid capsular surface (*curved arrow*), and central calcification (*arrowhead*). On pathology evaluation, the tumor focally extended beyond the thyroid border.

prevalence of malignancy associated with macrocalcifications in one study was 17.2% for clumped calcification within the nodule and 19.5% for peripheral calcifications.[52] Peripheral calcification can obscure the internal composition and echogenicity of the nodule, and ACR TI-RADS suggests these nodules should be scored as solid and isoechoic in the algorithm. Peripheral calcifications that are interrupted with protruding soft tissue have higher rates of malignancy,[53] and the margin of this soft tissue can be characterized as lobulated.[5]

Punctate echogenic foci (PEF) are nonshadowing, echogenic foci measuring less than 1 mm and should be assessed for posterior features and composition of surrounding nodule material. The term "microcalcification" should be avoided, as colloid and microcyst wall interfaces have similar appearance. Cystic fluid that contains PEF with large comet-tail artifact, or triangular or V-shaped echoes extending more than 1 mm posterior to the PEF, are highly likely to be benign[52] (see **Fig. 12**). Similarly, small echogenic foci within spongiform nodules are not suspicious, as they likely represent reflectors at the backwalls of tiny cysts. PEF found in solid nodule components with small (<1 mm) or no posterior artifact are suspicious, as they may represent the psammomatous calcifications found in papillary carcinoma[27] and have a 15% prevalence of malignancy[52] (see **Figs. 8** and **15**; **Fig. 19**). In a recent study, PEF had a positive predictive value of only 45% to 48% for the presence of psammomatous calcifications, as dystrophic calcifications and colloid also can give this appearance.[54]

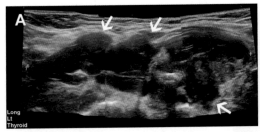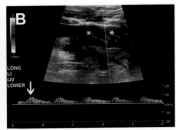

Fig. 18. A 59-year-old woman with metastatic follicular carcinoma with Hurthle cell features. (*A*) Longitudinal gray-scale extended view image shows a large (11 cm) hypoechoic left thyroid mass (*calipers*) with irregular margins and extrathyroidal extension (*arrows*). (*B*) Longitudinal spectral Doppler of the left lower internal jugular vein demonstrates an intraluminal hypoechoic solid mass (*asterisk*) with arterial flow (*arrow*) indicating tumor invasion into the left internal jugular vein.

Features Not Part of the American College of Radiology Thyroid Imaging, Reporting and Data System Scoring Algorithm

Nodule vascularity is not part of ACR TI-RADS lexicon, as lesion vascularity has not been found to consistently correlate with papillary thyroid cancer; however, there is an association with follicular cancers.[5,23,35] Color Doppler can be helpful to differentiate solid tissue from debris or hemorrhage within a cystic nodule, or delineate a subtle isoechoic nodule.

Nodule size does not contribute to suspicion of malignancy in the ACR TI-RADS algorithm, but size is used as part of the decision to biopsy or follow the nodule once the level of suspicion has been determined.[5] Nodule size is not a specific feature of malignancy and the various society guidelines have different size thresholds when combined with morphologic features, other patient factors such as comorbidities, and shared decision making with the patient to guide decision to perform nodule FNA, nodule imaging follow-up frequency, and duration or no follow-up at all.

There is general agreement that nodules smaller than 1.0 cm should not undergo FNA.[5,32–40,55]

The ACR TI-RADS documents do not specifically address nodules with increased [^{18}F]fluorodeoxyglucose (^{18}FDG) activity on PET studies. In patients undergoing PET examinations, 1.6% to 2.5% of patients have focal hypermetabolic activity in the thyroid, and a range of 11% to 35% of these nodules are subsequently diagnosed as malignant.[56–58] The ATA guidelines recommend FNA of hypermetabolic nodules ≥1 cm independent of other ultrasound features.[23]

Although cervical lymph nodes are not part of the ACR TI-RADS system, the thyroid ultrasound examination should include survey of neck lymph nodes in levels I to VI and documentation of size and location of any suspicious nodes.[59] Suspicious features include round or globular shape, short axis measurement ≥1 cm, loss of echogenic hilum, peripheral instead of hilar flow, cystic areas, and PEF[5] (**Figs. 20** and **21**).

Summary of Features Suspicious for Thyroid Malignancy

In summary, features suspicious for malignancy include hypoechoic and very hypoechoic echogenicity, taller-than-wide shape, irregular margins, PEF in solid nodules, macrocalcifications, and focal increased ^{18}FDG activity on PET imaging.[5,23,46,47,52] In addition, risk factors for thyroid cancer should be considered when evaluating patients with nodules (**Box 5**).[23] The overall degree of suspicion in the ultrasound report and the decision to biopsy will depend on the thyroid algorithm used by the radiologists, which can be selected in consensus with the referring clinicians to ensure clear and consistent communication within the care team.

Because the prevalence of benign thyroid nodules is so high, the risk-stratification systems aim to reduce unnecessary biopsies with benign

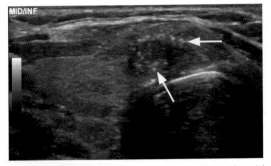

Fig. 19. A 39-year-old woman with papillary thyroid carcinoma confirmed by FNA after transverse gray-scale ultrasound demonstrated a hypoechoic nodule with multiple PEF (*arrows*).

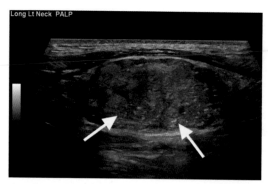

Fig. 20. A 30-year-old man with slowly enlarging left neck mass, with biopsy results of metastatic papillary thyroid carcinoma. Longitudinal gray-scale ultrasound showed an enlarged lymph node with loss of echogenic hilum and multiple PEF (*arrows*).

TI-RADS[37] to 3422 nodules with diagnostic FNA. All nodules could be classified with ACR TI-RADS, but 3.9% with KSThR TI-RADS and 13.9% with ATA guidelines could not be classified. The application of ACR TI-RADS would have resulted in reduction in FNA of benign nodules of nearly 53%, compared with 22% reduction for the ATA guidelines, and 20% for the KSThR system.[61] Grani and colleagues[55] applied 5 international scoring systems (ATA,[23] the American Association of Clinical Endocrinologists,[38] ACR,[5] the European Thyroid Association,[39] and KSThR[37]) to evaluate 502 nodules ≥1.0 cm with diagnostic FNA. ACR TI-RADS had the greatest reduction in biopsies and lowest false negative rate.[55]

results. Several recent studies have shown ACR TI-RADS performs well to reduce biopsies with higher accuracy, when applied alone or when compared with other systems.[55,60–63] Hoang and colleagues[62] retrospectively compared individual practice patterns with ACR TI-RADS for 15 malignant and 85 benign nodules with reduction in recommended biopsies and improved accuracy by both private practice radiologists and expert consensus readers. Middleton and colleagues[61] applied ACR TI-RADS[5], ATA 2015 guidelines[23], and Korean Society of Thyroid Radiology (KSThR)

PITFALLS IN NODULE EVALUATION

Although cystic, almost completely cystic, and spongiform nodule compositions are consistently benign,[43,44] the nodule in its entirety must be carefully assessed to ensure no suspicious areas or overestimation of cystic or spongiform components. Spongiform nodules should have the appearance of a cut sponge or honeycomb with cyst fluid making up 50% or more of the nodule. The mixed cystic and solid nodules should be further characterized by features in the solid component, and FNA should target the solid

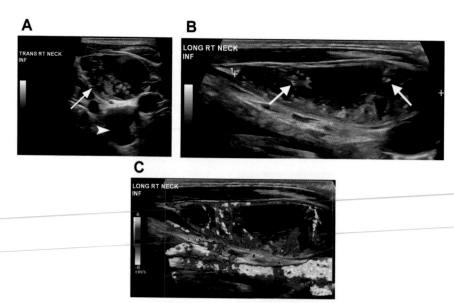

Fig. 21. A 20-year-old man presented with a right neck mass initially thought to be a branchial cleft cyst. Surgical excision revealed metastatic papillary thyroid cancer. (*A*) Transverse gray-scale ultrasound demonstrates 2 abnormal lymph nodes. The larger lymph node shows solid and cystic changes (*arrow*), and the smaller lymph node is entirely cystic (*arrowhead*). (*B*) Longitudinal gray-scale image demonstrates multiple PEF (*arrows*) in the solid component. (*C*) Color Doppler ultrasound shows hypervascularity within the solid portions of the metastatic lymph node.

> **Box 5**
> **Risk factors for thyroid malignancy**
>
> Total body radiation (ie, for bone marrow transplantation)
>
> Childhood or adolescent radiation exposure (ie, nuclear fallout or head and neck radiation therapy)
>
> Familial syndromes associated with thyroid cancer (ie, Cowden syndrome, familial adenomatous polyposis, multiple endocrine neoplasia 2)

component if that area meets criteria for sampling, as up to 7% of papillary thyroid cancers can have cystic components.[64]

Occasionally, cystic or almost completely cystic nodules can undergo degenerative changes over time with decreasing size, replacement of cyst fluid with hypoechoic or very hypoechoic solid material, ill-defined margins and PEF, resulting in a highly suspicious appearance. Similar changes may occur in nodules that have undergone previous aggressive sampling. Color Doppler may help differentiate debris from vascularized tissue. In isolation, these nodules will likely meet criteria for FNA; however, if a prior study can precisely confirm a previously benign cystic nodule in the same location, follow-up imaging may be sufficient.[65,66]

A diffuse thyroid disease can present as only focal nodular abnormalities. Subacute thyroiditis may have scattered focal hypoechoic regions. The typical reticular pattern of chronic lymphocytic thyroiditis can be variable within the gland, mimicking nodules. The echogenic "white knight" nodules in chronic lymphocytic thyroiditis are

benign[43] (**Fig. 22**); however, solid isoechoic and hypoechoic nodules should be evaluated by their morphologic criteria for possible FNA the same as nodules in a background of normal parenchyma[9] (see **Figs. 3** and **4**).

SUMMARY

Thyroid ultrasound with gray-scale and color Doppler can differentiate normal thyroid parenchyma from diffuse or nodular thyroid disease by assessing gland size, echogenicity, echotexture, margins, and vascularity. The various causes of diffuse thyroid disease often have overlapping sonographic imaging features. Most thyroid nodules result from benign hyperplastic changes or benign follicular adenoma, with a much smaller percentage that is malignant. A systematic approach to nodule morphology should include evaluation of composition, echogenicity, margin, shape, and any echogenic foci. Because the prevalence of benign thyroid nodules is so high, consistent use of a risk-stratification system can reduce unnecessary biopsies with benign results.

ACKNOWLEDGMENTS

The authors thank Dr Franklin N. Tessler, Professor Emeritus, Abdominal Imaging Section of the Department of Radiology at the University of Alabama at Birmingham, for reviewing the article.

DISCLOSURE

The authors have nothing to disclose.

REFERENCES

1. Langer JE. Sonography of the thyroid. Radiol Clin North Am 2019;57(3):469–83.
2. Kim DW, Eun CK, In HS, et al. Sonographic differentiation of asymptomatic diffuse thyroid disease from normal thyroid: a prospective study. AJNR Am J Neuroradiol 2010;31(10):1956–60.
3. Dighe M, Barr R, Bojunga J, et al. Thyroid ultrasound: state of the art part 1 - thyroid ultrasound reporting and diffuse thyroid diseases. Med Ultrason 2017;19(1):79–93.
4. Solbiati L, Charboneau W, Cantisani V, et al. The thyroid gland. In: Rumack CM, Wilson SR, Charboneau JW, et al, editors. Diagnostic ultrasound. 5th edition. Philadelphia: Elsiver; 2018. p. 697–731.
5. Tessler FN, Middleton WD, Grant EG, et al. ACR thyroid imaging, reporting and data system (TI-RADS): white paper of the ACR TI-RADS committee. J Am Coll Radiol 2017;14(5):587–95.

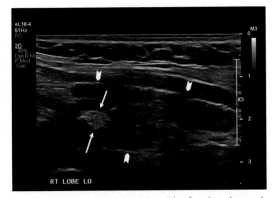

Fig. 22. A 13-year-old girl with focal echogenic nodule (*white arrows*) on gray-scale ultrasound; the "white knight" pattern is benign in the setting of Hashimoto disease (right lobe longitudinal plane). Arrowheads show the thyroid border.

6. Mete O, Rotstein L, Asa SL. Controversies in thyroid pathology: thyroid capsule invasion and extrathyroidal extension. Ann Surg Oncol 2010;17(2):386–91.

7. Ahn HS, Kim DW, Lee YJ, et al. Diagnostic accuracy of real-time sonography in differentiating diffuse thyroid disease from normal thyroid parenchyma: a multicenter study. AJR Am J Roentgenol 2018; 211(3):649–54.

8. Ragusa F, Fallahi P, Elia G, et al. Hashimotos' thyroiditis: epidemiology, pathogenesis, clinic and therapy. Best Pract Res Clin Endocrinol Metab 2019;33(6):101367.

9. Patel BN, Kamaya A, Desser TS. Pitfalls in sonographic evaluation of thyroid abnormalities. Semin Ultrasound CT MR 2013;34(3):226–35.

10. Brancato D, Citarrella R, Richiusa P, et al. Neck lymph nodes in chronic autoimmune thyroiditis: the sonographic pattern. Thyroid 2013;23(2):173–7.

11. Jones MR, Mohamed H, Catlin J, et al. The presentation of lymph nodes in Hashimoto's thyroiditis on ultrasound. Gland Surg 2015;4(4):301–6.

12. Kesireddy M, Lasrado S. Cancer, thyroid lymphoma. In: StatPearls. Treasure Island (FL): StatPearls Publishing LLC; 2020.

13. Omori N, Omori K, Takano K. Association of the ultrasonographic findings of subacute thyroiditis with thyroid pain and laboratory findings. Endocr J 2008;55(3):583–8.

14. Cappelli C, Pirola I, Gandossi E, et al. Ultrasound findings of subacute thyroiditis: a single institution retrospective review. Acta Radiol 2014;55(4):429–33.

15. Maqdasy S, Benichou T, Dallel S, et al. Issues in amiodarone-induced thyrotoxicosis: update and review of the literature. Ann Endocrinol (Paris) 2019;80(1):54–60.

16. Danzi S, Klein I. Amiodarone-induced thyroid dysfunction. J Intensive Care Med 2015;30(4):179–85.

17. Elnaggar MN, Jbeili K, Nik-Hussin N, et al. Amiodarone-induced thyroid dysfunction: a clinical update. Exp Clin Endocrinol Diabetes 2018;126(6):333–41.

18. Michot JM, Bigenwald C, Champiat S, et al. Immune-related adverse events with immune checkpoint blockade: a comprehensive review. Eur J Cancer 2016;54:139–48.

19. Fessas P, Possamai LA, Clark J, et al. Immunotoxicity from checkpoint inhibitor therapy: clinical features and underlying mechanisms. Immunology 2020;159(2):167–77.

20. Yamauchi I, Sakane Y, Fukuda Y, et al. Clinical features of nivolumab-induced thyroiditis: a case series study. Thyroid 2017;27(7):894–901.

21. Angell TE, Min L, Wieczorek TJ, et al. Unique cytologic features of thyroiditis caused by immune checkpoint inhibitor therapy for malignant melanoma. Genes Dis 2018;5(1):46–8.

22. Zakeri H, Kashi Z. Variable clinical presentations of Riedel's thyroiditis: report of two cases. Case Rep Med 2011;2011:709264.

23. Haugen BR, Alexander EK, Bible KC, et al. 2015 American Thyroid Association Management guidelines for adult patients with thyroid nodules and differentiated thyroid cancer: the American Thyroid Association guidelines task force on thyroid nodules and differentiated thyroid cancer. Thyroid 2016; 26(1):1–133.

24. Wilhelm S. Evaluation of thyroid incidentaloma. Surg Clin North Am 2014;94(3):485–97.

25. American Cancer Society: Cancer Statistics Center. Available at: https://cancerstatisticscenter.cancer.org/?_ga=2.40814946.1106973017.1578172910-250140191.1560095408#!/. Accessed January 04, 2020.

26. Thyroid Cancer - Cancer Stat Facts. 2020. Available at: https://seer.cancer.gov/statfacts/html/thyro.html. Accessed January 04, 2020.

27. Kumar V, Abbas AK, Aster JC. Endocrine system. In: Kumar V, Abbas AK, Aster JC, editors. Robbins basic pathology. 10th edition. Philadelphia: Elsevier, Ic; 2018. p. 749–96.

28. Cabanillas ME, McFadden DG, Durante C. Thyroid cancer. Lancet 2016;388(10061):2783–95.

29. Cibas ES, Ali SZ. The 2017 Bethesda system for reporting thyroid cytopathology. Thyroid 2017;27(11): 1341–6.

30. Nishino M, Nikiforova M. Update on molecular testing for cytologically indeterminate thyroid nodules. Arch Pathol Lab Med 2018;142(4):446–57.

31. Nixon IJ, Coca-Pelaz A, Kaleva AI, et al. Metastasis to the thyroid gland: a critical review. Ann Surg Oncol 2017;24(6):1533–9.

32. Frates MC, Benson CB, Charboneau JW, et al. Management of thyroid nodules detected at US: Society of Radiologists in Ultrasound consensus conference statement. Radiology 2005;237(3):794–800.

33. Horvath E, Majlis S, Rossi R, et al. An ultrasonogram reporting system for thyroid nodules stratifying cancer risk for clinical management. J Clin Endocrinol Metab 2009;94(5):1748–51.

34. Kwak JY, Han KH, Yoon JH, et al. Thyroid imaging reporting and data system for US features of nodules: a step in establishing better stratification of cancer risk. Radiology 2011;260(3):892–9.

35. Grant EG, Tessler FN, Hoang JK, et al. Thyroid Ultrasound Reporting Lexicon: White Paper of the ACR Thyroid Imaging, Reporting and Data System (TIRADS) Committee. J Am Coll Radiol 2015;12(12 Pt A):1272–9.

36. Na DG, Baek JH, Sung JY, et al. Thyroid imaging reporting and data system risk stratification of thyroid nodules: categorization based on solidity and echogenicity. Thyroid 2016;26(4):562–72.

37. Shin JH, Baek JH, Chung J, et al. Ultrasonography diagnosis and imaging-based management of thyroid nodules: revised korean society of thyroid radiology consensus statement and recommendations. Korean J Radiol 2016;17(3):370–95.

38. Gharib H, Papini E, Garber JR, et al. American Association of Clinical Endocrinologists, American College of Endocrinology, and Associazione Medici Endocrinologi Medical Guidelines for clinical practice for the diagnosis and management of thyroid nodules–2016 update. Endocr Pract 2016;22(5):622–39.

39. Russ G, Bonnema SJ, Erdogan MF, et al. European Thyroid Association guidelines for ultrasound malignancy risk stratification of thyroid nodules in adults: the EU-TIRADS. Eur Thyroid J 2017;6(5):225–37.

40. Rago T, Cantisani V, Ianni F, et al. Thyroid ultrasonography reporting: consensus of Italian Thyroid Association (AIT), Italian Society of Endocrinology (SIE), Italian Society of Ultrasonography in Medicine and Biology (SIUMB) and Ultrasound Chapter of Italian Society of Medical Radiology (SIRM). J Endocrinol Invest 2018;41(12):1435–43.

41. Ha EJ, Baek JH, Na DG. Risk stratification of thyroid nodules on ultrasonography: current status and perspectives. Thyroid 2017;27(12):1463–8.

42. Tessler FN, Middleton WD, Hoang JK. ACR TI-RADS Webinar Part II: Case Based Review & Frequently Asked Questions. 2018. Available at: https://www.acr.org/Clinical-Resources/Reporting-and-Data-Systems/TI-RADS#Webinars.

43. Bonavita JA, Mayo J, Babb J, et al. Pattern recognition of benign nodules at ultrasound of the thyroid: which nodules can be left alone? AJR Am J Roentgenol 2009;193(1):207–13.

44. Virmani V, Hammond I. Sonographic patterns of benign thyroid nodules: verification at our institution. AJR Am J Roentgenol 2011;196(4):891–5.

45. Tessler FN, Middleton WD, Hoang JK. ACR TI-RADS Webinar Part I: This Is How We Do It. 2018. Available at: https://www.acr.org/Clinical-Resources/Reporting-and-Data-Systems/TI-RADS#Webinars.

46. Kim EK, Park CS, Chung WY, et al. New sonographic criteria for recommending fine-needle aspiration biopsy of nonpalpable solid nodules of the thyroid. AJR Am J Roentgenol 2002;178(3):687–91.

47. Moon W-J, Jung SL, Lee JH, et al. Benign and malignant thyroid nodules: US differentiation—multicenter retrospective study. Radiology 2008;247(3):762–70.

48. Grani G, Lamartina L, Ramundo V, et al. Taller-than-wide shape: a new definition improves the specificity of TIRADS systems. Eur Thyroid J 2019;9(2):85–91.

49. Tessler FN, Middleton WD, Grant EG. Thyroid imaging reporting and data system (TI-RADS): a user's guide. Radiology 2018;287(3):1082.

50. Kamaya A, Tahvildari AM, Patel BN, et al. Sonographic detection of extracapsular extension in papillary thyroid cancer. J Ultrasound Med 2015;34(12):2225–30.

51. Shah JP, Loree TR, Dharker D, et al. Prognostic factors in differentiated carcinoma of the thyroid gland. Am J Surg 1992;164(6):658–61.

52. Malhi H, Beland MD, Cen SY, et al. Echogenic foci in thyroid nodules: significance of posterior acoustic artifacts. AJR Am J Roentgenol 2014;203(6):1310–6.

53. Park YJ, Kim JA, Son EJ, et al. Thyroid nodules with macrocalcification: sonographic findings predictive of malignancy. Yonsei Med J 2014;55(2):339–44.

54. Tahvildari AM, Pan L, Kong CS, et al. Sonographic-pathologic correlation for punctate echogenic reflectors in papillary thyroid carcinoma: what are they? J Ultrasound Med 2016;35(8):1645–52.

55. Grani G, Lamartina L, Ascoli V, et al. Reducing the number of unnecessary thyroid biopsies while improving diagnostic accuracy: toward the "right" TI-RADS. J Clin Endocrinol Metab 2019;104(1):95–102.

56. Soelberg KK, Bonnema SJ, Brix TH, et al. Risk of malignancy in thyroid incidentalomas detected by 18F-fluorodeoxyglucose positron emission tomography: a systematic review. Thyroid 2012;22(9):918–25.

57. Bertagna F, Treglia G, Piccardo A, et al. Diagnostic and clinical significance of F-18-FDG-PET/CT thyroid incidentalomas. J Clin Endocrinol Metab 2012;97(11):3866–75.

58. Makis W, Ciarallo A. Thyroid Incidentalomas on (18)F-FDG PET/CT: clinical significance and controversies. Mol Imaging Radionucl Ther 2017;26(3):93–100.

59. AIUM-ACR-SPR-SRU practice parameter for the performance and interpretation of a diagnostic ultrasound examination of the extracranial head and neck. J Ultrasound Med 2018;37(11):E6–12.

60. Middleton WD, Teefey SA, Reading CC, et al. Multi-institutional analysis of thyroid nodule risk stratification using the American College of Radiology Thyroid imaging reporting and data system. AJR Am J Roentgenol 2017;208(6):1331–41.

61. Middleton WD, Teefey SA, Reading CC, et al. Comparison of Performance Characteristics of American College of Radiology TI-RADS, Korean Society of Thyroid Radiology TIRADS, and American Thyroid Association Guidelines. AJR Am J Roentgenol 2018;210(5):1148–54.

62. Hoang JK, Middleton WD, Farjat AE, et al. Reduction in thyroid nodule biopsies and improved accuracy with American College of Radiology thyroid imaging reporting and data system. Radiology 2018;287(1):185–93.

63. Yoon SJ, Na DG, Gwon HY, et al. Similarities and differences between thyroid imaging reporting and data systems. AJR Am J Roentgenol 2019;213(2):W76–84.

64. Chan BK, Desser TS, McDougall IR, et al. Common and uncommon sonographic features of papillary thyroid carcinoma. J Ultrasound Med 2003;22(10):1083–90.

65. Lacout A, Chevenet C, Marcy PY. Mummified thyroid syndrome. AJR Am J Roentgenol 2016;206(4):837–45.

66. Ren J, Baek JH, Chung SR, et al. Degenerating thyroid nodules: ultrasound diagnosis, clinical significance, and management. Korean J Radiol 2019;20(6):947–55.

Computed Tomography and MR Imaging of Thyroid Disease

Katie Suzanne Traylor, DO

KEYWORDS

• CT • MR imaging • Thyroid • Cancer • Goiter • Thyroid nodules • Surgical implications

KEY POINTS

- Both CT and MR imaging are important imaging modalities that incidentally detect benign and malignant thyroid disease.
- Cross-sectional imaging is not typically the first-line imaging technique for thyroid nodule characteristics but is extremely beneficial for surgical staging.
- Staging of papillary thyroid cancer depends on a combination of imaging findings, histology, and the patient's age.
- Calcifications and/or cystic changes involving cervical lymph nodes are highly concerning for metastatic lymphadenopathy.

INTRODUCTION

Many benign and malignant disorders can occur in the thyroid. Some thyroid diseases can be subclinical; however, others present with structural (ie, thyroid goiter) or functional (ie, thyroiditis) abnormalities.[1,2] Thyroid cancer is the most common endocrine malignancy in the United States, affecting more than 400,000 people per year, with the incidence doubling between 2000 and 2009. This higher number of cases is likely due to increased usage of computed tomography (CT) and MR imaging. Incidental thyroid nodules are often found on neck/cervical spine imaging performed for a vast array of non–thyroid-related etiologies. Despite this overall increased incidence, patient mortality has not changed.[3] CT and MR imaging are especially important in the presurgical evaluation of thyroid diseases for extent of disease, involvement of the adjacent structures, and presence of distant disease.[4,5]

NORMAL ANATOMY AND IMAGING TECHNIQUE

The thyroid structure consists of 2 lobes, draped over the trachea and connected by the isthmus at midline.[6,7] The thyroid is hypervascular, part of the visceral space, and encapsulated by the middle layer of the deep cervical fascia. Typically, each lobe measures approximately $2.0 \times 3.0 \times 5.0$ cm (transverse $\times$ anteroposterior $\times$ craniocaudal) with isthmus measuring up to 0.3 cm.[6,7] The superior border of the thyroid extends to level of the mid-thyroid cartilage and extends inferiorly to the fifth or sixth tracheal ring. The thyroid wraps around the trachea and into the tracheoesophageal grooves (TEG), containing the recurrent laryngeal nerve (RLN).[7] The common carotid arteries (CCA) and internal jugular veins (IJV) are posterolateral, and the strap muscles are anterior to the thyroid (Fig. 1).[6] The thyroid is hypervascular and supplied mainly by superior thyroid artery from the external carotid artery and the inferior thyroid artery from the thyrocervical trunk. In a small percentage of patients, a thyroid IMA arises directly from the aorta. The esophagus is posterior and separated from the thyroid by the TEG (Fig. 2A). The lymphatic drainage for the thyroid is variable, including the internal jugular chain, paratracheal, mediastinal, and retropharyngeal regions.[7]

Neuroradiology Division, Department of Radiology, University of Pittsburgh Medical Center Presbyterian, 200 Lothrop Street, South Tower, 2nd Floor, Suite 200, Pittsburgh, PA 15213, USA
E-mail address: traylorks@upmc.edu

Radiol Clin N Am 58 (2020) 1059–1070
https://doi.org/10.1016/j.rcl.2020.07.004
0033-8389/20/© 2020 Elsevier Inc. All rights reserved.

Imaging Technique and Protocol		
	Computed Tomography	**MR Imaging**
Field of view	Skull base to the carina	Skull base to the carina
Patient positioning	Patient's arm at the side with neck in neutral position to slightly extended to mimic operating room positioning[a,1]	Patient's arm at the side with neck in neutral position to slightly extended to mimic operating room positioning[a,1]
Imaging acquired	• Soft tissue windows in axial at 2.5-mm slice thickness with coronal and sagittal reconstructions. • Axial bone window at 1.25-mm slice thickness	• Anterior neck coil centered over the thyroid • Unenhanced T1-weighted in axial and sagittal planes • Axial fast spin-echo T2-weighted with fat saturation (FS)[b] • Axial and coronal T1-weighted post contrast with FS[b]

[a] This positioning is necessary for thyroid goiters, as incorrect positioning can result in the thyroid having a lower apparent neck position resulting in a sternotomy rather than a simple low collar incision.[1]
[b] FS is mandatory to allow the thyroid lesions to be more conspicuous.[7,8]

IMAGING CHARACTERISTICS

The imaging appearance of the thyroid varies with the modality.[6] Many different modalities are used to evaluate the thyroid, including ultrasonography, nuclear medicine scintigraphy, CT, and MR imaging.[1]

On nonenhanced (NE) CT, the thyroid is intrinsically hyperdense (80–100 Hounsfield units) when compared with the musculature due to elevated iodine content (see **Fig. 1**A).[7] The thyroid is able to concentrate 25 to 50 times more iodine than serum. The thyroid attenuation directly correlates with thyroid function; therefore, the more decreased the thyroid function the less hyperdense the thyroid.[8] On contrast-enhanced (CE) CT, the thyroid avidly enhances due to hypervascularity (see **Fig. 1**B).[7] The thyroid on MR imaging has homogeneous signal intensity, slightly greater than that of the strap musculature on T1-weighted and T2-weighted imaging (**Fig. 2**A, B). After the administration of gadolinium, the thyroid homogeneously enhances (**Fig. 2**C).[7]

THYROID PATHOLOGY
Benign

Imaging has significantly increased over recent years, resulting in an increased number of incidental findings, unrelated to the examination indication.[9] Many incidental findings are benign thyroid nodules, identified on ultrasonography (9%–33%), cross-sectional scans (16%–18%), and PET (1%–2%).[6,9] Incidence of these nodules increase with age, and they occur more frequently in women. Not all incidental nodules need ultrasonography follow-up, given the overall indolent behavior of most thyroid cancers (**Table 1**). In addition, these nodules only have a 1% to 2% risk of malignancy. If, however, a nodule has focal fludeoxyglucose uptake on PET, fine needle aspiration needs to be performed, as there is a 26% to

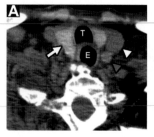 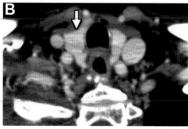

Fig. 1. Axial CT imaging of thyroid. (*A*) The thyroid is intrinsically hyperdense on unenhanced CT (*white arrow*). The common carotid artery (*gray arrowhead*) and internal jugular vein (*white arrowhead*) are posterolateral to the thyroid. Esophagus (E) is located posterior to the thyroid, whereas the trachea (T) is located anterior to the esophagus. (*B*) Contrast-enhanced CT shows avid enhancement of the thyroid (*white arrow*).

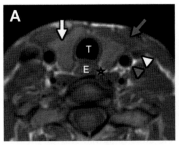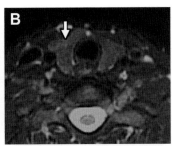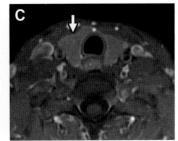

Fig. 2. MR imaging of thyroid. (*A*) T1-weighted axial MR image of thyroid (*white arrow*) is slightly hyperintense compared with adjacent strap muscles (*gray arrow*). Esophagus (E) is posterior to thyroid, and trachea (T) is anterior to the esophagus. Internal jugular vein (*white arrowhead*) is lateral to thyroid and common carotid artery (*gray arrowhead*). The tracheoesophageal groove (*star*) is the fat between the trachea, esophagus, and thyroid. (*B*) T2-weighted MR image shows that the thyroid (*white arrow*) is hyperintense to adjacent strap muscles (*gray arrow*). (*C*) T1-weighted, contrast-enhanced, fat-saturated axial MR image shows normal thyroid (*white arrow*) enhancement.

50% risk of primary thyroid malignancy.[1] Although thyroid nodules can be detected with CT and MR imaging, ultrasonography remains the best for nodule characterization.[6]

Incidental thyroid nodules

The goal of the evaluation for these incidental thyroid nodules is to determine malignancy risk, whereas most are benign. CT is often used in patients with head and neck cancer for operative planning, restaging, and follow-up; however, this is not necessarily true with thyroid cancer. Characterization of thyroid nodules on CT or MR imaging is largely nonspecific; however, these studies can help with large or retrosternal thyroid goiters (TGs), which are not adequately assessed on ultrasonography due to the trachea and sternum. CT also characterizes calcifications better than ultrasonography . Calcifications may be "egg-shell," rim-like, or curvilinear, and 22% of these types of calcifications are associated with malignancy.[10]

Thyroid goiter

TG occurs due to abnormal thyroid growth with or without substernal extension.[1] A simple TG occurs in the absence of autoimmune disease, thyroiditis, thyroid dysfunction, or thyroid malignancy.[11] Abnormal growth occurs over several years, most commonly in 50-year-old to 60-year-old women, and can be due to environmental and/or genetic factors. Functional (ie, hyperthyroidism) or structural abnormalities can cause a multitude of compressive symptoms (ie, dyspnea).[1] Multinodular TG is heterogeneous due to nodularity, hemorrhage, calcifications, cyst formation, and scarring (**Fig. 3**). There can be asymmetric hypertrophy of the thyroid with extension substernally or into the posterior mediastinum.[8] CT is important for presurgical evaluation, and there are specific details the surgeon needs to know: degree of substernal extension, displacement or compressed structures, symmetry of the vocal folds suggesting paralysis, and extrathyroidal extension suggesting superimposed malignancy. Imaging findings suggestive of malignancy include invasion of adjacent structures, rather than simple displacement or compression, and also the presence of cervical lymphadenopathy (**Fig. 4**).[1]

Thyroiditis

Thyroiditis is a benign inflammatory condition, often clinically apparent without need for imaging. However, Riedel's thyroiditis (RT) has fairly characteristic imaging findings. Although the etiology remains largely unknown, it is thought to be autoimmune. RT occurs due to a rare fibrotic condition

Table 1
Diagnostic criteria for managing incidental thyroid nodules on computed tomography or MR imaging[30]

Age, y	Nodule Size, cm	Recommendation
<35	<1	No additional imaging in low-risk patient
	≥1	Ultrasound advised
≥35	<1	No additional imaging in low-risk patient
	1–1.4	Additional imaging at providers discretion
	≥1.5	Ultrasound advised

From Hoang JK, Langer JE, Middleton WD, et al. Managing incidental thyroid nodules detected on imaging: white paper of the ACR Incidental Thyroid Findings Committee. J Am Coll Radiol 2015;12(2):143-50; with permission.

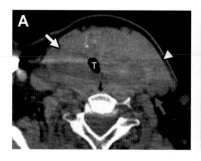

Fig. 3. Preoperative unenhanced CT for thyroid goiter. (A) Axial unenhanced CT at the level of the thyroid demonstrates massively enlarged, heterogeneous thyroid (*white arrow*) causing rightward tracheal (T) deviation with mild narrowing. Mass effect on the surrounding structures causes posterolateral displacement of the common carotid artery (*gray arrow*) and stretching/thinning of the strap muscles (*white arrowhead*). No findings of extrathyroidal extension or invasion of adjacent structures is seen. (B) Coronal unenhanced CT of the thyroid goiter demonstrates rightward tracheal deviation with mild narrowing (*white arrow*).

in which thyroid tissue is destroyed with infiltration of the adjacent soft tissues. This overgrowth of fibrosing connective tissue increases over time leading to a palpable, firm, painless enlarging thyroid mass with compressive symptoms (ie, dyspnea, dysphagia, hoarseness, aphonia). On clinical examination, the differential for RT includes malignancy, such as anaplastic thyroid cancer (ATC), lymphoma, and sarcoma. Definitive treatment of RT remains surgery to relieve the compressive symptoms.[12] RT can be suggested on MR imaging due to characteristic imaging features of fibrosis. The thyroid will be hypointense on T1/T2-weighted images (**Fig. 5**) with homogeneous enhancement. These imaging characteristics are in contradistinction to Hashimoto thyroiditis, thyroid carcinoma, and lymphoma, which are T2 hyperintense. RT also can be associated with mediastinal fibrosis, retroperitoneal fibrosis, and sclerosing cholangitis.[8]

Malignant

There are 4 predominant types of thyroid cancer: papillary (PTC), follicular (FTC), medullary (MTC), and ATC. Both PTC and FTC are considered well-differentiated thyroid cancers (DTC). DTCs have the best prognosis, with a 10-year survival rate greater than 95% for PTC and 85% for FTC.

MTC has a 10-year survival rate of approximately 75%, whereas ATC is the most aggressive with a mean survival of 9 weeks and poor 5-year survival of 7%.[1] When a large thyroid mass is discovered, DTC remains the most likely diagnosis, as DTCs encompass more than 90% of all thyroid malignancies. However, lymphoma, ATC, MTC, and metastatic disease should still be considered.[13] DTC can occur at any age, but the mean age is 49 years with approximately 39% diagnosed before age 45. Although most DTCs are sporadic, family history and prior neck radiation are known risk factors. Young patients have the best prognosis due to the more indolent histologic subtypes and better treatment response. In fact, patients with DTC who are ≤55 years old can only be stage I or II despite advanced disease, reflecting the improved prognosis.[14,15] When a patient is >55 years old with DTC, the patient can be staged I-IVa/b depending on tumor extent (T), lymph node metastasis (N), and distant metastatic disease (M). When the tumor is limited to the thyroid gland, ≤4 cm in size, without positive lymph nodes or distant metastatic disease, the patient is stage I. For thyroid disease that is limited to the thyroid but greater than 4 cm or with gross extrathyroidal extension invading only the strap muscles, the stage is II. In addition, any T of DTC

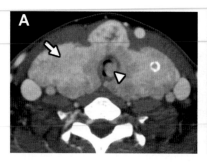

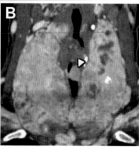

Fig. 4. A 32-year-old woman with known thyroid goiter, increasing size over the past 2 years with worsening dyspnea. (A) CECT axial image shows thyroid goiter (*white arrow*). Instead of simply compressing the trachea, a portion of the mass has invaded the trachea (*white arrowhead*), suggesting a more aggressive component. (B) CECT coronal image of the thyroid goiter demonstrates the site of tracheal invasion (*white arrowhead*). This portion of the mass was proven to be papillary thyroid cancer.

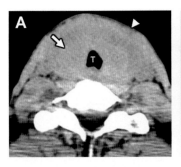 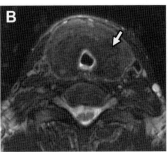

Fig. 5. A 42-year-old woman with a 5-month history of thyroid enlargement. At time of open biopsy, the thyroid was adherent to the strap muscles with preliminary pathology report being Riedel thyroiditis versus lymphoma. (*A*) Unenhanced CT axial image through thyroid demonstrates thyroidal enlargement with a smooth appearance (*white arrow*). No significant mass effect on the trachea (T) is seen. The strap muscles are stretched (*white arrowhead*). (*B*) T2-weighted, fat-saturated axial image shows diffusely T2-hypointense thyroid (*white arrow*) compared with **Fig. 2B**. Markedly decreased T2 signal suggests diagnosis of Riedel thyroiditis, which was later confirmed.

with lymph node metastasis is also stage II. For stage III, there can be any T or N of DTC with gross extrathyroidal extension and invasion of the subcutaneous soft tissues, larynx, trachea, esophagus, or RLN. Stage IVa can be any T or N with gross extrathyroidal extension invading the prevertebral fascia or with the presence of carotid artery or mediastinal vasculature encasement. Stage IVb occurs when there is any T or N stage with the presence of distant metastatic disease.[15]

Literature has shown that calcifications are more commonly found in thyroid malignancies over benign etiologies. For example, 26% to 79% of thyroid malignancies have calcifications, whereas benign etiologies have calcifications in only 8% to 39% of cases. CT is best for characterizing most calcifications versus ultrasonography , and these can be classified as macrocalcifications or microcalcifications. Microcalcifications have been found to have a higher association with thyroid malignancy; one study found that 70% of CT-detected microcalcifications were associated with malignancy, and 94% of these harbored PTC (**Fig. 6D**).[10]

Cervical lymphadenopathy from thyroid cancer can have calcification, hyperenhancement, internal proteinaceous components, hemorrhage, or may be cystic/necrotic.[1] Several studies have shown that the presence of lymphadenopathy in PTC leads to an increased risk of recurrence and an overall reduced survival. If there are calcifications within cervical lymph nodes, thyroid malignancy should be considered.[10]

DTCs rarely need CT or MR imaging for surveillance, and ultrasonography is less expensive and more accessible. In addition, iodinated contrast with CT is often contraindicated in thyroid cancer, as it could interfere and delay treatment with radioiodine due to false-negative radioiodine wholebody scans.[14] However, if it is determined that the addition of contrast will not delay treatment, CT neck with contrast and ultrasonography of the neck are usually appropriate in the presurgical

evaluation of DTC according to the American College of Radiology (ACR) Appropriateness Criteria (AC). In preoperative evaluation, MR imaging of the neck with or without contrast or CT neck without contrast may be appropriate.[16] CT is helpful in characterizing thyroid nodal metastases to evaluate for cystic components, rounded shape, or calcifications. The primary role of CT is in the postoperative setting where the thyroglobulin continues to rise but ultrasonography remains negative. CT chest is often needed, as the lungs are the most common location for metastasis after the neck.[14]

Papillary
PTC is most common type, accounting for 84% to 91% of all thyroid malignancies. It most commonly affects female adolescents and young adults (2.5:1.0 women:men), and has the best prognosis with more than 95% 5-year survival rate.[17] PTC has only a 1% to 2% mortality rate at 20 years after diagnosis.[18] Of all of the thyroid malignancies, PTC has the highest rate of cervical lymph node involvement, with involvement in up to 50% of cases. These lymph nodes may be cystic/necrotic, hypervascular, calcified, or hemorrhagic (**Fig. 6**).[19] PTC can also rarely occur in a thyroglossal duct cyst (TDC) (**Fig. 7**). Therefore, any nodularity or calcification noted within a TDC should be concerning for superimposed thyroid cancer, which is most commonly PTC.[20,21]

PTC does not typically invade the surrounding structures; however, if there is adjacent soft tissue involvement, a more aggressive component is suggested. PTC most commonly spreads to the regional lymph nodes, and if there is invasion of the upper aerodigestive tract or distant metastasis, there is a poorer prognosis with increased risk for recurrence.[17]

Follicular
FTC is the second most common type, accounting for 5% of cases. They are well differentiated, low

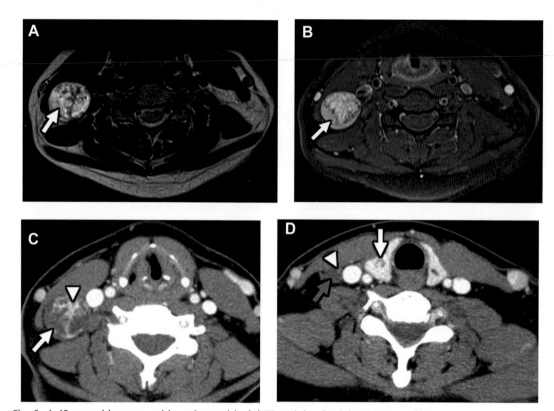

Fig. 6. A 43-year-old woman with optic neuritis. (*A*) T2-weighted axial MR image of the cervical spine was performed to look for demyelination; however, a partially cystic/necrotic right level III lymph node was discovered (*white arrow*). (*B*) T1-weighted, contrast-enhanced axial fat-saturated MR image shows same node avidly enhancing (*white arrow*). Given the young age, thyroid cancer was suggested and CECT was obtained. (*C*) CECT axial image through the level of the thyroid cartilage demonstrates a partially cystic/necrotic right level III lymph node (*white arrow*) with areas of enhancement/calcification (*white arrowhead*). (*D*) CECT axial image at the level of the thyroid. There is a largely cystic/necrotic right level IV lymph node (*gray arrow*) with a punctate calcification (*white arrowhead*). Pathology showed papillary thyroid cancer with the primary cancer being located in the right thyroid lobe (*white arrow*).

grade, and often found in the setting of iodine deficiency. FTC tends to be solitary and are slightly more aggressive than PTC. On pathologic evaluation, they have capsular and vascular invasion. Spread occurs via lymphatics, thus most commonly spreading to lung and bone. In the past decade, there have been many new studies showing that noninvasive encapsulated follicular variant PTC has virtually no risk of recurrence, metastasis, or death; however, the presence of more invasive components worsens prognosis. Although these tumors concentrate iodine less than PTC, radioiodine imaging may remain helpful.[22–24]

Medullary

MTC arises from the parafollicular C cells in the thyroid, accounting for 1% to 2% of all thyroid cancers. C cells secrete calcitonin, and the thyroid contains less than 0.01% to 0.1% of these cells.

MTCs are typically sporadic, but approximately 25% are associated with hereditary causes such as multiple endocrine neoplasia - type 2A or 2B syndromes or other familial causes linked to the Ret Proto-Oncogene.[25]

At presentation, approximately 48% of the patients have localized disease, 35% have disease extending beyond the thyroid or regional lymphadenopathy, and 13% have metastatic disease to the lung, liver, or bone (**Fig. 8**).[25] MTC often requires a multitude of imaging to evaluate the full extent of disease to best direct management; initially, imaging of the neck is preferred.[16,25] However, if there are elevated tumor markers or symptoms that are concerning for disease recurrence in other parts of the body, these areas are individually imaged. In the asymptomatic patient, imaging is dependent on the calcitonin levels.[16] The current American Thyroid Association guidelines suggest imaging to exclude metastatic disease in

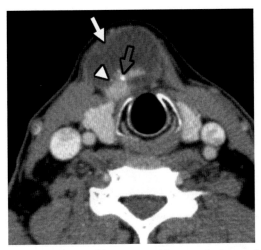

Fig. 7. A 35-year-old woman with an anterior neck mass. Unenhanced CT at the level of the thyroid demonstrates a TDC (*white arrow*) located at midline. Within the cyst, there is nodular, enhancing soft tissue (*white arrowhead*) with a punctate calcification (*gray arrow*). Pathology confirmed papillary thyroid cancer within a TDC.

pretreated patients with a calcitonin greater than 500 pg/mL (1836 pmol/L).[26] Postsurgical patients need imaging to exclude metastatic disease when serum calcitonin is >150 pg/mL (551 pmol/L).[27]

Most patients initially presenting with a palpable neck mass in the fifth or sixth decade of life have a sporadic case of MTC. These tumors are most likely located in the posterior thyroid resulting in compression or invasion of the adjacent structures leading to hoarseness, dysphagia, or respiratory impairment. Ultrasonography typically has nonspecific findings; therefore, CT and MR imaging are used for larger (>3 cm) nodules and to determine substernal extension or structural invasion. When the primary tumor is >1 cm, there is an increased risk for ipsilateral nodal involvement. Smaller thyroid malignancies may be first assessed with ultrasonography, with increased attention to the ipsilateral neck; however, there remains a 36% false-negative rate with these studies. CECT is often used to detect and characterize cervical and mediastinal lymphadenopathy, as well as to evaluate for pulmonary disease (see **Fig. 8B–C**). Although sclerotic or lytic lesions can be detected on CT, evaluation for bone marrow infiltration, spinal canal, and soft tissue is limited; therefore, further evaluation with MR imaging may be necessary.[25]

Surgery remains the only curative treatment in MTC, so detection of distant metastatic disease is critical. At the time of diagnosis, there is 35% to 50% nodal involvement and 10% to 15% distant disease.[25]

Anaplastic

ATC accounts for 1% to 2% of all thyroid malignancies; however, it accounts for more than 50% of all of the thyroid cancer deaths and continues to have the worst prognosis of all thyroid malignancies despite continued improvements in treatment. The mean survival rate remains at approximately 5 months, with the 1-year survival being 20%, and 2-year survival being 10%. ATC has been found to either occur de novo or via dedifferentiation of superimposed DTC. In contradistinction to all of the other thyroid malignancies, all cases of ATC are staged by the American Joint Committee on Cancer TNM stage as Stage IV due to its aggressiveness. Stage IVA is surgically resectable with tumor contained within the thyroid, stage IVB has extrathyroidal extension without distant disease, and stage IVC has distant metastatic disease. Surgical treatment is altered by presence of carotid encasement, vascular involvement, mediastinal extension, lymphadenopathy, distant disease, and invasion of the trachea, larynx, or esophagus.[13]

Typically, ATC presents with a rapidly enlarging neck mass in older patients, as the doubling rate can be as rapid as 1 week. There is a female predominance (1.5:1.0, women:men) with an overall characteristic of significant local invasion and soft tissue necrosis. Despite ultrasonography being the most common study for thyroid disease, these patients frequently undergo CECT due to the rapid neck enlargement. Typically, significant invasion of the adjacent structures occurs, involving the larynx, strap muscles, trachea, esophagus, and TEG. At diagnosis, approximately 40% have nodal spread, and 43% have distant disease. The most common sites of metastatic disease in decreasing order are lung, adrenals, liver, and brain. Death usually occurs from degree of pulmonary disease followed in frequency by airway compromise, hemorrhage, and cardiac arrest. Initial workup of these patients typically includes a high-quality CECT of the neck, whole-body PET-CT, brain MR imaging, and CT chest due to extent of distant disease at diagnosis.[13]

CECT for ATC characteristically shows a large necrotic thyroid mass with ill-defined margins, extrathyroidal extension, and invasion of the adjacent structures, versus DTCs, which are smaller and present with a solid, homogeneous, hypoattenuating nodule. Calcifications are commonly found in both PTC and AT; however, a higher incidence are found with ATC (62%) versus PTC (32%). Lymphoma and ATC can both present

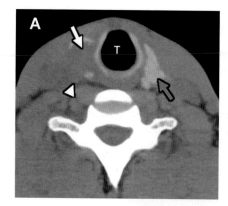
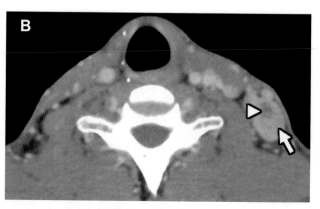
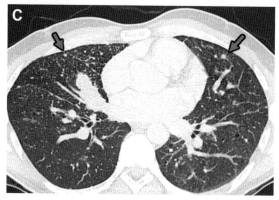

Fig. 8. A 33-year-old man with 2-year history of diarrhea and palpable anterior neck mass. Calcitonin level was 26,000. (*A*) Unenhanced CT axial image at level of thyroid shows ill-defined hypodense mass located in posterior right thyroid (*white arrow*). No definite invasion of the trachea (T) or significant mass effect on the right common carotid artery (*white arrowhead*) is seen. Left thyroid is normal and hyperdense due to the intrinsic iodine (*gray arrow*). (*B*) CECT axial image after total thyroidectomy demonstrates metastatic cervical lymphadenopathy. The enhancing node (*white arrow*) has small central area of necrosis (*white arrowhead*). (*C*) Axial CT of chest demonstrates military pattern of thyroid metastatic disease (*gray arrows*). Patient also had extensive necrotic mediastinal lymphadenopathy and disease in spine and liver.

with a rapidly enlarging neck mass, and distinction of the 2 is extremely important for treatment and diagnosis (flow cytometry is needed for lymphoma). Lymphoma also tends to typically have homogeneous enlargement, no calcifications, and no necrosis. Metastatic ATC also tends to be necrotic, whereas DTC typically is more homogeneously enhancing or solid, but occasionally also can be cystic.[13]

Lymphoma

Lymphoma is rare and accounts for 1.8% to 8.0% of all thyroid malignancies with a strong association with Hashimoto thyroiditis. The typical patient is an elderly woman with a rapidly enlarging thyroid with compressive symptoms. The presentation is very similar to AT; however, ATC is not associated with Hashimoto. On CT, lymphoma can demonstrate low-attenuation masses affecting either a large portion or the entire thyroid (**Fig. 9**). The 5-

year survival rate for stage IE is 75% to 89%, with stage IIE falling to 25% to 40%. Lymphoma must be diagnosed early, and the prognosis is largely dependent on the initial stage. Although CT imaging characteristics with clinical symptoms are suggestive of the diagnosis, biopsy remains mandatory and should be targeted to the solid portion of the tumor.[28]

TREATMENT IMPLICATIONS

CT and MR imaging are not routinely used for preoperative evaluation of thyroid cancer because ultrasonography is typically sufficient.[1] However, the recently revised thyroid cancer guidelines and the ACR AC have included a strong recommendation for the preoperative utilization of CT.[5,16] CT and MR imaging are complementary and yield important information especially in the preoperative assessment of advanced and recurrent thyroid

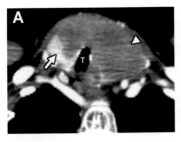
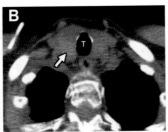

Fig. 9. A 68-year-old woman with long-standing history of Hashimoto thyroiditis with progressed swelling over past 5 days. (A) CECT axial image shows thyroidal enlargement with decreased enhancement of most of the thyroid (white arrowhead) with small noninvolved, normally enhancing thyroid tissue (white arrow). Minimal tracheal (T) narrowing and rightward deviation is present. (B) On unenhanced CT axial image after treatment, the thyroid is significantly decreased in size (white arrow) without residual tracheal (T) deviation.

carcinoma post-thyroidectomy. Cross-sectional imaging studies also aid in the evaluation of lymphadenopathy, especially in regions more difficult to assess with ultrasonography (ie, retropharyngeal region, mediastinum, low-level IV nodal station). The surgeon must know the extent of both thyroid and nodal disease. Invasion of the surrounding tissues can also be assessed on CT or MR imaging with attention to the paraspinal musculature, esophagus, trachea, larynx, and vasculature.[29]

The primary treatment in patients with thyroid cancer is total thyroidectomy followed by radioiodine, unless only microscopic disease is present.[7] In the past, NECT has been emphasized in thyroid cancer before radioiodine to not cause iodine overload before treatment; however, CECT has been found to be a good adjunct to ultrasonography when advanced disease is suspected, including invasive primary tumor and clinically apparent bulky lymphadenopathy.[4,5] Iodinated contrast is typically cleared from the residual thyroid tissue within 4 to 6 weeks, and thus should not have a significant negative impact on subsequent radioactive iodine analysis or treatment.[5] In the postoperative setting of thyroid cancer, the ACR AC states the utilization of thyroid ultrasonography is usually appropriate, whereas Iodine[123]/Iodine[131] whole-body scan, CT neck with contrast, and MR imaging neck with and without contrast may be appropriate.[16]

CT and MR imaging are necessary with a high clinical suspicion for local invasion, which may preclude curative intent or result in a more complicated surgery. The radiologist should focus on the thyroid and adjacent structures within the visceral space, including the trachea, esophagus, larynx, pharynx, and RLN. Imaging findings that raising concern for invasion include encasement of the trachea/esophagus greater than 180°, lumen deformity (see Fig. 4), focal mucosal irregularity, mucosal thickening, and effacement of the TEG fat with signs of vocal fold dysfunction.[1] T4a disease is diagnosed in the presence of invasion of any of these central

structures.[7] After these more central structures are assessed, the vascular structures, strap muscles, and prevertebral space should be interrogated. If there is any deformation of the CCA, there is a much higher likelihood of arterial invasion. A less specific sign for arterial invasion, is ≥180° of soft tissue encasement of the CCA. The CCA is the most commonly invaded artery; however, the mediastinal vessels also need to be assessed (Fig. 10).[1] If there is more than 270° of encasement of the mediastinal or carotid arteries, the mass is likely to be unresectable. T4b disease occurs in the presence of vascular invasion.[7] Invasion of the strap muscles is suspected once the mass has extended beyond the external surface of these muscles. Prevertebral muscle involvement is more challenging because the mass can compress the muscle resulting in MR imaging signal changes without actual invasion. Last, metastatic disease should be assessed. PTC and MTC both more typically spread to the regional lymph nodes, whereas FTC more commonly spreads to the lung and bones. ATC is very locally aggressive, but it can also spread to lymph nodes and lung. Thyroid cancer nodal disease typically involves level VI first, followed by levels II-V. Despite these more common nodal levels, metastasis from thyroid cancer also can go to the retropharyngeal nodes (Fig. 11), retroesophageal nodes, and the superior mediastinal nodes.[1]

Thyroid malignancy can also result in occlusion or effacement of the IJV; however, this does not influence the surgically resectability or stage. The IJV is easily compressible and thus can be occluded or effaced without invasion. Also, the presence of venous occlusion is not a reliable finding to suggest invasion.[7]

DIFFERENTIAL DIAGNOSIS

- Rapidly enlarging thyroid: lymphoma, ATC
- Palpable, firm, enlarging thyroid: lymphoma, ATC, thyroid sarcoma, Riedel thyroiditis

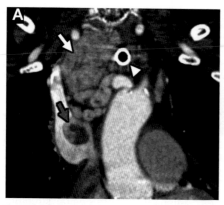
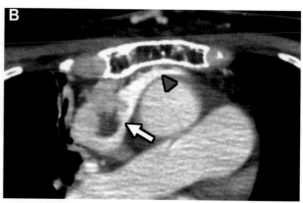

Fig. 10. A 74-year-old woman with papillary thyroid cancer and components of poorly differentiated thyroid cancer presenting with increasing shortness of breath. (*A*) CECT coronal image shows thyroidal enlargement enlarged thyroid (*white arrow*) with leftward tracheal deviation with endotracheal tube in place (*white arrowhead*). Inferior extension of thyroid into superior mediastinum is present with invasion of the superior vena cava (*gray arrow*). (*B*) CECT axial image at the level of the brachiocephalic vein (*gray arrowhead*) as it enters the superior vena cava shows the mass invades the adjacent vein (*white arrow*), rather than just compressing.

- Cystic lymphadenopathy: thyroid or human papillomavirus squamous cell carcinoma metastatic disease
- Calcifications in lymph nodes: thyroid carcinoma, granulomatous disease, treated lymphoma

- Cystic cervical lymph nodes in a young woman: consider thyroid carcinoma
- There can be ectopic thyroid tissue from the level of the foramen cecum to the thyroid bed, and this tissue can have same ailments as the normally positioned thyroid

PEARLS, PITFALLS, VARIANTS

- Presence of calcifications is nonspecific but can suggest malignancy
  - Punctate calcifications more likely to be due to PTC
- Retropharyngeal lymph node: think of nasopharyngeal, sinonasal, and thyroid carcinoma

WHAT THE REFERRING PHYSICIAN NEEDS TO KNOW

- Degree of substernal extension
- Deviation/compression of the adjacent structures ± suspected invasion
- Vocal fold asymmetry
- Cervical lymphadenopathy

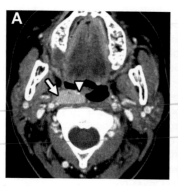
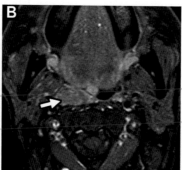
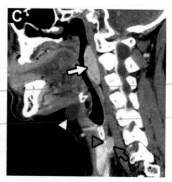

Fig. 11. A 39-year-old woman with an enlarging central neck mass for 1 year. (*A*) CECT axial image demonstrates an avidly enhancement right retropharyngeal lymph node (*white arrow*) with punctate calcification (*white arrowhead*). (*B*) T1-weighted contrast-enhanced, fat-saturated, axial MR image demonstrates enhancing retropharyngeal lymphadenopathy (*white arrow*). (*C*) CECT sagittal image shows the retropharyngeal lymph node (*white arrow*) positive for metastatic papillary thyroid cancer. Primary thyroid malignancy is in right thyroid (*gray arrow*) with a punctate calcification (*gray arrowhead*). Palpable central neck mass (*white arrowhead*) was a ruptured dermoid cyst.

- Suspicion of malignancy and whether biopsy is required

SUMMARY

Evaluation of thyroid disorders has continued to evolve; in the past, cross-sectional imaging was not used as it is currently. CT and MR imaging have become important in the preoperative assessment of benign etiologies such as thyroid goiter but are also important in the initial evaluation of thyroid malignancies and recurrent disease. It is important to discuss in the imaging report the substernal extent of the thyroid, extrathyroidal extension of disease, compression/displacement of the surrounding structures, and whether there is invasion of the adjacent structures as these findings can alter the surgical plan.

DISCLOSURE

The authors have nothing to disclose.

REFERENCES

1. Hoang JK, Sosa JA, Nguyen XV, et al. Imaging thyroid disease: updates, imaging approach, and management pearls. Radiol Clin North Am 2015;53(1): 145–61.
2. Cox AE, LeBeau SO. Diagnosis and treatment of differentiated thyroid carcinoma. Radiol Clin North Am 2011;49(3):453–62, vi.
3. Hoang JK, Choudhury KR, Eastwood JD, et al. An exponential growth in incidence of thyroid cancer: trends and impact of CT imaging. AJNR Am J Neuroradiol 2014;35(4):778–83.
4. Haugen BR, Alexander EK, Bible KC, et al. 2015 American Thyroid Association management guidelines for adult patients with thyroid nodules and differentiated thyroid cancer: The American Thyroid Association Guidelines Task Force on Thyroid Nodules and Differentiated Thyroid Cancer. Thyroid 2016;26(1):1–133.
5. Haugen BR. 2015 American Thyroid Association management guidelines for adult patients with thyroid nodules and differentiated thyroid cancer: what is new and what has changed? Cancer 2017; 123(3):372–81.
6. Nachiappan AC, Metwalli ZA, Hailey BS, et al. The thyroid: review of imaging features and biopsy techniques with radiologic-pathologic correlation. Radiographics 2014;34(2):276–93.
7. Bin Saeedan M, Aljohani IM, Khushaim AO, et al. Thyroid computed tomography imaging: pictorial review of variable pathologies. Insights Imaging 2016; 7(4):601–17.
8. Loevner LA, editor. Anatomy and pathology of the thyroid and parathyroid glands. 5th edition. St Louis (MO): Mosby, Inc., an affliate of Elseiver Inc.; 2011.
9. Farrá JC, Picado O, Liu S, et al. Clinically significant cancer rates in incidentally discovered thyroid nodules by routine imaging. J Surg Res 2017;219: 341–6.
10. Wu CW, Dionigi G, Lee KW, et al. Calcifications in thyroid nodules identified on preoperative computed tomography: patterns and clinical significance. Surgery 2012;151(3):464–70.
11. Rallison ML, Dobyns BM, Meikle AW, et al. Natural history of thyroid abnormalities: prevalence, incidence, and regression of thyroid diseases in adolescents and young adults. Am J Med 1991;91(4): 363–70.
12. Hennessey JV. Clinical review: Riedel's thyroiditis: a clinical review. J Clin Endocrinol Metab 2011;96(10): 3031–41.
13. Ahmed S, Ghazarian MP, Cabanillas ME, et al. Imaging of anaplastic thyroid carcinoma. AJNR Am J Neuroradiol 2018;39(3):547–51.
14. Johnson NA, LeBeau SO, Tublin ME. Imaging surveillance of differentiated thyroid cancer. Radiol Clin North Am 2011;49(3):473–87, vi.
15. Manzardo OA, Cellini M, Indirli R, et al. TNM 8th edition in thyroid cancer staging: is there an improvement in predicting recurrence? Endocr Relat Cancer 2020. https://doi.org/10.1530/ERC-19-0412.
16. Hoang JK, Oldan JD, Mandel SJ, et al. ACR appropriateness criteria. J Am Coll Radiol 2019;16(5S): S300–14.
17. Aslam W, Shakespeare A, Jones S, et al. Massive hemoptysis: an unusual presentation of papillary thyroid carcinoma due to tracheal invasion. BMJ Case Rep 2019;12(8). https://doi.org/10.1136/bcr-2019-229330.
18. Song B, Wang H, Chen Y, et al. Magnetic resonance imaging in the prediction of aggressive histological features in papillary thyroid carcinoma. Medicine (Baltimore) 2018;97(26):e11279.
19. Som PM, Brandwein M, Lidov M, et al. The varied presentations of papillary thyroid carcinoma cervical nodal disease: CT and MR findings. AJNR Am J Neuroradiol 1994;15(6):1123–8.
20. Alatsakis M, Drogouti M, Tsompanidou C, et al. Invasive thyroglossal duct cyst papillary carcinoma: a case report and review of the literature. Am J Case Rep 2018;19:757–62.
21. Glastonbury CM, Davidson HC, Haller JR, et al. The CT and MR imaging features of carcinoma arising in thyroglossal duct remnants. AJNR Am J Neuroradiol 2000;21(4):770–4.
22. Franssila KO, Ackerman LV, Brown CL, et al. Follicular carcinoma. Semin Diagn Pathol 1985;2(2): 101–22.

23. Hay ID. Papillary thyroid carcinoma. Endocrinol Metab Clin North Am 1990;19(3):545–76.

24. Borda A, Zahan AE, Piciu D, et al. A 15 year institutional experience of well-differentiated follicular cell-derived thyroid carcinomas; impact of the new 2017 TNM and WHO Classifications of Tumors of Endocrine Organs on the epidemiological trends and pathological characteristics. Endocrine 2020;67(3):630–42.

25. Kushchayev SV, Kushchayeva YS, Tella SH, et al. Medullary thyroid carcinoma: an update on imaging. J Thyroid Res 2019;2019:1893047.

26. Wells SA, Asa SL, Dralle H, et al. Revised American Thyroid Association guidelines for the management of medullary thyroid carcinoma. Thyroid 2015; 25(6):567–610.

27. Raue F, Frank-Raue K. Long-term follow-up in medullary thyroid carcinoma. Recent Results Cancer Res 2015;204:207–25.

28. Takashima S, Ikezoe J, Morimoto S, et al. Primary thyroid lymphoma: evaluation with CT. Radiology 1988;168(3):765–8.

29. Sanchez RB, vanSonnenberg E, D'Agostino HB, et al. Ultrasound guided biopsy of nonpalpable and difficult to palpate thyroid masses. J Am Coll Surg 1994;178(1):33–7.

30. Hoang JK, Langer JE, Middleton WD, et al. Managing incidental thyroid nodules detected on imaging: white paper of the ACR Incidental Thyroid Findings Committee. J Am Coll Radiol 2015;12(2):143–50.

Parathyroid Imaging

Malak Itani, MD*, William D. Middleton, MD

KEYWORDS

- Parathyroid • Imaging • Radiology • Hyperparathyroidism • Ultrasound • Sestamibi
- Four-dimensional CT

KEY POINTS

- In patients with primary hyperparathyroidism, imaging of parathyroid glands plays an important role in localization of parathyroid adenomas prior to minimally invasive parathyroid resection.
- PHPT is caused by a single adenoma in 80% of cases, double adenomas in 5%, and multigland hyperplasia in 15%.
- Ultrasound and sestamibi scans are first-line imaging modalities with sensitivities of 80% and 84%, respectively.
- 4DCT is particularly valuable in cases of nondiagnostic or discordant ultrasound and sestamibi, or after failed neck operation.

INTRODUCTION

Primary hyperparathyroidism (PHPT) is an endocrine disorder defined by an elevated or inappropriately normal parathyroid hormone (PTH) level. Secondary hyperparathyroidism is elevated PTH in response to a metabolic alteration in patients with chronic kidney disease, typically due to high blood phosphorus levels, low levels of active vitamin D, or low blood calcium levels. With chronic elevation in PTH levels, true autonomy of the parathyroid glands occurs, leading to tertiary hyperparathyroidism. The role of imaging in hyperparathyroidism is to guide minimally invasive surgical interventions for PHPT.[1] Medical therapy remains the mainstay of management in secondary and tertiary hyperparathyroidism; therefore, the focus of this review is related to PHPT.

The prevalence of PHPT is 1 to 7 cases per 1000 individuals, with higher incidence among female and Black individuals, and the older population.[2] The highest prevalence of PHPT is among postmenopausal women and is estimated to be as high as 3%.[3] Sporadic PHPT is associated with exposure to ionizing radiation in childhood and with chronic lithium use.[4] The clinical presentation is usually nonspecific, and classically summarized as "stones, bones, groans, and moans" in reference to kidney stones, bone pain, abdominal groans from gastrointestinal symptoms, and psychiatric moans from central nervous system effects. Although this remains the clinical presentation in developing countries, the most common presentation in the United States and Europe is incidental asymptomatic hypercalcemia on routine laboratory analysis.[5] Normocalcemic hyperparathyroidism is a variant of PHPT recognized in 2009, usually diagnosed during investigations for low bone mineral density.[6] PHPT is caused by a single enlarged adenoma in 80% of cases, double adenomas in 5% to 10% of cases, multigland hyperplasia in 10% to 15% of cases (usually in familial endocrinopathies), and parathyroid carcinoma in less than 1% of cases.[1]

The parathyroid glands develop from the pharyngeal pouches in the fifth and sixth weeks of gestation and migrate caudally. The superior glands descend only a short distance, and thus their final location is less variable. They are typically located posterior to the thyroid, between the junction of the upper and middle thirds of the thyroid gland, and close to the inferior margin of the cricoid cartilage. The inferior glands migrate for a longer distance, more medially and inferiorly,

Mallinckrodt Institute of Radiology, Washington University in St. Louis School of Medicine, 510 South Kingshighway Boulevard, Campus Box 8131, St Louis, MO 63110, USA
* Corresponding author.
E-mail address: mitani@wustl.edu

Radiol Clin N Am 58 (2020) 1071–1083
https://doi.org/10.1016/j.rcl.2020.07.006
0033-8389/20/© 2020 Elsevier Inc. All rights reserved.

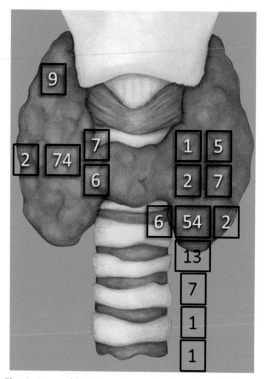

Fig. 1. Normal location of superior (patient right) and inferior (patient left) parathyroid glands. Previously published materials unchanged from the source. (*From* Mellnick VM, Middleton WD, Parathyroid Sonography. *Ultrasound Clinics* 2014; 9:339-350; with permission.)

and are thus more variable in location, and can be found anywhere from the angle of the mandible to the superior pericardium[7,8] (**Fig. 1**). Their classic location is directly posterior to the inferior margin of the thyroid gland (50% of cases) or 1 cm below it (15% of cases).[9] Ectopic locations for either superior or inferior glands include the tracheoesophageal groove, retroesophageal space, and rarely within the thyroid. Additional locations for ectopic superior parathyroid glands include retropharyngeal locations and posterior mediastinum, whereas ectopic inferior glands also can be found within the thymic capsule (38% of ectopic glands), carotid sheath, submandibular region, and down into the mediastinum.[1,10] Normal glands are very small in size, measuring 5 × 3 × 1 mm with estimated weight of 15 to 45 mg,[11] and are usually not visualized on imaging.[12] Most people have 4 parathyroid glands, although 2.5% to 15.0% have supernumerary glands[7] that can be located adjacent to the normal parathyroid glands or in the mediastinum and thymic capsule.[1]

IMAGING PROTOCOLS

Imaging modalities used for localizing parathyroid adenomas include ultrasound, 4-dimensional computed tomography (4DCT) and nuclear medicine scintigraphy. Imaging protocols are summarized in **Table 1**.

Ultrasound provides the advantages of being relatively inexpensive, using nonionizing radiation, delivering superb image quality in thin patients,

Table 1
Optimized imaging protocols for parathyroid adenoma detection

Protocol parameter	Ultrasound	4DCT	Scintigraphy
Scan range	Hyoid bone to thoracic inlet	Angle of mandible to carina	Parotid glands to lower heart
Patient positioning	Supine with neck hyperextension	Supine	Supine
Contrast or radiopharmaceutical	–	100 mL Omnipaque 350 at 5–6 mL/s	20 mCi Tc-99m sestamibi
Timing	–	Noncontrast Arterial phase (25 s) Venous phase (82 s)	Immediate at 5 min; delayed at 2 h
Acquisition	Linear high-frequency transducer	Slice thickness 0.75 mm	Immediate planar Delayed planar and SPECT/CT
Reconstruction	–	Axial, coronal, and sagittal 2-mm soft tissue windows	Axial, coronal, and sagittal typically at acquired thickness

Abbreviations: 4DCT, 4-dimensional CT; CT, computed tomography; SPECT, single-photon emission CT.

Table 2
Typical imaging features of parathyroid adenomas

Ultrasound	Solid well-circumscribed homogeneously hypoechoic ovoid structure Craniocaudal orientation of the long axis Variable internal vascularity
Scintigraphy	Persistent radiopharmaceutical retention on delayed images Extrathyroidal radiotracer uptake on SPECT images Tracer-avid soft tissue nodule on fused SPECT/CT images
4DCT	Early arterial enhancement Early washout on venous-phase images

Abbreviations: 4DCT, 4-dimensional CT; CT, computed tomography; SPECT, single-photon emission CT.

having a low carbon footprint, and especially providing concomitant evaluation of the thyroid gland. Its primary disadvantages are poor image quality in obese patients and operator dependency. It is typically performed after placing a pillow under the patient's shoulders so that there is hyperextension of the neck. A high-frequency linear transducer is used to allow for higher resolution. Additional evaluation of the superior mediastinum can be attempted with a high-frequency curved array transducer, such as the ones used for neonatal head or transvaginal ultrasound. Color Doppler or power Doppler can also help in the diagnosis. The examination initially focuses on the region posterior and inferior to the thyroid gland. Visualization of the paratracheal and paraesophageal regions is improved by turning the patient's head to the contralateral side and scanning from a lateral approach. When an enlarged parathyroid gland is not detected in the typical locations, survey of potentially ectopic locations also should be performed.[13,14]

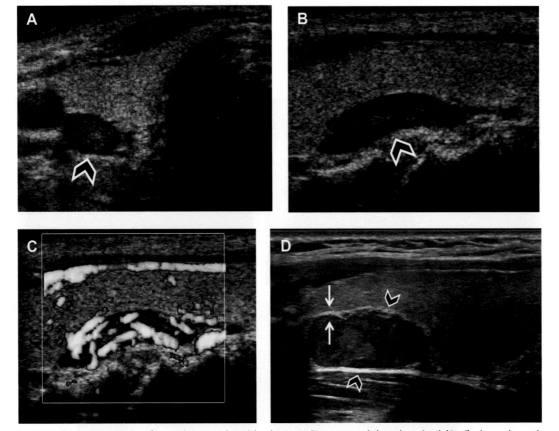

Fig. 2. Typical appearance of superior parathyroid adenoma. Transverse (*A*) and sagittal (*B, C*) views show the typical grayscale and power Doppler appearance of a superior parathyroid adenoma (*arrowheads*). It is a solid, ovoid, well-defined, hypoechoic nodule immediately posterior to the thyroid gland with increased internal vascularity. (*D*) Sagittal view in a different patient shows another superior parathyroid adenoma (*arrowheads*). The white line (*arrows*) that separates the parathyroid adenoma from the thyroid helps distinguish this nodule from a thyroid nodule.

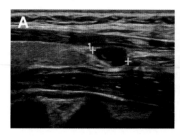
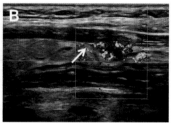

Fig. 3. Typical appearance of inferior parathyroid adenoma. Sagittal views show the typical grayscale (A) and color Doppler (B) appearance of an inferior parathyroid adenoma (cursors in A). It is a solid, ovoid, well-defined, hypoechoic nodule immediately inferior to the thyroid gland with increased internal vascularity and a polar vessel (arrow in B) exiting the superior border of the nodule.

Nuclear scintigraphy for parathyroid adenoma localization is usually performed with a single radiotracer (Tc-99m sestamibi). Immediate and 2-hour delayed planar images are obtained, in addition to an immediate or a delayed single-photon emission computed tomography (SPECT) or SPECT/CT acquisition. Because the most common cause for a false positive diagnosis of parathyroid adenoma on scintigraphy is a thyroid adenoma, a dual tracer subtraction technique can provide a way to characterize the latter. In the dual tracer technique, an additional imaging acquisition is performed with a thyroid imaging agent, such as Tc-99m pertechnetate or I-123, then subtracted from the sestamibi images.

4DCT is another major technique for localizing parathyroid adenomas. It was introduced as a multiphase CT with 4 phases (noncontrast, arterial, venous, and delayed), thus referred to as 4D, the fourth dimension being time. The fourth delayed phase is no longer considered necessary because the 3-phase protocol provides a good balance between radiation exposure and diagnostic performance.[15]

IMAGING FINDINGS/PATHOLOGY
Diagnostic Criteria

The diagnostic criteria for parathyroid adenomas are listed in **Table 2**. On ultrasound, the typical

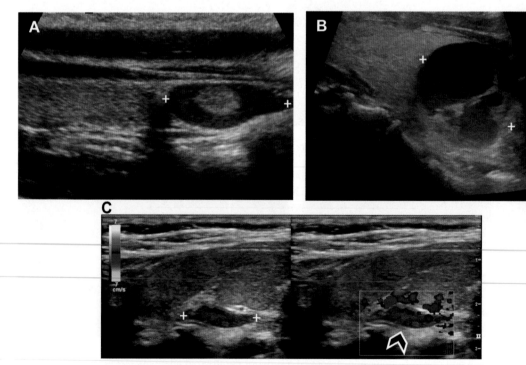

Fig. 4. Examples of atypical sonographic appearance of parathyroid adenomas (cursors) in different patients containing (A) internal echogenic components, (B) cystic spaces, and (C) minimal detectable internal flow (arrowhead), as seen on side-by-side grayscale and color Doppler images.

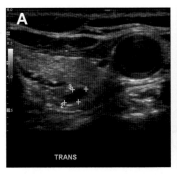
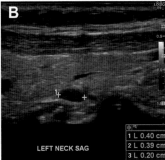

Fig. 5. Advantage of ultrasound in patients with thin neck. Transverse (*A*) and sagittal (*B*) grayscale images show a small superior parathyroid adenoma (*cursors*).

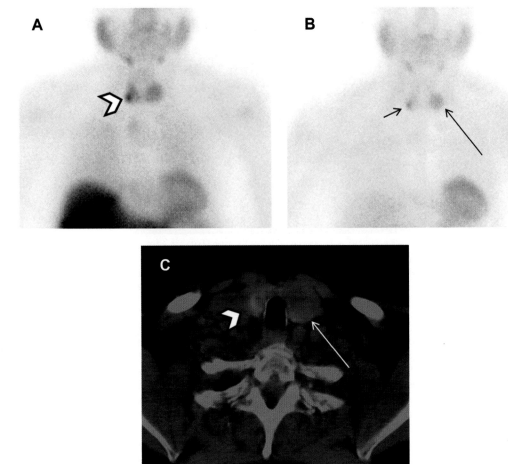

Fig. 6. Parathyroid adenoma on sestamibi scan. (*A*) Immediate and (*B*) delayed anterior images of Tc-99m sestamibi demonstrate a focus of intense uptake inferior to the right thyroid lobe (*arrowhead*) that becomes more conspicuous on the delayed 2-hour images (*short arrow*). Round area of focal uptake in the left thyroid on delayed images was confirmed histologically to be benign nodular hyperplasia (*long arrow*). (*C*) Axial fused SPECT/CT images localize the area of increased uptake to a small soft tissue nodule consistent with parathyroid adenoma. Again noted is the left thyroid lesion.

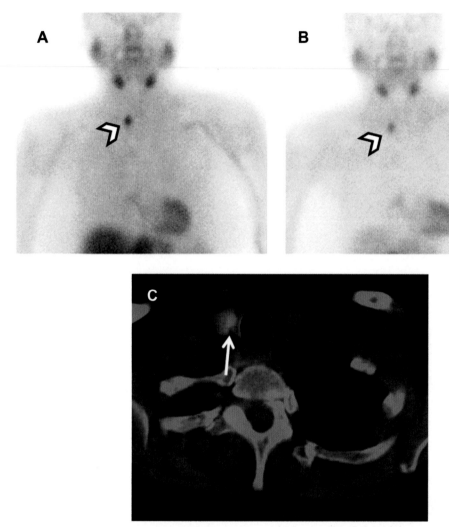

Fig. 7. Parathyroid adenoma on sestamibi scan. (*A*) Immediate and (*B*) delayed anterior images of Tc-99m sesta-mibi in a 73-year-old woman with prior thyroidectomy. A focus of increased uptake (*arrowheads*) in the right inferior neck is very clearly visualized given lack of uptake in the thyroid bed. (*C*) Fused axial SPECT/CT images localize the area of increased uptake to a small soft tissue nodule, consistent with parathyroid adenoma (*arrow*).

appearance for an enlarged parathyroid is a solid, well-circumscribed homogeneously hypoechoic ovoid structure, with its long axis oriented cranio-caudally (**Figs. 2** and **3**). Less commonly, parathy-roid adenomas can be isoechoic to the thyroid, contain focal hyperechoic areas, demonstrate internal heterogeneity, or contain cystic spaces (**Fig. 4**). Adenomas usually have detectable internal vascularity that may be less than, equal to, or greater than thyroid vascularity. However, when adenomas are small and deep, there may be no detectable flow. In some cases, there is a dominant peripheral vessel inserting or exiting at its pole. A large size of more than 3 cm, lobulated or irregular margins, extensive heterogeneity, or

calcifications should raise concern for parathyroid carcinoma, particularly when the patient has more severe symptoms and laboratory abnormalities. The sensitivity of ultrasound for detecting parathy-roid adenomas has been reported to range be-tween 65% and 97%, with one meta-analysis concluding an overall sensitivity of 80%.[16] In another meta-analysis, ultrasound had a pooled sensitivity of 76.1% and positive predictive value (PPV) of 93.2% for detecting parathyroid ade-nomas.[15] Sensitivity for detection of small parathy-roid adenomas is particularly good in patients with thin necks (**Fig. 5**). Sensitivity, however, decreases in obese patients, with multigland disease, after prior neck surgeries, and in the presence of

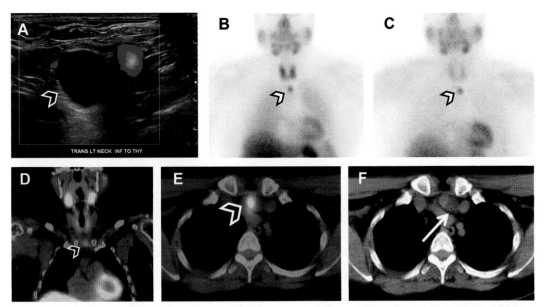

Fig. 8. Ectopic parathyroid adenoma on sestamibi scan. (*A*) Neck ultrasound identified a cyst (*arrowhead*) inferior to the left thyroid lobe. Sestamibi scan confirmed radiotracer uptake in the superior mediastinum on (*B*) immediate images, with persistent uptake on (*C*) 2-hour delay images (*arrowheads*). Findings were confirmed on SPECT/CT as seen on fused (*D*) coronal and (*E*) axial images (*arrowheads*), and on (*F*) correlative CT, which demonstrates the partial cystic component (*arrow*). On surgery, the patient was found to have a cystic parathyroid adenoma in the superior mediastinum (of which the cystic component was only partially visualized on neck ultrasound).

thyromegaly.[15,17] Due to lack of an acoustic window, ultrasound also has limited sensitivity in detecting ectopic mediastinal parathyroid glands.

On sestamibi scan, parathyroid adenomas demonstrate early and intense uptake of sestamibi due to their increased mitochondrial activity, which may be obscured by similar level of tracer uptake in the thyroid gland. Approximately 60% of parathyroid adenomas demonstrate persistent tracer uptake, due to slower washout rate than the thyroid, and are detected as a focus of increased radiotracer on 2-hour delayed planar images[18] (**Figs. 6** and **7**). A second variant of parathyroid adenoma demonstrates early washout of tracer similar to the thyroid gland; these are harder to appreciate but can be detectable as a focal bulge in the contour of the thyroid gland on the immediate planar images. In addition, some adenomas demonstrate more intense uptake of tracer than the thyroid gland on early-phase images, which can aid in their detection. It is important to mention all focal abnormalities when reporting sestamibi scans and to correlate them with anatomic imaging of the thyroid gland. In some cases, there is persistent radiotracer uptake within the thyroid gland on delayed phase images, commonly seen in elderly individuals or in patients with diffuse thyroid disease; an even more delayed acquisition, such as a 4-hour delay, to allow for better clearance of the radiopharmaceutical from the thyroid gland, can be beneficial. SPECT images can be performed directly after the immediate planar images or at the 2-hour delay time point, and they increase sensitivity for detection of parathyroid adenomas due to 3-dimensional images that improve visualization of superimposed structures. Availability of CT images for localization can further increase sensitivity and diagnostic confidence in parathyroid adenomas and can facilitate comparison with other imaging studies and assist the surgeon in finding the adenoma. The diagnostic performance of scintigraphy with SPECT is generally comparable to ultrasound,

Box 1
Differential considerations
Lymph node
Exophytic thyroid nodule
Lipoma/fat lobule
Vascular structures
Metastatic thyroid cancer
Other cervical and mediastinal lesions

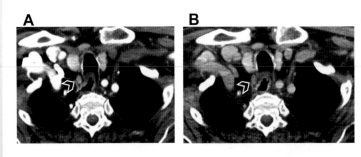

Fig. 9. Typical appearance of a parathyroid adenoma on 4DCT. Axial (*A*) arterial-phase image demonstrates an enhancing soft tissue nodule (*arrowheads*) in the tracheoesophageal groove with (*B*) venous-phase rapid washout, consistent with parathyroid adenoma. Patient underwent selective exploration of the right neck, and intraoperative parathyroid hormone levels dropped from 88 to 34 pg/mL.

with added benefit for detecting mediastinal adenomas (**Fig. 8**). In a recent meta-analysis, the sensitivity ranged between 57% and 100% with a pooled sensitivity of 84%.[16] In another meta-analysis of planar, SPECT, and SPECT/CT with Tc-99m sestamibi for detecting parathyroid adenomas, the pooled sensitivities were 63%, 66%, and 84%, and the PPVs were 90%, 82%, and 95%, respectively.[19] It is important to note that combining scintigraphy with ultrasound provides an incremental value in diagnostic accuracy of parathyroid adneomas.[4,15]

On 4DCT images, parathyroid adenomas are most conspicuous on arterial-phase images where they demonstrate avid enhancement, with rapid washout on venous-phase images (**Figs. 9** and **10**). The main concern with 4DCT is the radiation exposure; thus, it is reserved for cases in which

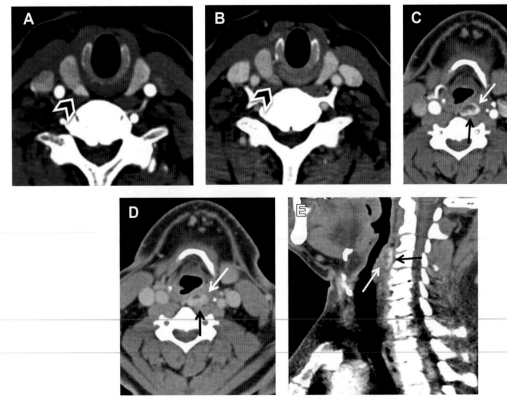

Fig. 10. Superior parathyroid adenoma on 4DCT. Typical appearance of a right superior parathyroid adenoma (*arrowheads*) seen on (*A*) arterial and (*B*) venous-phase images as a hyperenhancing soft tissue nodule directly posterior to the thyroid gland, with rapid washout. (*C, D, E*) Ectopic parathyroid adenoma (*arrows*) detected as a retropharyngeal nodule just anterior to the cervical spine, demonstrating peripheral (*C*) arterial hyperenhancement, with peripheral washout but central filling on the (*D*) venous phase, suspicious for parathyroid adenoma. This adenoma was causing mass effect on the posterior wall of the hypopharynx on sagittal reconstruction (*E*).

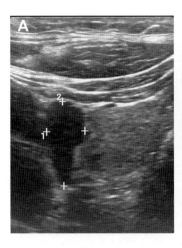
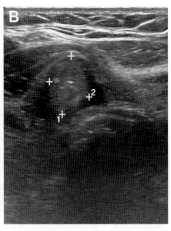

Fig. 11. Parathyroid adenoma and incidental papillary thyroid cancer. (A) Transverse grayscale image shows a parathyroid adenoma (cursors) adjacent to the right lobe of the thyroid. (B) Transverse view of the isthmus shows a solid, isoechoic, taller-than-wide nodule (cursors) with punctate echogenic foci. This TR5 nodule by American College of Radiology Thyroid Imaging, Reporting and Data System criteria measured 1.1 cm and was histologically confirmed to be a papillary thyroid cancer.

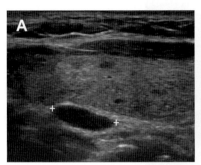
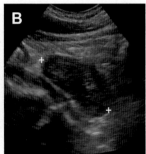

Fig. 12. Multigland adenomas. (A) Longitudinal grayscale view of the right neck shows superior parathyroid adenoma (cursors) posterior to the right thyroid. (B) An additional view of the low right neck obtained with a transvaginal probe shows a second parathyroid adenoma (cursors) of the inferior gland.

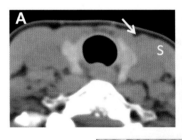
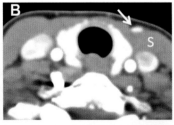
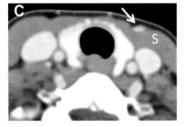
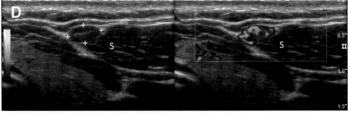

Fig. 13. Reimplanted parathyroid. A 56-year-old woman status post parathyroidectomy with reimplantation of one gland presents with recurrent hyperparathyroidism. (A–C) 4DCT images demonstrate a small nodule (arrows) anterior to the sternocleidomastoid muscle (S) that enhances avidly in the (B) arterial phase and washes out in the (C) venous phase, typical of a parathyroid adenoma. (D) Preoperative ultrasound was performed for marking the reimplanted gland, and demonstrates an enlarged parathyroid gland (cursors) superficial to the most medial aspect of the left sternocleidomastoid muscle (S) with intense hypervascularity.

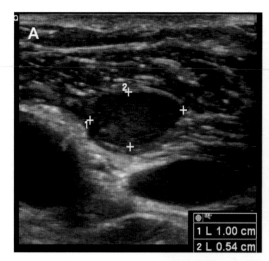

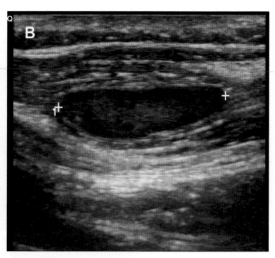

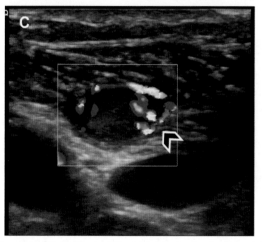

Fig. 14. Ectopic parathyroid adenoma. (*A*) Axial and (*B*) sagittal B-mode and (*C*) axial color Doppler images in a 45-year-old man with prior history of papillary thyroid cancer status post thyroidectomy and parathyroidectomy 19 years ago, with parathyroid reimplantation in the left forearm presents with persistent elevated calcium and elevated parathyroid hormone level of 120 pg/mL (reference range 14–64). Neck ultrasound images demonstrate a hypoechoic nodule (*cursors* in *A* and *B*) along the cervical lymph node chain at level 3 overlying the great vessels with internal vascularity (*arrowhead* in *C*) and a prominent feeding vessel. The radiologic differential considerations were recurrent metastatic lymph node versus ectopic parathyroid adenoma. Thyroglobulin levels in the serum and in the nodule aspirate were undetectable (<0.1 ng/mL). Cytology and surgical pathology were consistent with parathyroid adenoma.

ultrasound and sestamibi were nonlocalizing or discordant, or for patients with persistent or recurrent hyperparathyroidism after neck exploration.[20,21] In addition, 4DCT demonstrates higher sensitivity for detecting multigland disease.[21] Compared with ultrasound and SPECT, a 4DCT might provide a similar to slightly improved performance with sensitivity of 73.0% to 89.4%.[15,17] A cost-utility analysis in 2011 demonstrated that surgeons use ultrasound and scintigraphy as first-line modalities for localization and reserve 4DCT for more challenging or reoperative cases.[1]

Differential Diagnosis

A variety of cervical and superior mediastinal structures can be mistaken for a parathyroid adenoma (**Box 1**). On ultrasound, differential considerations for parathyroid adenomas include well-defined cervical nodules, such as lymph nodes, which are typically differentiated by their location along lymph node chains and an echogenic fatty hilum with hilar vascularity. Consequentially, morphologically abnormal lymph nodes with loss of the fatty hilum or peripheral vascularity can be harder to differentiate from parathyroid adenomas

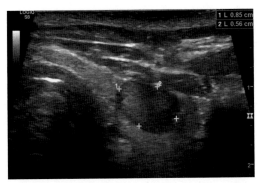

Fig. 15. Intrathyroid parathyroid adenoma. Transverse sonogram of the left thyroid shows a solid, hypoechoic intrathyroidal nodule (*cursors*). FNA showed a PTH tissue washout level of 8832 pg/mL, consistent with an intrathyroidal parathyroid adenoma.

than morphologically benign nodes. If the nodule is located lateral to the common carotid artery, it is very unlikely to be a parathyroid adenoma. Other differential considerations include exophytic

thyroid nodules or separate thyroid lobulations in which a prominent thin hyperechoic septum is seen between 2 portions of the thyroid gland. This is most often along the posterior border of the mid to lower portion of the thyroid and is due to an anatomic variant known as the tubercle of Zuckerkandl. This can be differentiated on ultrasound by examining the entire margins of the nodule; a prominent lobulation or exophytic nodule typically has a thin portion that is still communicating with the thyroid gland. An anechoic fluid-filled esophageal diverticulum or a vascular structure might be mistaken for a very hypoechoic parathyroid adenoma; in these scenarios, color Doppler and varying manual pressure with the transducer can aid in the diagnosis.

On sestamibi scan, a thyroid adenoma can be differentiated from a parathyroid adenoma with a dual tracer study in which a thyroid adenoma demonstrates uptake of Tc-99m pertechnetate or I-123 but a parathyroid adenoma remains photopenic (cold). Alternatively, correlation with ultrasound

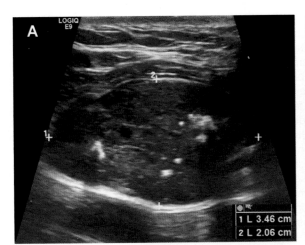
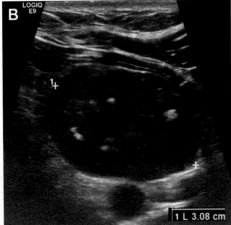
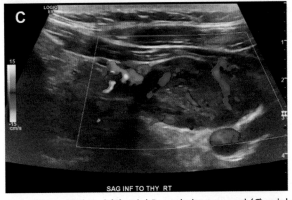

Fig. 16. Parathyroid carcinoma. (*A*) Sagittal and (*B*) axial B-mode images and (*C*) axial color Doppler images in a 38-year-old man with primary hyperparathyroidism demonstrate an enlarged parathyroid with internal calcifications (*cursors* in *A* and *B*). Pathology was consistent with parathyroid carcinoma with negative surgical margins.

can establish the diagnosis of a thyroid rather than a parathyroid nodule. Other causes of false positive sestamibi uptake in the neck are rare and include malignancies such as lung, breast, and papillary thyroid cancer, in addition to reactive and metastatic lymph nodes.[11]

On 4DCT, causes of false positive findings include arterial hyperenhancing lesions, such as vascular structures, neuroendocrine tumors, and pathologic lymph nodes such as those metastatic from hypervascular primary malignancies, namely papillary thyroid cancer. It is important to perform noncontrast CT as part of the 4DCT protocol to differentiate hyperenhancement from hyperdense lesions such as ectopic thyroid nodules and mildly calcified lymph nodes.

Pearls, Pitfalls, and Variants

A major advantage of parathyroid sonography is its ability to evaluate thyroid nodules. Because these patients are typically going to the operating room to resect an abnormal parathyroid gland, it is also important to know whether there is a thyroid nodule that needs attention. Any suspicious thyroid nodule should either undergo fine needle aspiration (FNA) before surgery or should be resected during the parathyroid operation (Fig. 11). Parathyroid adenomas are most often solitary, but approximately 5% to 10% of patients will have involvement of 2 glands. It is important not to fall for the "happy eye syndrome" once a single adenoma is identified (Fig. 12). In addition, 4-gland hyperplasia can be seen in the subset of patients with secondary or tertiary hyperparathyroidism who are referred for surgical resection in cases of severe osteopenia, uncontrolled symptoms, calciphylaxis, or very high parathyroid hormone levels; preoperative imaging is not routinely performed in these patients, but it can be useful to identify ectopic gland location or asymmetric gland hyperplasia.[22] In these patients, a portion of a gland can be reimplanted in the forearm, or anterior to abdominal wall musculature or sternocleidomastoid muscle (Fig. 13).

Lymph nodes are typically differentiated from parathyroid adenomas by their location and their morphologic features, but ectopic parathyroid adenomas may present in the expected location of cervical lymph nodes, rendering their diagnosis more challenging (Fig. 14). In these cases, additional passes can be performed during the FNA for determining PTH levels in the nodule.

Another diagnostic challenge arises with intrathyroid parathyroid adenomas (Fig. 15), especially in patients with a multinodular thyroid gland. Determining PTH levels in the nodule is also crucial

in these cases because it is harder to differentiate a parathyroid adenoma from a thyroid nodule on cytology than it is to differentiate a parathyroid adenoma from a lymph node.

List: Pearls and Pitfalls

　Look for a fatty hilum to differentiate lymph nodes from adenomas

　Given that intrathyroidal parathyroid adenomas are rare, if you suspect one, then consider sampling for PTH levels before surgery

　Always look for multigland disease

List: Variants

　Ectopic locations of parathyroid adenomas

　Internal cystic spaces in cystic adenomas

　Focal hyperechoic areas or internal heterogeneity

WHAT THE REFERRING PHYSICIAN NEEDS TO KNOW

Bilateral neck exploration has been the classic surgical approach for parathyroidectomy; however, with preoperative localization imaging studies, a minimally invasive technique is possible in a large subset of patients, providing improved cosmesis, shorter operation time, shorter hospital stay, lower cost of care, lower morbidity, and high cure rates.[1] For the surgeon, when localization with ultrasound and sestamibi is concordant, a minimally invasive technique can be performed, with intraoperative confirmation of normalized PTH levels. The information relayed to the referring provider should include the accurate size and location of the parathyroid adenoma, as well as presence of any features concerning for carcinoma, such as unusually large size, invasion of the adjacent vessels or of the thyroid capsule, irregular margins, or calcifications (Fig. 16).

It is obvious that the presence of multiple enlarged glands should be conveyed, as it might alter the surgical approach. If a suspected parathyroid nodule has atypical sonographic features, FNA can be performed to confirm the diagnosis, especially if scintigraphy was discordant. In patients with challenging surgery, such as those with prior neck radiation or multiple prior neck surgeries, microwave or alcohol ablation of parathyroid adenomas can be offered as a therapeutic procedure.[23–25]

List: What the Referring Physician Needs to Know

  Location of parathyroid adenoma: side, inferior, superior, ectopic

  Multiplicity of adenomas

  Presence of any features concerning for carcinoma

  Need for PTH sampling for confirmation of atypical or intrathyroid nodule

  Amenability to alcohol ablation, especially in poor surgical candidates

SUMMARY

Imaging plays an important role in management of PHPT, particularly in localizing parathyroid adenomas and helping select patients who are eligible for minimally invasive surgery. Ultrasound and sestamibi scan remain the first line of imaging, with 4DCT reserved for more challenging cases.

REFERENCE

1. Mallick R, Chen H. Diagnosis and management of hyperparathyroidism. Adv Surg 2018;52(1):137–53.

2. Yeh MW, Ituarte PH, Zhou HC, et al. Incidence and prevalence of primary hyperparathyroidism in a racially mixed population. J Clin Endocrinol Metab 2013;98(3):1122–9.

3. Macfarlane DP, Yu N, Leese GP. Subclinical and asymptomatic parathyroid disease: implications of emerging data. Lancet Diabetes Endocrinol 2013;1(4):329–40.

4. Walker MD, Silverberg SJ. Primary hyperparathyroidism. Nat Rev Endocrinol 2018;14(2):115–25.

5. Silverberg SJ, Clarke BL, Peacock M, et al. Current issues in the presentation of asymptomatic primary hyperparathyroidism: proceedings of the Fourth International Workshop. J Clin Endocrinol Metab 2014;99(10):3580–94.

6. Corbetta S. Normocalcemic hyperparathyroidism. Front Horm Res 2019;51:23–39.

7. Taslakian B, Trerotola SO, Sacks B, et al. The essentials of parathyroid hormone venous sampling. Cardiovasc Intervent Radiol 2017;40(1):9–21.

8. Gilmour JR. The gross anatomy of the parathyroid glands. J Pathol Bacteriol 1938;46(1):133–49.

9. Policeni BA, Smoker WR, Reede DL. Anatomy and embryology of the thyroid and parathyroid glands. Semin Ultrasound CT MR 2012;33(2):104–14.

10. Lyden ML, Wang TS, Sosa JA. Surgical anatomy of parathyroid glands. In: Carty SE, Chen W, editors. Uptodate; 2019. Available at: https://www.uptodate.com/contents/surgical-anatomy-of-the-parathyroid-glands.

11. Vaz A, Griffiths M. Parathyroid imaging and localization using SPECT/CT: initial results. J Nucl Med Technol 2011;39(3):195–200.

12. Mellnick VM, Middleton WD. Parathyroid sonography. Ultrasound Clin 2014;9(3):339–49.

13. Devcic Z, Jeffrey RB, Kamaya A, et al. The elusive parathyroid adenoma: techniques for detection. Ultrasound Q 2013;29(3):179–87.

14. Kamaya A, Quon A, Jeffrey RB. Sonography of the abnormal parathyroid gland. Ultrasound Q 2006;22(4):253–62.

15. Treglia G, Trimboli P, Huellner M, et al. Imaging in primary hyperparathyroidism: focus on the evidence-based diagnostic performance of different methods. Minerva Endocrinol 2018;43(2):133–43.

16. Nafisi Moghadam R, Amlelshahbaz AP, Namiranian N, et al. Comparative diagnostic performance of ultrasonography and 99mtc-sestamibi scintigraphy for parathyroid adenoma in primary hyperparathyroidism; systematic review and meta- analysis. Asian Pac J Cancer Prev 2017;18(12):3195–200.

17. Cheung K, Wang TS, Farrokhyar F, et al. A meta-analysis of preoperative localization techniques for patients with primary hyperparathyroidism. Ann Surg Oncol 2012;19(2):577–83.

18. Eslamy HK, Ziessman HA. Parathyroid scintigraphy in patients with primary hyperparathyroidism: 99mTc sestamibi SPECT and SPECT/CT. Radiographics 2008;28(5):1461–76.

19. Wei WJ, Shen CT, Song HJ, et al. Comparison of SPET/CT, SPET and planar imaging using 99mTc-MIBI as independent techniques to support minimally invasive parathyroidectomy in primary hyperparathyroidism: a meta-analysis. Hell J Nucl Med 2015;18(2):127–35.

20. Machado NN, Wilhelm SM. Diagnosis and evaluation of primary hyperparathyroidism. Surg Clin North Am 2019;99(4):649–66.

21. Tian Y, Tanny ST, Einsiedel P, et al. Four-dimensional computed tomography: clinical impact for patients with primary hyperparathyroidism. Ann Surg Oncol 2018;25(1):117–21.

22. Pitt SC, Sippel RS, Chen H. Secondary and tertiary hyperparathyroidism, state of the art surgical management. Surg Clin North Am 2009;89(5):1227–39.

23. Singh Ospina N, Thompson GB, Lee RA, et al. Safety and efficacy of percutaneous parathyroid ethanol ablation in patients with recurrent primary hyperparathyroidism and multiple endocrine neoplasia type 1. J Clin Endocrinol Metab 2015;100(1):E87–90.

24. Kitaoka M. Ultrasonographic diagnosis of parathyroid glands and percutaneous ethanol injection therapy. Nephrol Dial Transplant 2003;18(Suppl 3):ii27–30.

25. Liu F, Yu X, Liu Z, et al. Comparison of ultrasound-guided percutaneous microwave ablation and parathyroidectomy for primary hyperparathyroidism. Int J Hyperthermia 2019;36(1):835–40.

Neck Procedures: Thyroid and Parathyroid

Nirvikar Dahiya, MD*, Maitray D. Patel, MD, Scott W. Young, MD

KEYWORDS

- Ultrasonography • Sonography • Fine needle • Core biopsy • Thyroid

KEY POINTS

- Multiple variations of fine-needle aspirations exist. Using needles between 23-gauge and 27-gauge and making 4 to 6 passes achieves the best results for most nodules.
- Visualization of the biopsy needle in plane with the transducer is the preferred method.
- Parathyroid biopsies have higher sensitivity and specificity if they include needle washout samples to estimate the parathyroid hormone (PTH) concentration.

INTRODUCTION

Ultrasonography is commonly used to guide diagnostic sampling procedures in the neck, primarily targeting thyroid nodules with sonographic findings raising suspicion for thyroid carcinoma. Lymph node diagnostic sampling using sonographic guidance has also been widely adopted and has supplanted surgical excisional biopsy in the evaluation of physically enlarged or image-detected suspicious lymph nodes in patients with known or suspected malignancy at risk for neck nodal metastases. In general, imaging-detected parathyroid adenomas can be reliably characterized based on scintigraphic and sonographic findings, so presurgical diagnostic sampling of hyperparathyroid patients with parathyroid adenomas is reserved for those infrequent instances in which the diagnosis is unclear. However, advances and improvements in ablation technique have allowed ablation treatment of parathyroid adenomas in some patients. Similarly, ablative techniques can be applied to papillary thyroid carcinoma recurrences in the thyroid surgical bed or in neck nodes. This article discusses important practical considerations in performing diagnostic sampling and ablative procedures in the neck in the context of endocrine tumors. Although most of the discussion would also be pertinent to the evaluation of other head and neck masses (including those in the parotid/salivary glands, those related to squamous cell carcinoma and other head and neck primary tumors, those related to lymphoma, and those related to soft tissue lumps and bumps), these other potential diagnostic sampling and therapeutic ablation targets are not addressed here, in keeping with the theme of endocrine imaging. After providing an overview of fine-needle sampling terminology and efficacy, including a review of the role of core biopsy for thyroid nodules, this article goes into practical details regarding our technique for performing thyroid nodule fine-needle sampling, articulates pitfalls and pearls in the application of that technique, and subsequently describes special considerations when this technique is applied to possible parathyroid adenomas or thyroid gland lymphomas. The article concludes by examining emerging ablative techniques applied to thyroid and parathyroid tumors.

FINE-NEEDLE SAMPLING: TERMINOLOGY, EFFICACY, AND QUALITY ASSESSMENT

Although the term fine-needle aspiration (FNA) has become the standard way to describe fine-needle

Department of Radiology, Mayo Clinic, 5777 East Mayo Boulevard, Phoenix, AZ 85054, USA
* Corresponding author.
E-mail address: dahiya.nirvikar@mayo.edu

Radiol Clin N Am 58 (2020) 1085–1098
https://doi.org/10.1016/j.rcl.2020.07.005

sampling of thyroid nodules and other targets, it is important to understand that this broad term applies to 2 different variations in method, and unfortunately 1 of the variations shares the same name. When first introduced, the term aspiration biopsy reflected the method in which the operator applies suction (ie, aspiration) using a syringe, sometimes with a special syringe holder, as a fine needle is moved through a target to draw up cellular material that can then be plated out on a slide for histologic evaluation; this has been termed fine-needle aspiration sampling (FNAS) or fine-needle aspiration cytology (FNAC). A modification of this technique without using aspiration was pioneered in France in the 1980s and first described for thyroid lesions by Santos and Leiman[1] in 1988; this has been termed fine-needle capillary sampling or fine-needle nonaspiration cytology (FNNAC). The use of the term capillary instead of aspiration is unfortunate, because it implies that capillary action is the mechanism by which the cellular material is drawn up into the needle[2]; in fact, the cellular material is pushed into the needle by the scraping effect of the beveled needle edge combined with the repeated excursions in the tissue,[3] and capillary forces serve only to keep the material in the needle bore when the needle is removed. It is likely that this scraping action that loosens cellular material from the nodule architecture also plays a primary role when aspiration is applied, with the aspiration not loosening the material itself but only serving to help draw the material scraped off by the repeated needle excursions into the needle bore. In any case, the broader term fine-needle aspiration and its abbreviation FNA are commonly used to refer to either method, and this broader meaning is implied by the use of the abbreviation FNA in this article unless otherwise specified.

Comparison between the efficacy of FNAC and FNNAC has been a subject of considerable investigation. The principal problem with FNAC is that the application of aspiration increases the chance of bloody smears, which impair cytologic interpretation; this is particularly an issue with thyroid nodules, which tend to yield bloody samples with aspiration. In contrast, the principal problem with FNNAC is that operators may not scrape enough cells into the needle, either because of suboptimal technique or because of fibrotic nodules. There have been several studies that purport to compare the efficacy of FNAC and FNNAC in evaluating thyroid nodules, and a meta-analysis of those studies that eventually reviewed 1842 individual patients with 2221 samples collected by both FNAC and FNNAC showed that both techniques can be useful. The analysis concluded that the method performed likely depends on operator preference,[2]

but acknowledged that a combination approach might be best. The Consensus Statement on Thyroid FNA put forward by the Korean Society of Thyroid Radiology advocates that operators start with the FNNAC technique and continue with that technique if samples seem to be adequate, switching to the FNAC technique if initial passes yield only minimal material.[4]

Another factor that can influence the efficacy of fine-needle sampling is needle size. Recognition that the cellular material is scraped off and not sucked out of the nodule when FNA is performed helps to understand why there is usually worse performance of FNA with larger needle size. Larger needles (larger than 23 gauge), especially when used with the aspiration method, only increase the amount of contaminating blood drawn into the needle without significantly increasing the amount of scraped cells.[5] In contrast, as needles get thinner (smaller than 27 gauge), they may be harder to direct through overlying soft tissues and may be less effective in scraping material off the nodule, particularly if there is calcification. As a result, using a needle between 23 gauge and 27 gauge is likely to achieve the best results for most nodules.

Immediate cytopathology assessment of samples to establish sampling adequacy can positively influence FNA efficacy but has workflow drawbacks. Usually in this workflow, a cytopathologist or cytopathology technologist is requested to come with the necessary equipment (microscope) to the room in which the FNA procedure is being performed to evaluate samples as they are collected; after each sampling pass, time is taken for the cytopathologist to review the material, telling the operator to stop taking samples once sample adequacy has been confirmed. This process requires cytopathology resources that are not always available; moreover, resource coordination becomes more challenging in that the FNA procedure cannot begin until the cytopathologist is in the room, introducing workflow delays. In addition, the time taken by the cytopathologist to review the material after each pass adds time to the procedure. In contrast, a nondiagnostic result caused by specimen inadequacy adds considerably more cost because the patient may then return for another procedure or may end up going to surgical evaluation for a nodule that may prove to be benign. A study performed by Zhu and Michael[6] revealed interesting data that highlight how procedural technique can be altered to substantially reduce nondiagnostic thyroid nodule FNA outcomes when immediate assessment of cytologic adequacy is not pursued. The nondiagnostic rate of thyroid nodule FNA for patients subdivided into groups by the number of passes taken proved to be a function of the number passes, with increasing success rates as the number of passes approached 6 (**Table 1**). In the group of patients in whom 6 passes were made, the nondiagnostic rate was 1.4%, and this rate did not change significantly for groups with more than 6 passes.

This recognition that operators should optimally take 6 passes when not using immediate assessment of cytologic adequacy is important to consider when trying to understand the role of core needle biopsy (CNB) for thyroid nodules. For example, a team of Korean investigators has published several articles touting the role of CNB in the diagnosis of thyroid malignancy, concluding that core biopsy may even have a role as an initial diagnostic procedure for thyroid nodules instead of FNA.[7,8] In part, this team makes this conclusion because their analysis presumes a nondiagnostic FNA rate of 22.6%, which itself is based on practice in which operators take 3 or fewer FNA samples.[9] With such sparse sampling practice, it is no wonder that FNA compares poorly with CNB; their 22.6% nondiagnostic rate for FNA is concordant with that predicted by the data from Zhu and Michael[6] when taking so few samples (see **Table 1**). A more robust meta-analysis shows that there is no demonstrable role for core biopsy before FNA in the evaluation of thyroid nodules.[10] Core biopsy might play a role in further evaluation of nodules in which initial FNA outcome is that the nodule has atypia of undetermined significance/follicular lesion of undetermined significance, but evidence suggests that using CNB instead of a second FNA for such lesions does not meaningfully change patient care, because patients typically move on to diagnostic lobectomy anyway.[11]

THYROID AND PARATHYROID FINE-NEEDLE ASPIRATION: OUR APPROACH

Every ultrasonography practice has site-specific variations in how patients are selected for thyroid nodule FNA and how the procedure is performed, reflecting institutional framework and resources, referring clinician desires, patient expectations, and radiologist preferences. Because it can be useful to understand how other practices perform these procedures, this article highlights our approach at Mayo Clinic Arizona.

- Patient selection: it is important to communicate with referring providers when selecting which nodules to sample. Although there has been wide adoption of the American College of Radiology (ACR) Thyroid Imaging Reporting and Data System (TI-RADS) algorithm to stratify the malignancy risk of thyroid nodules using sonographic features,[12] the scheme used at Mayo Clinic Arizona (as articulated in Ask-MayoExpert) varies in some ways because it represents a collaboration with other stakeholders at our institution who do not agree completely with the ACR model. A full discussion of the exact algorithm in use at Mayo Clinic Arizona is beyond the scope of this article; much of the algorithm is similar to the ACR TI-RADS approach, and it uses the ACR lexicon. The important concept to convey is that ultrasonography practices should try to work with their referring providers and should communicate whatever system they are using in their reports. In our practice, we include a link to the AskMayoExpert guidelines, as well as the ACR lexicon.
- Scheduling notes: we have an agreement with our referring providers to schedule patients for thyroid ultrasonography and FNA when a nodule is clinically suspected. If we find a nodule that meets FNA criteria, we proceed with a biopsy without spending additional time in trying to get the order from the physician for the biopsy. This arrangement is extremely helpful to expedite evaluation of the thyroid nodule and a biopsy, if needed, efficiently.
- Anticoagulation status: in our estimation, thyroid FNA is safe and can be performed on patients who are anticoagulated or on aspirin. This opinion is in accordance with the Society of Interventional Radiology guidelines for quality improvement related to percutaneous

Table 1
Correlation between number of fine-needle aspiration passes and nondiagnostic fine-needle aspiration rates

FNA Passes Taken	Number of Patients	Number of Nondiagnostic Results	Nondiagnostic Rate (%)
≤3	20	5	25.0
4	100	11	11.0
5	115	6	5.2
6	67	1	1.4
≥7	141	2	2.1

From Zhu W, Michael CW. How important is on-site adequacy assessment for thyroid FNA? An evaluation of 883 cases. Diagn Cytopathol. 2007 Mar;35(3):183-6; with permission.

needle biopsy.[13] Anticoagulation does not significantly reduce the success rate for thyroid FNA.[14]

- Patient position: in general, mild hyperextension of the neck is useful and can be achieved by using a small pillow or towel under the shoulders of the patient in a supine position. The patient's face is turned to the opposite direction in relation to the planned biopsy site (head to left for biopsy of a nodule in right lobe and vice versa). Adequate positioning helps in stretching of the skin surface and pushes the thyroid more anteriorly, thus reducing the depth of the biopsy target (Fig. 1).
- Transducer: thyroid biopsies are preferred to be performed with a high-frequency, small-footprint, hockey-stick transducer (we use a L8-18i-D transducer). This transducer lends itself well to the subtle manipulations required for adequate trajectory establishment. Sometimes a larger-footprint linear transducer may also be used. We prefer the latter when we need to use part of the transducer to exert pressure on the neck to fix a calcified or fibrous nodule that moves (sideways) when we attempt to insert the FNA needle into the nodule.
- Approach: some operators always prefer a trajectory to the nodule that has a medial to lateral approach (from the tracheal side to the sternocleidomastoid muscle side), whereas others prefer a lateral to medial approach (arguing that a pathway through the hypoechoic sternocleidomastoid muscle helps visualize the needle better). Irrespective of the personal preference, the trajectory

chosen should be the shortest and the safest access to the nodule.[15]

- Biopsy tray setup: the equipment required for a thyroid nodule FNA is simple. The biopsy tray we use includes the following items (Fig. 2):
  ○ Disposable 10-mL plastic syringes
  ○ Disposable 25-gauge and 22-gauge needles, 3.8 cm (1.5 inches) long
  ○ Glass slides for preparation of cytology smears
  ○ Sterile gauze pads
  ○ Lidocaine (1% lidocaine buffered with 8.4% sodium bicarbonate)
  ○ ChloraPrep: 2% weight per volume chlorhexidine gluconate and 70% volume per volume isopropyl alcohol
  ○ Koplin jar with alcohol
  ○ Sterile transducer cover
  ○ Sterile drape with a hole
- Procedure technique: before beginning the procedure, a time-out is performed to verify the patient's name and date of birth and to confirm the biopsy target as per the requisition. Once the ultrasonography transducer is selected, it is wiped with an alcohol-based swab, and a short sterile transducer cover is used for covering the transducer and maintaining sterility during the procedure (Fig. 3). After disinfecting the skin with an antiseptic agent (we use ChloraPrep), a sterile drape is used to cover the neck while centering the hole in the drape over the planned biopsy trajectory mark. A small amount of local anesthesia is injected at the point of entry, and a wheal is created on the dermis. This stage is

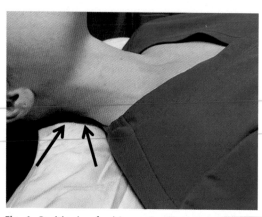

Fig. 1. Positioning for biopsy. A pillow under the upper back and lower neck allows for hyperextension (*arrows*) of the neck, pushing the thyroid anteriorly and also fixing it by stretching the soft tissues.

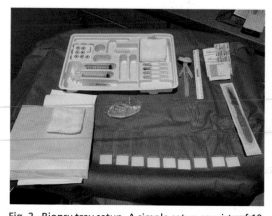

Fig. 2. Biopsy tray setup. A simple setup consists of 10-mL plastics syringes, disposable 25-gauge and 22-gauge needles, glass slides for cytology smears, sterile gauze pads, sterile drape with the hole, ChloraPrep, and transducer cover.

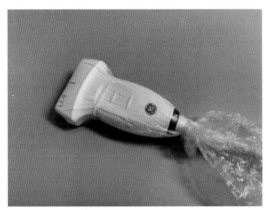

Fig. 3. Covering the transducer with a sterile sheath before the biopsy.

followed by a deeper infiltration of the soft tissues to the thyroid capsule (Fig. 4). Although the wheal on the skin is performed without the use of the transducer, the deeper anesthesia of the subcutaneous fat planes and muscles is obtained by directing the needle under ultrasonography guidance. At our institution, we use a 25-gauge needle to sample the nodule. Most of the time, the scraping effect of the beveled needle edge combined with the repeated excursions in the tissue is enough to procure the cells needed for the diagnosis. In some instances when the nodule is more fibrotic, a syringe may be attached to the needle to apply suction during the procedure. Rarely, a larger-gauge needle, such as 22 to 23 gauge, may be used to obtain adequate material. Very rarely, a longer needle (a spinal needle) may be used if the target lesion is deep in the neck or the patient has a bulky large neck. The visualization of the needle should be oriented in the long-axis plane because the needle is visualized in its entire

trajectory (Fig. 5). It makes for good habit to track the needle from its insertion into the skin, its advancement through the soft tissues, and its ultimate entry into the target nodule. In rare situations, a short-axis approach may be performed, wherein the needle is inserted in the short axis along the middle of the transducer. In this instance, only the tip of the needle is visualized and the entire trajectory path is not visualized (Fig. 6). The latter technique has found increased use in interventional radiology for vascular access and is mentioned in this article as an alternate methodology. The authors strongly recommend using the former technique for neck biopsies (ie, the method that visualizes the needle in the long-axis plane in its entire trajectory; see Fig. 5). The process of traversing the nodule with the needle is a skill that has a learning curve. Slow, deliberate excursions of the needle within the nodule are observed in real time. Some experts perform rotation of the needle as the sample is being taken. Conceivably, the rotation of the sharp beveled needle helps scrape more relevant material for cytology. Cystic or necrotic areas within the nodule are best avoided during the FNA. The advantages of using only the needle for procuring the cellular material are the flexibility in manipulation of the needle by holding it from the hub and easier visualization of the appearance of aspirate in the hub as an end point. Attaching a 5-mL or 10-mL syringe to the needle can also help to better control the needle and the ejection of the material after sampling. Adopting 1 of the 2 methods (syringe aspiration or not) is also a matter of personal preference and does not matter as long as the eventual outcome is the procurement of a high-yield aspirate. It is important to keep an eye on the hub of the

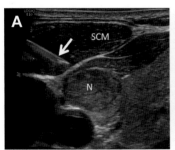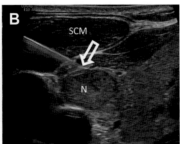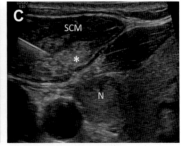

Fig. 4. FNA of the right thyroid nodule (N). Transverse images through the right thyroid. (A) The path of the lidocaine infiltration needle (arrow) through the sternocleidomastoid (SCM) muscle. (B) The infiltration of the lidocaine to the thyroid capsule (open arrow). (C) Retraction of the lidocaine needle with continuous infiltration of the anesthetic into the muscle making it hyperechoic (asterisk).

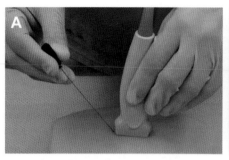
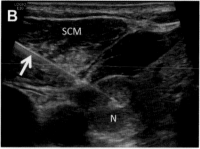

Fig. 5. Technique of needle visualization. (A) The alignment of the needle along the long axis of the transducer. (B) The entire trajectory of the biopsy needle (arrow) through the SCM) into the thyroid nodule (N) in a longitudinal plane.

needle as you perform the excursions. When we see a drop of blood in the hub of the needle, we do not perform further excursions. Excessive blood within the hub of the needle only increases the contamination of the specimen with red blood cells without increasing cellular material. Once the material is obtained, we smear the material on a slide. In addition to the smear, we also flush the needle with Cytolyte solution so that a cell block (cells coalesced using a centrifuge) is available for the cytopathologist for further evaluation if needed. We try to do at least 5 passes to obtain adequate material. In our practice, the smear is prepared by the radiologist performing the procedure. In other practices, the smear may be prepared by a cytology technician or an on-site pathologist. In some instances, the on-site pathologist confirms the presence of adequate cellular material after the first or second pass, thus limiting the total number of passes needed. The slides are sent to the laboratory, usually placed in alcohol; in some cases, air-dried slides can be of diagnostic value.

- Use of thyroglobulin (Tg) assay: in patients who have had prior thyroidectomy for thyroid

cancer, sampling of morphologically abnormal lymph nodes or small nodules in the paratracheal postsurgical bed can be useful to evaluate for recurrent neoplasm. In addition to the FNA samples obtained in a similar fashion to thyroid nodule biopsy, additional needle washout samples are sent for measurement of Tg levels. The process of acquisition of samples for Tg assay may vary in some laboratories, but we generally perform the following:

1. After an FNA has been done with a 25-gauge needle and the material in the needle has been expelled onto a slide for cytologic analysis, attach the used FNA needle to an empty 10-mL syringe.
2. Place the needle tip into the pool of saline, apply suction to the syringe, and withdraw a small amount of saline up through the needle until the saline starts to fill the hub of the needle or end of the syringe (probably only 0.125–0.25 mL of fluid).
3. Expel this fluid forcefully back through the needle, into a separate test tube. This is the needle washing used for analysis.
4. Repeat for each needle pass of the biopsied site (usually 3–6 needle passes),

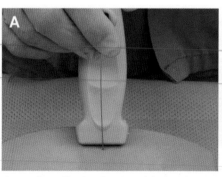
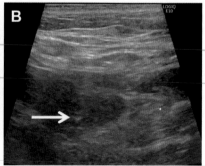

Fig. 6. Technique of needle visualization. (A) The alignment of the needle along the short axis of the transducer. (B) Only the tip of the biopsy needle (arrow) into the lymph node in a longitudinal plane.

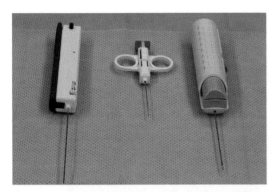

Fig. 7. Types of core biopsy needles. Full-core biopsy needle with end-fire mechanism (*left*), a hemicore biopsy needle with a slotted mechanism (*right*), and a semiautomatic biopsy needle with slotted mechanism that allows more control of the deployment of the inner stylet (*center*).

and empty into the same test tube, accumulating a total of about 0.5 to 1.0 mL of fluid to be sent to the laboratory.

Tg level less than 1 ng per FNA is considered normal. Tg level between 1 and 10 ng per FNA is indeterminate, and the chance that the sample target is related to recurrent disease is based on the degree of suspicion from the morphology of the sonographic findings. Tg level more than 10 ng per FNA is consistent with recurrent malignancy.

- Core biopsy needle and technique: core biopsies of the thyroid are generally avoided secondary to increased vascularity of the thyroid gland. In some instances in which repeat FNA sampling is suboptimal or inadequate and the concern for malignancy is high, core biopsy may be performed. If the differential diagnosis includes thyroid lymphoma, a core biopsy may be performed to obtain more tissue material for a definitive diagnosis. The core biopsy needles are usually 18 gauge and can use devices with an end-fire

mechanism, which yields a full core sample, or slotted mechanism, which yields a hemicore sample (**Fig. 7**). A discussion on the different types of core biopsy needles is beyond the scope of this article; the slotted mechanism devices may allow more control of the deployment of the inner stylet, but yield less tissue. The example shown in **Fig. 8** was anaplastic carcinoma that underwent a core biopsy with an 18-gauge needle. Unlike FNA, the core biopsy tissue samples are sent to the laboratory in formalin.

- Pitfalls and special situations:
  - Rim calcified nodules are harder to biopsy. It can help to identify a break in the rim calcification and allow use of that break as the point of entry for the FNA (**Fig. 9**).
  - Thyroid nodules in the isthmus can be mobile during the FNA, and pressure from the transducer can be used from the opposite direction to limit movement of the thyroid nodule (**Fig. 10**).
  - If a nodule is positioned on posterior aspect of the thyroid, particularly on the left, make sure that you exclude an esophageal diverticulum masquerading as nodule. A simple maneuver of swallowing by the patient can help differentiate between the two: the diverticulum shows air within the lumen (**Fig. 11**).
  - The tubercle of Zuckerkandl can simulate the presence of the nodule. Scan in both planes; usually the images in the longitudinal plane show a connection of the structure with the thyroid body (**Fig. 12**).
- Parathyroid adenoma: FNA of a parathyroid gland that is enlarged or a parathyroid nodule has similar technique to FNA being performed for the thyroid nodule, but usually requires additional techniques because the cytologic features of a parathyroid adenoma can be indistinguishable from a benign thyroid

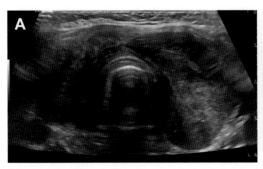
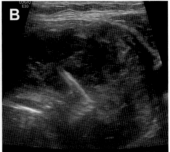

Fig. 8. Core biopsy. (*A*) A large infiltrative mass lesion involving both the lobes of the thyroid gland. (*B*) The trajectory of an 18-gauge core biopsy needle.

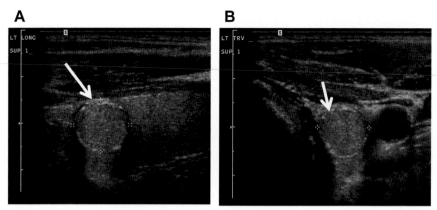

Fig. 9. Rim calcified nodule. Longitudinal (*A*) and transverse (*B*) images of a rim calcified nodule. Biopsy can be attempted through the small breaks in the calcifications along the rim (*arrows*) in either plane.

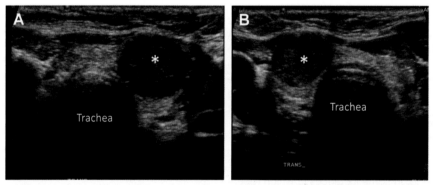

Fig. 10. Mobile nodule in isthmus. Transverse images from the neck. (*A*) A thyroid nodule (*asterisk*) on the left of the trachea. (*B*) The same nodule displaced to the right of the trachea. Transducer pressure from one side can limit the mobility of the nodule.

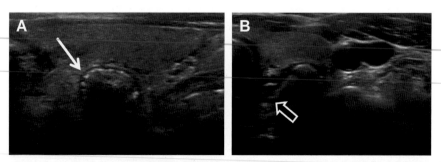

Fig. 11. Esophageal diverticulum. Longitudinal (*A*) and transverse (*B*) images through the left thyroid. (*A*) An echogenic lesion (*arrow*) posterior to the thyroid simulating a rim calcified thyroid nodule. (*B*) Medial extension of this echogenic lesion toward the esophagus (*open arrow*).

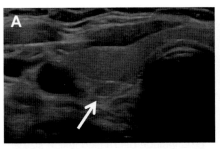
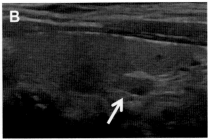

Fig. 12. Tubercle of Zuckerkandl. Transverse (*A*) and longitudinal (*B*) images through the right thyroid show an isoechoic nodule (*arrows*) in posterior aspect of the thyroid. The longitudinal plane image clearly shows the connection of the structure to the body of the thyroid posteriorly.

adenoma. In addition to samples obtained for making cytologic smears, additional samples are obtained to estimate the parathyroid hormone (PTH) concentration in needle washout. This PTH analysis in the rinse material obtained during the FNA procedure helps differentiate thyroid tissue from enlarged parathyroid glands. A positive cutoff value for PTH washout is usually higher than the serum PTH level.[16] The utility of this technique has specificity and sensitivity ranging from 91% to 100%. The FNA needle is rinsed with a small volume of normal saline solution immediately after a specimen for cytologic examination has been expelled from the needle for a smear. Specimen collection is critical for the performance of the assay, and the needle should be rinsed with a minimal volume of saline. Each FNA needle from a single biopsied area is washed with 0.1 to 0.5 mL of normal saline. The washes from a single area are pooled (final volume 1–1.5 mL). PTH levels are measured in the saline wash. This process is similar to the one described for Tg assay.

- Postprocedure: following a thyroid sampling procedure, there is usually no need to hold the patient in the nursing area. Compression of the biopsy spot for few minutes, followed by an adhesive bandage, is sufficient before discharging the patient. In some instances, providing the patient with an ice pack to hold over the biopsy site for 15 to 20 minutes helps with the healing process and decreases the extent of the bruise.

ULTRASONOGRAPHY-GUIDED ABLATIONS IN THE HEAD AND NECK
Ablation of Thyroid and Local Thyroidal Metastatic Disease

Several ablative technologies have been investigated for hyperfunctioning, benign or malignant, and cystic or solid thyroid masses.

Ethanol ablation (EA) has been used since the late 1980s for the treatment of thyroid nodules in patients not desiring surgical intervention, particularly for high-surgical-risk patients or for cosmetic outcome concerns.[17] Local instillation or infiltration leads to cellular apoptosis by inducing cell membrane lysis, protein denaturation, and vascular thrombosis.[18] EA has been used for both benign or malignant and cystic or solid masses. However, the advent of more complete ablative technologies, such as radiofrequency ablation (RFA), has largely segregated the role of EA to cystic thyroid nodules (50% or greater cystic component) that either have mass effect on adjacent structures, particularly the esophagus and trachea, or create a visible neck mass. Such masses are ideal candidates for EA because the procedure yields no cosmetic injury, is technically simple, is low risk, and uses very-low-cost materials.[19]

Protocols for cystic thyroid nodule ablation vary, but one technique is to access the cystic component of the nodule with a 20-gauge to 22-gauge needle or angiocatheter of a length appropriate to the depth of the nodule under sterile conditions, after local anesthesia of the skin and subcutaneous tissue with 1% lidocaine. Care is taken to avoid puncturing the deep wall of the cyst. If the liquid component is too viscous for aspiration with a 22-gauge catheter, a needle or catheter up to 20-gauge can be used. The entire cystic component is aspirated and the volume noted. Absolute ethanol is then slowly instilled up to 50% of the aspirated volume. If the patient expresses any discomfort during the slow instillation, the injection should be stopped. Dwell times vary from 5 to 20 minutes in the literature. In our practice, we allow the ethanol to dwell for 5 minutes, aspirate it completely, and then reinstill the same quantity of fresh ethanol into the cavity, on the theory that thyroid nodules typically rapidly refill with fluid when aspirated and the potential dilution of the first aliquot may impair the activity of the ethanol on the cyst wall. A second dwell time of 5 to 10 minutes is typical. Patients should be monitored for discomfort. Patients typically report no pain during the procedure, and skin discomfort should raise concern for leakage of ethanol along the needle or catheter path. When the dwell time is complete, the ethanol is aspirated completely, the tissue is compressed to coapt the walls for a few minutes, and a simple skin bandage is then applied. A typical treatment response is an 80% reduction in the cystic volume of the lesion at 3-month follow-up.[19] If satisfactory results are not achieved or the cystic component recurs, the procedure may be repeated as needed. An example of the technique is shown in **Fig. 13.** Other cystic lesions of the neck (in particular, thyroglossal duct cysts and nonhyperfunctioning parathyroid cysts) can be similarly ablated.[20,21]

EA is also a useful alternative to surgical resection for nodal recurrence of differentiated thyroid cancer (DTC). EA is usually reserved for patients who are unwilling or unable to undergo surgical resection. Elderly patients and others with significant comorbidities or patients who have had multiple nodal recurrences in whom extensive scarring may make additional resection difficult or disfiguring are ideal candidates. Goals of EA for nodal DTC include decreased lesion size and serum Tg level, absent color flow, and increased lesion echogenicity. Ample direct comparison with surgical intervention is lacking, but a success rate of 87.5%, compared with 94.8% for surgery, and a low complication rate were shown in a pooled analysis.[22,23]

Patient preparation is similar to routine thyroid FNA. Skin anesthesia is achieved with 1% lidocaine. Deep perilesional anesthesia is usually avoided, especially for central compartment (level

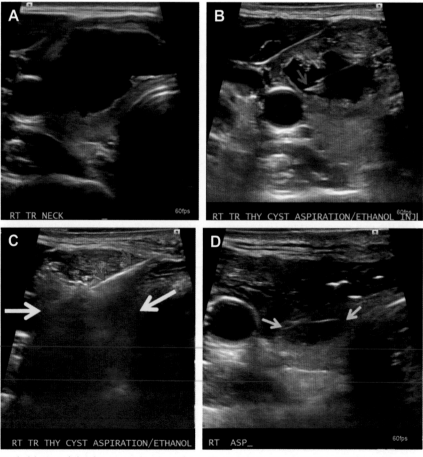

Fig. 13. Ethanol ablation. (*A*) A large predominantly cystic nodule in the right thyroid lobe. (*B*) Aspiration from a transisthmus approach with a 22-gauge needle (*red arrow at tip*). (*C*) Ethanol instillation with the indwelling needle (*red arrows*) and reverberation artifact related to ethanol interacting with the cyst wall, creating gas (*yellow arrows*). (*D*) Greater than 80% reduction in cyst volume after 2 sessions, 3 months later (*green arrows*).

VI) nodes, to preserve patient feedback regarding sudden increases in pain, which can indicate leakage of ethanol from the target nodule. If hydrodissection is desired to increase the distance from critical structures such as the esophagus or recurrent laryngeal nerve, saline instillation can be performed.

Ethanol is instilled in the node using a 22-gauge or 25-gauge needle. A 1-mL (tuberculin) syringe allows careful deposition of small aliquots within the target. For small lesions, such as those 5 mm or less, central deposition is usually adequate. For larger lesions, ethanol deposition should begin with the deepest part of the lesion, moving to more superficial areas as the lesion becomes echogenic, obscuring the needle tip. Intermittent imaging with color flow is helpful to determine the adequacy of vascular thrombosis. If an area still shows flow, the operator can wait a few minutes until the hyperechogenicity subsides and the needle can be repositioned accurately. For large nodes (>1 cm), the proceduralist should try to locate the area of color inflow and directly inject

into the inflow within the periphery of the node. This technique can result in a rapid devascularization of the node. Our protocol brings the patient back 1 to 2 days later for a reassessment of color flow in the target node or nodes, and additional EA is performed as needed. Typically, between 1 and 4 nodes are treated in each paired session. For large or deeply situated nodes, contrast-enhanced ultrasonography or microvascular flow settings can be helpful to augment flow detection, may provide better feedback to the operator, and could improve response. Future trials are needed in this area. EA of a level IV lymph node with subsequent devascularization in a patient with metastatic papillary thyroid carcinoma is shown in Fig. 14.

Ultrasonography-guided RFA of thyroid nodules is a safe and feasible alternative to surgery for DTC in high-surgical-risk patients or patients not desiring surgery when active surveillance is not desired or medically appropriate.[24] A straight, 1-cm active tip, 17-gauge internally cooled RFA device used at low wattage (typically 30 W) provides

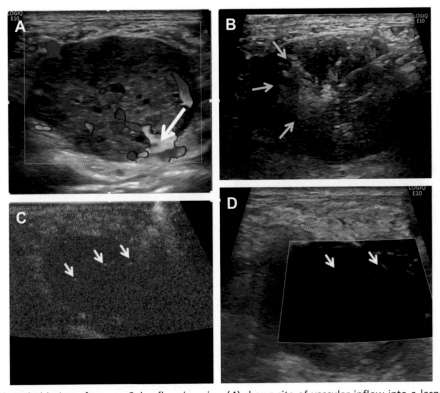

Fig. 14. Ethanol ablation of tumor. Color flow imaging (A) shows site of vascular inflow into a large, level IV, proven papillary thyroid nodal metastasis. Injection of 0.2 mL of absolute ethanol (*white arrow*) led to a rapid devascularization of the node. (B) Additional ethanol is injected (*red arrows* show needle trajectory) in small (typically 0.1-mL) aliquots throughout the node with echogenic dispersal through the lesion (*green arrows*). Contrast-enhanced (C) and microvascular flow (D) settings show minimal residual flow 2 days later (*white arrows*). Additional ethanol was injected in these areas targeted by flow detection.

appropriate control of the ablation field to avoid adjacent tissue injury. Under appropriate anesthesia, the RFA device is initially placed in the deepest, most medial portion of the nodule, usually from a transisthmus approach. Owing to this location's proximity to the recurrent laryngeal nerve and esophagus, this is the most critical part of the technique. The RFA device is activated at 30 W and continuously monitored until hyperechogenicity is noted surrounding the device; subsequently, it is immediately deactivated, and the device tip is repositioned in an unablated section of the nodule, working from posteromedial to anterolateral (**Fig. 15**). If the hyperechoic effect of ablation is not achieved at 30 W, gradually higher wattage can be applied. Longer ablation times can be tolerated toward the center of the nodule if it is large. This moving-shot technique allows careful but adequate coverage of benign or malignant nodules.[25,26] The operator should remain mindful that the risk of clinically relevant DTC morbidity is low, especially in older individuals, and that great care should be taken to avoid thermal injury to surrounding structures, even if this means that the edges of the tumor are suboptimally treated. This technique, therefore, differs from the goals of solid organ tumor ablation in the abdomen, where 5-mm to 10-mm ablative margins are the standard goal.

This RFA technique can be applied to large or growing benign thyroid nodules with mass effect achieving volume reduction between 50% and 80%.[27–30] Ablation of hyperfunctioning thyroid

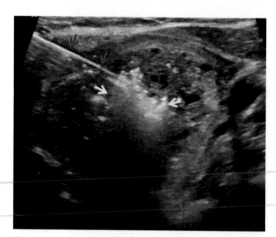

Fig. 15. Percutaneous RFA of a large benign thyroid nodule for symptomatic compression. Red arrows indicate the straight-tipped RFA antenna. Echogenic gas (*yellow arrows*) surrounds and obscures the antenna tip during the moving-shot technique. The peripheral 5 mm of the lesion are intentionally spared when treating benign symptomatic nodules to avoid thermal injury to adjacent structures.

nodules, using EA or RFA, is also performed but has not made its way into mainstream US practice, likely owing to the efficacy and low-risk profile of radioiodine ablation (RIA), despite the potential advantage of improved targeting using RFA compared with RIA. RIA is well established and remains the American Thyroid Association intervention of choice for most patients.[31]

Microwave ablation (MWA) is a more powerful ablative technology with a larger field effect; therefore, its use near thermally sensitive critical structures in the neck has been limited compared with RFA. Continuous hydrodissection to protect the surrounding structures has been advocated, along with the moving-shot technique with safe and effective results in the treatment of large thyroid nodules.[32]

Parathyroid and other nonthyroidal sites

Sparse literature exists for ablative head and neck procedures outside the thyroid and DTC-related nodal disease. However, cryoablation has been advocated for locally aggressive thyroidal and nonthyroidal head and neck malignancies that cannot undergo resection.[33] Ultrasonography guidance is useful in the positioning of cyroprobes, but monitoring of the resulting ablation is most appropriately performed with computed tomography or magnetic resonance, because the cryozone creates dense specular reflection, obscuring sonographic visualization of deep structures. Cryoablation is effective for local tumor and pain control in bone metastases, including those related to thyroid and other head and neck malignancies.[31,34]

EA, RFA, and MWA have all been described as having a potential role in the nonsurgical treatment of hyperfunctioning parathyroid adenoma in centers outside the United States.[35–37] However, the safety and efficacy of these treatments have not yet been established in US practice.

DISCLOSURE

The authors have nothing to disclose.

REFERENCES

1. Santos JE, Leiman G. Nonaspiration fine needle cytology. Application of a new technique to nodular thyroid disease. Acta Cytol 1988;32(3):353–6.
2. Song H, et al. Comparison of fine needle aspiration and fine needle nonaspiration cytology of thyroid nodules: a meta-analysis. Biomed Res Int 2015; 2015:796120.
3. Ramachandra L, Kudva R, Rao BH, et al. A comparative study of fine needle aspiration cytology (FNAC) and fine needle non-aspiration

cytology (FNNAC) technique in lesions of thyroid gland. Indian J Surg 2011;73(4):287–90.

4. Lee YH, Baek JH, Jung SL, et al. Ultrasound-guided fine needle aspiration of thyroid nodules: a consensus statement by the korean society of thyroid radiology. Korean J Radiol 2015;16(2):391–401.

5. Degirmenci B, et al. Sonographically guided fine-needle biopsy of thyroid nodules: the effects of nodule characteristics, sampling technique, and needle size on the adequacy of cytological material. Clin Radiol 2007;62(8):798–803.

6. Zhu W, Michael CW. How important is on-site adequacy assessment for thyroid FNA? An evaluation of 883 cases. Diagn Cytopathol 2007;35(3):183–6.

7. Chung SR, Suh CH, Baek JH, et al. The role of core needle biopsy in the diagnosis of initially detected thyroid nodules: a systematic review and meta-analysis. Eur Radiol 2018;28(11):4909–18.

8. Suh CH, et al. The role of core-needle biopsy for thyroid nodules with initially nondiagnostic fine-needle aspiration results: a systematic review and meta-analysis. Endocr Pract 2016;22(6):679–88.

9. Suh CH, et al. The role of core-needle biopsy in the diagnosis of thyroid malignancy in 4580 patients with 4746 thyroid nodules: a systematic review and meta-analysis. Endocrine 2016;54(2):315–28.

10. Kim SY, et al. Fine-needle aspiration versus core needle biopsy for diagnosis of thyroid malignancy and neoplasm: a matched cohort study. Eur Radiol 2017;27(2):801–11.

11. Yoon JH, Kwak JY, Moon HJ, et al. Ultrasonography-guided core needle biopsy did not reduce diagnostic lobectomy for thyroid nodules diagnosed as atypia of undetermined significance/follicular lesion of undetermined significance. Ultrasound Q 2019;35(3):253–8.

12. Middleton WD, et al. Multiinstitutional analysis of thyroid nodule risk stratification using the american college of radiology thyroid imaging reporting and data system. AJR Am J Roentgenol 2017;208(6):1331–41.

13. Gupta S, et al. Quality improvement guidelines for percutaneous needle biopsy. J Vasc Interv Radiol 2010;21(7):969–75.

14. Denham SL, Ismail A, Bolus DN, et al. Effect of anticoagulation medication on the thyroid fine-needle aspiration pathologic diagnostic sufficiency rate. J Ultrasound Med 2016;35(1):43–8.

15. Crockett JC. The thyroid nodule: fine-needle aspiration biopsy technique. J Ultrasound Med 2011;30(5):685–94.

16. Abdelghani R, Noureldine S, Abbas A, et al. The diagnostic value of parathyroid hormone washout after fine-needle aspiration of suspicious cervical lesions in patients with hyperparathyroidism. Laryngoscope 2013;123(5):1310–3.

17. Yasuda K, et al. Treatment of cystic lesions of the thyroid by ethanol instillation. World J Surg 1992;16(5):958–61.

18. Gelczer RK, Charboneau JW, Hussain S, et al. Complications of percutaneous ethanol ablation. J Ultrasound Med 1998;17(8):531–3.

19. Iniguez-Ariza NM, Lee RA, Singh-Ospina NM, et al. Ethanol ablation for the treatment of cystic and predominantly cystic thyroid nodules. Mayo Clin Proc 2018;93(8):1009–17.

20. Chung MS, et al. Treatment efficacy and safety of ethanol ablation for thyroglossal duct cysts: a comparison with surgery. Eur Radiol 2017;27(7):2708–16.

21. Sung JY. Parathyroid ultrasonography: the evolving role of the radiologist. Ultrasonography 2015;34(4):268–74.

22. Fontenot TE, Deniwar A, Bhatia P, et al. Percutaneous ethanol injection vs reoperation for locally recurrent papillary thyroid cancer: a systematic review and pooled analysis. JAMA Otolaryngol Head Neck Surg 2015;141(6):512–8.

23. Heilo A, et al. Efficacy of ultrasound-guided percutaneous ethanol injection treatment in patients with a limited number of metastatic cervical lymph nodes from papillary thyroid carcinoma. J Clin Endocrinol Metab 2011;96(9):2750–5.

24. Zhang M, et al. Ultrasound-guided radiofrequency ablation versus surgery for low risk papillary thyroid micro-carcinoma: results of over 5 years follow-up. Thyroid 2020. https://doi.org/10.1089/thy.2019.0147.

25. Baek JH, Jeong HJ, Kim YS, et al. Radiofrequency ablation for an autonomously functioning thyroid nodule. Thyroid 2008;18(6):675–6.

26. Jeong WK, et al. Radiofrequency ablation of benign thyroid nodules: safety and imaging follow-up in 236 patients. Eur Radiol 2008;18(6):1244–50.

27. Cesareo R, et al. Prospective study of effectiveness of ultrasound-guided radiofrequency ablation versus control group in patients affected by benign thyroid nodules. J Clin Endocrinol Metab 2015;100(2):460–6.

28. Hamidi O, et al. Outcomes of radiofrequency ablation therapy for large benign thyroid nodules: a mayo clinic case series. Mayo Clin Proc 2018;93(8):1018–25.

29. Kim YS, Rhim H, Tae K, et al. Radiofrequency ablation of benign cold thyroid nodules: initial clinical experience. Thyroid 2006;16(4):361–7.

30. Spiezia S, et al. Thyroid nodules and related symptoms are stably controlled two years after radiofrequency thermal ablation. Thyroid 2009;19(3):219–25.

31. Haugen BR, et al. 2015 American Thyroid Association Management Guidelines for Adult

Patients with Thyroid Nodules and Differentiated Thyroid Cancer: The American Thyroid Association Guidelines Task Force on Thyroid Nodules and Differentiated Thyroid Cancer. Thyroid 2016;26(1):1–133.

32. Li J, Liu Y, Liu J, et al. Ultrasound-guided percutaneous microwave ablation versus surgery for papillary thyroid microcarcinoma. Int J Hyperthermia 2018;34(5):653–9.

33. Gangi A, et al. "Keeping a cool head": percutaneous imaging-guided cryo-ablation as salvage therapy for recurrent glioblastoma and head and neck tumours. Cardiovasc Intervent Radiol 2019. https://doi.org/10.1007/s00270-019-02384-6.

34. Auloge P, et al. Complications of percutaneous bone tumor cryoablation: a 10-year experience. Radiology 2019;291(2):521–8.

35. Hu Z, Han E, Chen W, et al. Feasibility and safety of ultrasound-guided percutaneous microwave ablation for tertiary hyperparathyroidism. Int J Hyperthermia 2019;36(1):1129–36.

36. Korkusuz H, Wolf T, Grunwald F. Feasibility of bipolar radiofrequency ablation in patients with parathyroid adenoma: a first evaluation. Int J Hyperthermia 2018;34(5):639–43.

37. Shenoy MT, et al. Radiofrequency ablation followed by percutaneous ethanol ablation leading to long-term remission of hyperparathyroidism. J Endocr Soc 2017;1(6):676–80.

Imaging of Adrenal-Related Endocrine Disorders

Ceren Yalniz, MD[a], Ajaykumar C. Morani, MD[a],
Steven G. Waguespack, MD[b], Khaled M. Elsayes, MD[a],*

KEYWORDS

- Endocrine disorders • Endocrine abnormality • Adrenal pathologies • Imaging
- Excess hormone secretion

KEY POINTS

- Endocrine disorders associated with adrenal pathologies can be caused by insufficient adrenal gland function or excess hormone secretion.
- Excess hormone secretion may result from adrenal hyperplasia or hormone-secreting (ie, functioning) adrenal masses.
- Based on the hormone type, functioning adrenal masses can be classified as cortisol-producing tumors, aldosterone producing tumors, and androgen-producing tumors, which originate in the adrenal cortex, as well as catecholamine-producing pheochromocytomas, which originate in the medulla.
- Nonfunctioning lesions can cause adrenal gland enlargement without causing hormonal imbalance.
- Evaluation of adrenal-related endocrine disorders requires clinical and biochemical workup followed by imaging evaluation to reach a diagnosis and guide management.

INTRODUCTION

A wide spectrum of pathologies can affect the adrenal gland, including a range of functioning benign and malignant masses that secrete increased amounts of adrenal hormones as well as nonfunctioning tumors that do not affect hormone levels. Functioning tumors or hyperplasia of the adrenal cortex can cause Cushing syndrome (CS) from cortisol excess, Conn syndrome from aldosterone overproduction, or hyperandrogenism from androgen excess. Pheochromocytomas are tumors that arise from the adrenal medulla and secrete catecholamines. The other well-known adrenal pathology is adrenal insufficiency, which is characterized by low levels of adrenal hormones, and may result from adrenalectomy, autoimmune disorders, granulomatous diseases, hemorrhage, bilateral adrenal metastases, or infections causing adrenal gland destruction and hypofunction. The diagnosis of adrenal-related endocrine disorders is usually based on physical examination and biochemical workup, followed by imaging evaluation. Proper management of endocrine disorders, especially those that are neoplastic, requires a multidisciplinary team collaboration among endocrinologists, radiologists, pathologists, and surgeons. In this review, we focus on adrenal disorders associated with an endocrine abnormality and will not include nonfunctioning adrenal tumors.

[a] Department of Abdominal Imaging, Division of Diagnostic Imaging, The University of Texas MD Anderson Cancer Center, 1400 Pressler Street, Houston, TX 77030, USA; [b] Department of Endocrine Neoplasia and Hormonal Disorders, The University of Texas MD Anderson Cancer Center, 1400 Pressler Street, Houston, TX 77030, USA
* Corresponding author.
E-mail address: kmelsayes@mdanderson.org

Radiol Clin N Am 58 (2020) 1099–1113
https://doi.org/10.1016/j.rcl.2020.07.010

IMAGING EVALUATION

Imaging evaluation guides the appropriate management of adrenal-related endocrine disorders. Computed tomography (CT) with adrenal mass–dedicated protocol is the reference standard imaging modality for assessment of adrenal gland pathologies. An adrenal CT is performed with 2.5 to 3 mm thin slices, before and after intravenous administration of 100 to 150 mL of iodinated contrast material.[1] The adrenal mass protocol includes density measurement of the mass on noncontrast CT. An unenhanced attenuation value less than 10 Hounsfield units (HU) is characteristic of a lipid-rich adenoma. However, for adrenal masses with attenuation values greater than 10 HU, the absolute percentage of enhancement washout is calculated by measuring the unenhanced attenuation, the enhanced attenuation at 60 seconds, and attenuation 15 minutes after contrast injection to show rapid enhancement and rapid washout.

CT is often the first-line modality for adult adrenal imaging due to its wide availability, reproducibility, good temporal resolution and better spatial resolution than MR imaging.[2] Adrenal abnormalities can be detected and characterized using contrast-enhanced CT with or without noncontrast images, as mentioned previously.

Other imaging modalities, such as MR imaging and PET with fluorodeoxyglucose (FDG) or other specialized radioactive tracers such as gallium-68 DOTATATE are useful as adjuncts to CT when CT is negative or inconclusive.[3] Ultrasonography can be considered as an imaging modality for adrenal lesions in neonates and young children[4]; however, because the echogenicity of adrenal glands is close to the echogenicity of retroperitoneal fat, it is a challenge to visualize adrenal glands on ultrasound in older children and adults. In addition, ultrasound has limitations in identifying small lesions, and overlying bowel gas can be an impediment to adequate visualization.

MR imaging, which is discussed in greater detail later in this article, is often used as problem solver, especially when CT is contraindicated or inconclusive. MR imaging has a particular advantage of the lack of ionizing radiation. Chemical shift in-phase and opposed-phase are the most important MR imaging pulse sequences for characterizing adrenal masses by detecting intracytoplasmic lipid, high level of which is most often indicative of benign adrenal adenoma, with some exceptions such as lipid-containing metastases, collision tumors, or adrenocortical cancers. Ultimately, CT has been found to have the upper hand, compared with MR imaging, for differentiating between lipid-poor adrenal adenomas,[5] which show characteristic delayed postcontrast washout without detectability of lipid on chemical shift MR imaging, and other indeterminate adrenal masses. T2-weighted MR imaging may be helpful in the diagnosis of pheochromocytoma, which demonstrates marked hyperintensity; also known as "lightbulb sign."[6]

Nuclear medicine imaging modalities such as MIBG and indium-111 octreotide and gallium-68 DOTATATE PET are commonly used to evaluate pheochromocytoma. FDG-PET shows promise in the differentiation of malignant cortical lesions from benign masses. Malignant lesions show increased FDG uptake, and FDG-PET has been shown to have 94% to 100% sensitivity and 80% to 100% specificity in the detection of malignant masses.[3]

OVERVIEW OF ADRENAL-RELATED ENDOCRINE DISORDERS

Endocrine disorders associated with adrenal pathologies may be subclinical or clinical and can be classified into hypofunctioning disorders, such as adrenal insufficiency, or hyperfunctioning disorders, such as hyperaldosteronism, hypercortisolism, catecholamine excess, and hyperandrogenism.

Adrenal Insufficiency

Primary adrenal insufficiency occurs due to partial or complete destruction of the adrenal cortex, and patients with this condition may present with hyponatremia, hyperkalemia, fatigue, muscle weakness, hypotension, weight loss, abdominal pain, and hyperpigmentation. Common etiologies of primary adrenal insufficiency are autoimmune disease (ie, Addison disease), granulomatous diseases such as tuberculosis, other infections, neoplasms such as metastases and lymphoma, adrenal gland hemorrhage, adrenoleukodystrophy, and congenital adrenal hyperplasia.[7–9]

Screening tests for adrenal insufficiency include morning cortisol and adrenocorticotropic hormone (ACTH) levels or a high-dose cosyntropin (synthetic ACTH) stimulation test. Cortisol levels that fail to rise after ACTH stimulation and remain lower than 20 μg/dL indicate adrenal insufficiency.[10,11] In primary adrenal insufficiency, the synthesis and release of adrenocortical hormones are impaired.[11] The next step after the diagnosis of primary adrenal insufficiency is to check adrenal autoantibodies for autoimmune adrenal insufficiency. If autoantibodies are negative, very long chain fatty acids can be tested for adrenoleukodystrophy, serum 17-hydroxyprogesterone level can be measured for congenital adrenal hyperplasia, and CT can be performed to detect adrenal hemorrhage, infection, infiltration, or malignancy.[11] In adrenoleukodystrophy, very long chain fatty acids are accumulated in tissue and body fluids, and the clinical manifestations can be seen as central nervous system demyelination and primary adrenal insufficiency. Adrenal insufficiency is usually associated with cerebral adrenoleukodystrophy or adrenomyeloneuropathy involving the spinal cord and peripheral nerves, but in 8% of cases adrenal insufficiency is the only clinical manifestation.[12] Loes and colleagues[13] described 5 different MR imaging patterns of cerebral adrenoleukodystrophy, and the radiologic finding indicative of adrenal involvement is adrenal cortex atrophy.[12] In congenital adrenal hyperplasia, bilateral enlarged adrenal glands, wrinkled surface, and cerebriform pattern are characteristic ultrasound findings; however, the adrenal glands may also appear normal.[14] Therefore, ultrasonography should only be used as an adjunct to CT or MR imaging when adrenal hyperplasia is suspected.

CT imaging findings of primary adrenal insufficiency depend on the etiology and course of the disease. For instance, adrenal hemorrhage can present as a high-attenuation mass in the acute stage, then decrease in attenuation with aging of the hematoma.[15]

Infectious diseases and autoimmune and granulomatous disorders can cause bilateral enlargement of the glands[16] in the acute/subacute stage, with atrophy and often calcification of adrenal glands in the chronic stage. For example, Addison disease is considered subacute when present for less than 2 years, and in these cases, CT usually shows bilateral enlarged adrenal glands with occasional central necrosis and peripheral rim enhancement due to adrenalitis.[17,18]

In the chronic stage of adrenal insufficiency, CT shows bilateral adrenal gland atrophy. Calcifications are seen in 50% of cases of primary adrenal insufficiency secondary to tuberculosis; however, calcifications due to tuberculosis cannot be distinguished radiologically from other causes of calcifications, such as prior hemorrhage or idiopathic calcifications. Clinical and hormonal correlation is the key in such cases.[19–21]

Adrenal hemorrhage can result from blunt trauma, anticoagulation therapy, sepsis, or stress following surgery or severe burns, or it can be a complication of adrenal venous sampling.[22] In the setting of trauma, adrenal hemorrhage usually occurs in trauma of higher severity, and isolated adrenal hemorrhage is rare. Hemorrhage can also be seen in both benign and malignant masses such as adenomas, adrenal cortical carcinomas, myelolipomas, and pheochromocytomas.[23] Bilateral involvement can be seen in 20% of adrenal hemorrhage cases.[22] The most common imaging feature of hemorrhage, a high-attenuating adrenal mass, is seen in 83% of cases on unenhanced CT (Fig. 1). On MR imaging, adrenal hemorrhage shows intermediate signal intensity on T1-weighted images and low signal intensity on T2-weighted images in the acute stage and high signal intensity on both T1-weighted and T2-weighted images in the subacute stage. The typical appearance of chronic adrenal hemorrhage includes high signal intensity on T1-weighted images and hypointense peripheral rim on T2-weighted images. The high signal intensity on T1-weighted images can be due to methemoglobin, and hypointense peripheral rim on T2-weighted images is seen due to hemosiderin. Hematomas gradually decrease in size and may completely resolve or develop calcifications within a few months.[24]

Granulomatous infections such as tuberculosis or histoplasmosis account for 10% to 30% of primary adrenal insufficiency cases.[21] CT findings in the acute stage are bilateral adrenal enlargement, central necrosis, and peripheral rim enhancement. In the subacute and chronic stages, the adrenal glands become atrophic and calcified.

Other causes of adrenal insufficiency include lymphoma (Fig. 2) and metastases (Fig. 3). Lymphomatous adrenal lesions are usually homogeneous and large, but they can also be heterogeneous due to necrosis or hemorrhage. Adrenal lymphoma is bilateral in 50% of cases and is usually accompanied by retroperitoneal lymphadenopathy.[25] On CT, adrenal lymphoma usually demonstrates soft tissue attenuation and shows mild progressive enhancement.[26] On MR imaging, adrenal lymphoma typically exhibits low signal intensity on T1-weighted images and high signal intensity on T2-weighted images, with mild to moderate enhancement.[27]

The adrenal glands are a common site for hematogenous metastases because of their abundant blood supply, and most patients with adrenal metastases have a history of cancer. In a study by Song and colleagues,[28] not a single malignant lesion was found in 1049 patients without a history of malignancy who had adrenal nodules incidentally discovered at imaging. It is also rare to find an incidental adrenal metastasis at the initial presentation of an unknown primary malignancy. In a series of 1639 patients with unknown primary malignancy, the adrenal glands were involved in only 6%, and involvement was limited to the adrenal glands in only 0.2%; furthermore, all of the

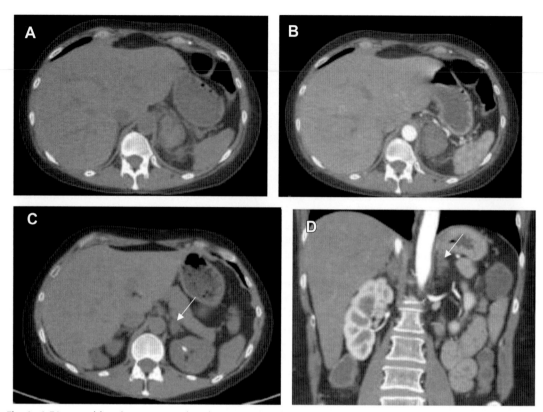

Fig. 1. A 51-year-old patient presented to the emergency department with abdominal pain. Axial unenhanced CT (*A*) and axial image of contrast-enhanced CT (*B*) demonstrate a well-circumscribed, rounded 3.2 × 4.2 cm mass involving the left adrenal gland with attenuation of 51 HU and no significant postcontrast enhancement, suggestive of hematoma. In the following 3 months, the patient had adrenal insufficiency symptoms in the form of fatigue, abdominal pain, and weakness. The workup for adrenal bleeding showed a heterozygous factor V Leiden mutation. Axial unenhanced CT (*C*) and coronal reformatted images of contrast-enhanced CT (*D*) performed 3 months later for follow-up showed interval resolution of the hematoma with diffuse left adrenal gland thickening (*arrow*).

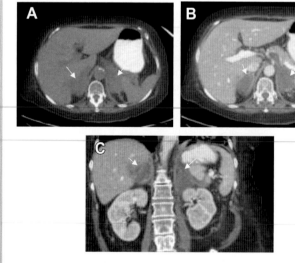

Fig. 2. A 70-year-old patient with a history of Burkitt lymphoma presented with adrenal insufficiency due to lymphomatous involvement of the bilateral adrenal glands. Axial unenhanced CT (*A*), and axial (*B*) and coronal (*C*) enhanced CT demonstrate bilateral enhancing adrenal masses (*arrows*).

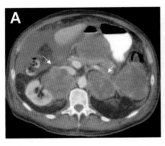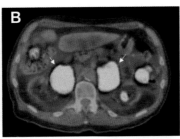

Fig. 3. A 76-year-old patient with adenocarcinoma of the lung with metastases to the bilateral adrenal glands, kidneys, bones, and mesentery presented with adrenal insufficiency. Axial enhanced CT (*A*) demonstrates bilateral adrenal masses (*arrows*), with the right adrenal mass indenting the right kidney collecting system. PET/CT (*B*) demonstrates increased FDG uptake in the bilateral adrenal glands (*arrows*). Biopsy of the right adrenal gland showed metastatic non–small cell carcinoma.

adrenal lesions were 6 cm or larger, and 75% of the patients had bilateral involvement.[29] Metastases to the adrenal glands most commonly originate from lung, breast, liver, kidney, and gastric cancers.[24] On CT, adrenal metastases usually have attenuation values greater than 10 HU on unenhanced series, and they show irregular peripheral or heterogeneous enhancement on contrast-enhanced series. Unlike adenomas, metastases enhance rapidly but do not exhibit enhancement washout, with the exception of some hypervascular metastatic lesions from primary tumors such as renal cell carcinoma and hepatocellular carcinoma, which can show rapid washout and hence can be misdiagnosed as adenomas.[30] Similarly, the presence of intracellular fat is highly specific for benign adenoma; however, some metastases, such as those from renal cell or hepatocellular carcinoma, can rarely contain intracellular lipid and mimic adrenal adenomas.[31–33] Associated hemorrhage and calcifications have been also described within these lesions. On MR imaging, metastatic masses typically demonstrate high signal intensity on T2-weighted images and low signal intensity on T1-weighted images and with heterogeneous postcontrast enhancement.

Hyperaldosteronism

Hyperaldosteronism can be primary, also known as Conn syndrome (the classic description of which is that of an aldosterone-producing adenoma), or secondary depending on the renin level. Whereas aldosterone levels in both primary and secondary hyperaldosteronism are high, the renin level is low in primary and high in secondary hyperaldosteronism (such as seen with a renin-secreting tumor or renovascular hypertension). Hyperaldosteronism presents with hypertension (typically refractory to multidrug therapy), hypokalemia (which is not always present), metabolic alkalosis, muscle cramps/weakness, headache, increased thirst, and frequent urination.

Common etiologies of secondary hyperaldosteronism are congestive heart failure, cirrhosis, nephrotic syndrome, renal artery stenosis, renin-secreting tumors, or diuretic use. Adrenal lesions in primary hyperaldosteronism can be unilateral or bilateral adrenal adenoma(s) (**Fig. 4**), adrenal hyperplasia, or adrenal carcinoma. Conn syndrome is caused by an aldosterone-producing adenoma in 35% of cases and bilateral idiopathic hyperplasia in 60% of cases.[34,35]

Screening tests for hyperaldosteronism include measuring the plasma renin activity (PRA) and plasma aldosterone concentration (PAC). Primary aldosteronism is suggested if the PAC:PRA ratio is greater than 20, and PAC levels greater than 20 ng/dL and PRA less than1 ng/mL per hour in the setting of spontaneous hypokalemia confirm the diagnosis. If both PRA and PAC are elevated, etiologies for secondary hyperaldosteronism should be further investigated. On the other hand, decreased PRA and PAC levels should prompt an investigation of other etiologies such as exogenous mineralocorticoids (eg, licorice ingestion) and CS.[36]

For confirmation of primary aldosteronism, measuring 24-hour aldosterone levels after oral sodium loading, measuring aldosterone response to intravenous saline infusion, and fludrocortisone suppression and captopril challenge tests may be used.[37] Aldosterone level higher than 10 ng/dL in a saline infusion test and direct renin concentration lower than 24 mIU/mL and PRA lower than 2 ng/mL hour in fludrocortisone suppression test are confirmatory results.[36]

After the biochemical confirmation of primary hyperaldosteronism, adrenal imaging should be pursued. If the patient has a unilateral adrenal adenoma on imaging and is younger than 40 years, unilateral adrenalectomy is the recommended treatment because the likelihood of this representing an incidental nonfunctional adrenal adenoma is only 1% to 2%.[38] Patients older than 40 years with a unilateral adrenal adenoma and patients with

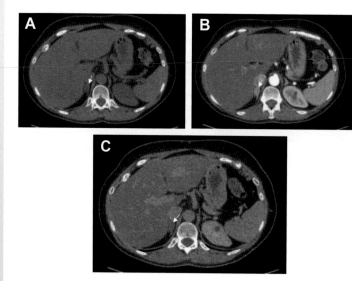

Fig. 4. A 53-year-old woman with a 14-year history of hypertension requiring multiple medications and hypokalemia with occasional muscle weakness and fatigue was referred to the endocrinology clinic while being treated for her breast cancer. Primary hyperaldosteronism was suspected. Axial unenhanced CT (*A*) demonstrates a well-circumscribed 1.5-cm oval mass involving the right adrenal gland with an attenuation of 19 HU. Contrast-enhanced CT in the portovenous phase (*B*) shows contrast uptake of the lesion, with attenuation of 106 HU. Delayed 15-minute axial CT (*C*) shows contrast washout with attenuation of 42 HU, yielding an absolute enhancement washout of 74%, characteristic of a lipid-poor adenoma (*arrow*).

normal glands or equivocal findings should be further investigated with selective adrenal venous sampling, which is the reference standard test for differentiating unilateral from bilateral adrenal disease.[39] A coincidental nonfunctioning neoplasm should be considered if adenomas are larger than 2 cm, because aldosteronomas are usually smaller than 1.5 cm.[40] If imaging shows bilateral adrenal gland thickening or micronodular changes, the diagnosis is bilateral adrenal hyperplasia or idiopathic hyperaldosteronism. If adrenal venous sampling confirms bilateral aldosterone production, medical management with an aldosterone receptor antagonist should be undertaken.[36] In addition, glucocorticoid-remediable aldosteronism, wherein aldosterone secretion is under the control of ACTH, also presents with nonlocalizing venous sampling test results.[41]

In this setting, adenomas can be detected on CT in only 70% of hyperaldosteronism cases. Aldosteronomas are typically homogeneous hypoattenuating nodules with attenuation less than 10 HU (if lipid-rich) and homogeneous contrast enhancement on CT, and they rarely show calcifications. Because the average diameter of aldosteronomas is less than 2 cm (approximately 20% measure <1 cm),[42] CT should be performed with a slice thickness of 5 mm or less. On MR imaging, they are iso- or hypointense relative to the liver on T1-weighted images and slightly hyperintense on T2-weighted images, with decrease in signal intensity on opposed-phase compared with in-phase pulse sequences.[42] It has been reported that aldosteronomas have the lowest attenuation values among hyperfunctioning adrenal adenomas.[42,43] As many as 50% of surgically proven aldosteronomas may be misdiagnosed as hyperplasia on CT.[44] Adrenal cortical hyperplasia is among the etiologies of patients presenting with excessive secretion of adrenal cortex hormones such as cortisol, aldosterone, and androgens, and 60% of hyperaldosteronism cases result from adrenal cortical hyperplasia. Adrenal cortical hyperplasia typically presents as smooth to slightly lobular, uniform enlargement, although macronodular morphology can be also seen. In diffuse hyperplasia, there is homogeneous enlargement of the entire gland, and the normal inverted V or Y configuration is maintained. The limbs of the adrenal glands usually measure more than 5 cm in length and more than 1 cm in thickness. The attenuation and signal intensity of cortical adrenal hyperplasia are usually similar to that of the normal gland (**Fig. 5**). In a small percentage of patients, low CT attenuation and signal drop on opposed-phased MR imaging can be seen, especially in cases with macronodules.[24,45,46]

Hypercortisolism

The chronic excess of cortisol causes CS, which presents with features that include obesity, moon facies, proximal muscle weakness, thin skin with easy bruising, violaceous striae, abnormal body fat distribution (ie, truncal obesity, fullness of the dorsal and supraclavicular fat pads), acne, hirsutism, hypertension, edema, low bone mass and fractures, amenorrhea, and impaired glucose tolerance. CS arises from exogenous glucocorticoid administration or endogenous overproduction of cortisol, which is either mediated by ACTH (ACTH-dependent CS) or caused by the neoplastic hypersecretion of cortisol from the

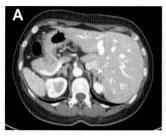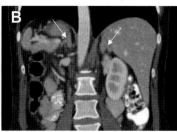

Fig. 5. A 43-year-old woman with situs inversus totalis and a history of Cushing disease due to a pituitary macroadenoma resected 7 years previously was referred to the endocrinology clinic for recurrent signs and symptoms of hypercortisolism. Axial contrast-enhanced CT (A) and coronal reformatted images of contrast-enhanced CT (B) show bilateral diffuse thickening of the adrenal glands (arrows), consistent with bilateral ACTH-driven adrenal hyperplasia.

adrenal cortex (ACTH-independent CS). ACTH-dependent hypercortisolism accounts for 80% of cases and is typically caused by an ACTH-producing pituitary tumor (Cushing disease) or more rarely by an ectopic ACTH-producing neuroendocrine tumor (NET) or a corticotropin-releasing hormone (CRH) producing tumor. The most likely source of ectopic ACTH production is a thoracic tumor (eg, bronchopulmonary NET, small cell lung cancer, thymic NET), but ectopic ACTH secretion can also occur in pancreatic NETs and, more rarely, pheochromocytomas and medullary thyroid carcinomas. CRH-producing tumors account for fewer than 1% of the cases.[5] ACTH-dependent CS can present with bilateral diffuse and uniform adrenal enlargement (see Fig. 5), which in time becomes nodular in appearance, and this is known as multinodular hyperplasia. Occasionally these ACTH-dependent macronodules grow larger and become autonomous, an entity called massive macronodular hyperplasia.[16,47]

ACTH-independent CS can result from an adrenal adenoma, carcinoma, primary pigmented nodular adrenocortical disease (PPNAD) or ACTH-independent macronodular adrenocortical hyperplasia (Fig. 6), also known as bilateral macronodular adrenal hyperplasia. Adenomas account for 60% of adrenal-related CS cases, and the remaining 40% adrenal-related CS cases are caused by adrenocortical carcinoma.[5]

A clinical suspicion of CS should be followed by screening tests, which include a 24-hour urinary free cortisol, serum cortisol level after 1 mg dexamethasone administration at 11 PM the prior evening, and/or a late-night salivary cortisol level. If cortisol levels are not elevated but the clinical suspicion is high, repeat screening tests intermittently should be considered because CS can be cyclic in nature. ACTH levels should be evaluated after a diagnosis of CS is made. Whereas normal or overly elevated ACTH levels are consistent with ACTH-dependent disease, low normal or overtly low

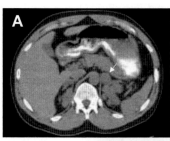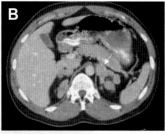

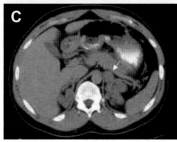

Fig. 6. A 33-year-old man with a 1-month history of hypertension and 20-pound weight gain, mostly abdominal, over the past 2 years and bilateral adrenal nodules was referred to the endocrinology clinic. He had an elevated 24-hour urinary free cortisol level, not suppressed by dexamethasone, and low ACTH concentration. ACTH-independent macronodular adrenal hyperplasia was suspected. Axial unenhanced CT (A) demonstrates bilateral well-circumscribed oval masses in the adrenal glands, the largest one measuring 2.7 cm in the left adrenal gland (arrow) with an attenuation of 38 HU. Contrast-enhanced CT in the portovenous phase (B) shows contrast uptake of the lesion with attenuation of 110 HU, and delayed 15-minute axial CT (C) shows contrast washout with attenuation of 59 HU, yielding an absolute enhancement washout of 71%, characteristic of a lipid-poor adenoma (arrow).

ACTH levels should prompt further evaluation of the adrenals. Pituitary MR imaging with and without contrast is performed once ACTH-dependent disease is identified. If MR imaging is negative for a pituitary cause or only a small pituitary lesion is detected, bilateral inferior petrosal sinus sampling can be considered. If inferior petrosal sinus sampling documents a peripheral source of ACTH secretion, additional imaging should be performed to evaluate for an ectopic ACTH-producing tumor.[5,48–51]

In the case of ACTH-independent CS, either CT or MR imaging should be performed to assess for an adrenal neoplasm. If adrenal imaging shows normal adrenal glands or micronodules, the Liddle test can be considered because patients with PPNAD show a paradoxic increase in cortisol secretion after the administration of dexamethasone.[52,53] In addition, adrenal venous sampling can be considered to determine laterality in selected cases.[54]

Adrenal adenomas are well-circumscribed round or ovoid lesions with homogeneous or slightly heterogeneous enhancement, measuring 1 to 5 cm.[55] A cortisol-secreting adenoma should be suspected when there is a focal mass in one adrenal gland and the other adrenal is smaller than normal, but there are no other reliable imaging findings that can discriminate the functionality of an adrenal adenoma. Low attenuation of adenomas due to their intracellular lipid content are diagnosed by unenhanced CT using a threshold of 10 HU, with high specificity of 98%. However, 30% of adenomas are lipid-poor and measure 10 HU or more on unenhanced CT.[56] Chemical shift imaging has been found to be sensitive in the differentiation of adenomas and other lesions with attenuation between 10 and 30 HU[57]; however, it has also been shown that chemical shift imaging is less sensitive than dynamic CT in lesions with attenuation less than 20 HU.[58] Diffusion-weighted imaging also has not been successful in the diagnosis of adenomas because of the overlap in apparent diffusion coefficient values among different adrenal masses.[59] Adenomas usually show fast and avid enhancement on early imaging (65–70 seconds) and fast washout. An absolute enhancement washout of more than 60% (100% × [attenuation in portal venous phase − attenuation in delayed phase]/[attenuation in portal venous phase − unenhanced attenuation]) or a relative enhancement washout of 40% (100% × [attenuation in portal venous phase − attenuation in delayed phase]/attenuation in portal venous phase) is highly sensitive and specific for the diagnosis of adrenal adenomas (Fig. 7).[56,60–62] On MR imaging, adrenal adenomas are homogeneous rounded lesions with low T1-weighted imaging signal, and they are isointense on T2-weighted imaging, with uniform early enhancement. A signal intensity index greater than 16.5%, which is calculated as 100 × ([in-phase signal intensity − opposed-phase signal intensity]/in-phase signal intensity), is highly specific for adrenal adenomas that contain intracellular lipid.[63]

Adrenocortical carcinoma is a rare tumor that can present as a palpable abdominal mass or abdominal/back pain. Approximately 40% of patients present with hormonal manifestations such as CS; virilization or feminization secondary to androgen or estrogen excess, respectively; or Conn syndrome.[64] Adrenocortical carcinoma usually presents as a large (>6 cm) heterogeneous mass due to hemorrhage and central necrosis.[65,66] It can invade adjacent structures and show venous extension. Adrenocortical carcinoma can be bilateral in rare cases and usually metastasizes to regional lymph nodes, lungs, liver, and bones.[67] Vascular invasion and distant metastases are found frequently at initial diagnosis. Adrenocortical carcinomas have precontrast attenuation values greater than 10 HU because of their lack of intracellular fat, and they enhance heterogeneously like other neoplastic adrenal lesions. Adrenocortical carcinomas have lower relative and absolute washout rates compared with adenomas.[45,68] Even though adrenocortical carcinomas show early rapid enhancement like adrenal adenomas, they do not show fast contrast washout. Calcifications can be found in 30% of adrenocortical carcinomas, and very rarely these tumors can have intracytoplasmic lipid (Fig. 8).[69] Only a few published cases have reported adrenocortical carcinoma with macroscopic fat.[70–72] An American College of Radiology (ACR) White Paper recommends follow-up CT or MR imaging in 12 months for benign-appearing, indeterminate adrenal nodules that are smaller than 4 cm.[73] In addition, according to the ACR White Paper, an increase of more than 20% (or an absolute increase of 5 mm) in the diameter is a suspicious feature on follow-up. It is also acknowledged that surgical series have shown a 4-cm cutoff to be sensitive for malignant lesions; however, more clinical evidence is needed to confirm this cutoff size.[74,75]

Another rare cause of CS is PPNAD, which is mostly associated with the Carney complex. PPNAD appears grossly as multiple small (<6 mm) pigmented nodules with atrophy of the involved adrenal cortex.[76] Other accompanying findings of Carney complex are soft tissue myxomas, especially affecting the atria; spotty skin pigmentation; and Sertoli cell tumors of the

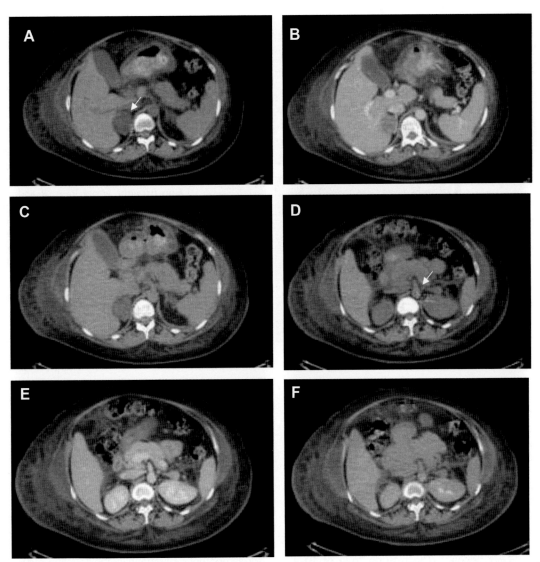

Fig. 7. A 28-year-old woman presented to the endocrinology clinic with recently diagnosed hypertension and elevated levels of testosterone during the second trimester of her pregnancy. An MR imaging from another center showed bilateral adrenal masses. Axial unenhanced CT after delivery (*A*) demonstrates a well-circumscribed oval mass measuring 4 cm involving the right adrenal gland (*arrow*) with an attenuation of 5 HU. Contrast-enhanced CT in the portovenous phase (*B*) shows contrast uptake of the lesion with attenuation of 56 HU. Delayed 15-minute axial CT (*C*) shows contrast washout with attenuation of 24 HU, yielding an absolute enhancement washout of 63%, characteristic of an adenoma. Axial unenhanced CT (*D*) demonstrates a well-circumscribed oval mass measuring 1.8 cm (*arrow*) involving the left adrenal gland with an attenuation of 15 HU. Contrast-enhanced CT in the portovenous phase (*E*) shows contrast uptake of the lesion with attenuation of 91 HU. Delayed 15-minute axial CT (*F*) shows contrast washout with attenuation of 40 HU, yielding an absolute enhancement washout of 67%, characteristic of a lipid-poor adenoma.

testes.[77] As previously mentioned, another cause of adrenal-related CS is ACTH-independent macronodular adrenal hyperplasia, which presents as bilateral enlarged adrenal glands with nodular contours on CT and hypodense lipid-containing nodules, ranging from 0.1 to 5.5 cm. On MR imaging, the nodules are hypointense relative to the liver on T1-weighted images and isointense to

hyperintense on T2-weighted images with signal drop on opposed-phase images due to lipid content.[78]

Catecholamine Excess

Catecholamine excess (overproduction of epinephrine/norepinephrine and their metabolites,

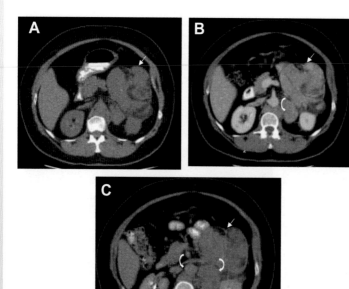

Fig. 8. A 42-year-old patient presented with an adrenal mass discovered at an outside facility. CT was performed for diagnostic workup of hypertension, diabetes mellitus, and hirsutism with elevated androgen and cortisol levels. Axial unenhanced CT (*A*), contrast-enhanced CT in the portovenous phase (*B*) and delayed 15-minute axial CT (*C*) demonstrate a large heterogeneous solid mass involving the left adrenal gland, measuring 13 cm in maximal dimension (*straight arrow* in *A*, *B* and *C*) with low attenuation areas, and speckles of calcifications with associated retroperitoneal lymphadenopathy (*curved arrows*). This mass was surgically resected and found to represent adrenocortical carcinoma.

metanephrine/normetanephrine) arises from secretory tumors of the adrenal medulla, including neuroblastoma and pheochromocytoma. Classic symptoms of catecholamine excess include hypertension, palpitations, headache, and sweating.

Pheochromocytomas are highly associated with hereditary disease, including multiple endocrine neoplasia types 2A and 2B (MEN2A and MEN2B), neurofibromatosis type 1, von Hippel-Lindau disease, and the group of familial paraganglioma syndromes due to mutations in the *SDHx* genes.[79] The historic "rule of 10 s," which suggested that 10% of pheochromocytomas are malignant, familial, extra-adrenal, diagnosed in children, or bilateral,[80] no longer holds true.[79] Pheochromocytomas can be multifocal and/or coexist with paragangliomas in 30% to 70% of cases, more so in familial cases or cases with a hereditary syndrome.[81] Pheochromocytomas are bilateral in 20% to 40% of cases, and up to 80% of those occurring in the pediatric population are associated with genetic mutation syndromes.[82] The incidence of pheochromocytoma in the hypertensive population is 0.1% to 0.6%, and the incidence in the general population is 0.05%, according to an autopsy series.[82]

In a patient clinically suspected to harbor a pheochromocytoma, free plasma metanephrines or 24-hour urinary metanephrines should be checked. If the metanephrine level is less than 2 times the normal level in a symptomatic patient, pheochromocytoma is highly unlikely. When the metanephrine level is 2 to 4 times higher than the normal level, repeat testing and an assessment of plasma or urine catecholamines should be pursued. When the metanephrine level is 4 times higher than the normal level, a pheochromocytoma can be diagnosed biochemically, and the next step should be imaging studies. If abdominal CT or MR imaging is negative, CT of the neck, chest, and pelvis should be considered to look for sympathetic paragangliomas.[83–87] If a mass is detected on anatomic imaging and there is no concern for multifocal disease, surgery can be performed after appropriate medical blockade. Genetic counseling and testing also should be pursued in all cases. If localizing studies are negative or there is a concern for multifocal disease (especially in cases of hereditary disease), functional imaging with 123I/131I MIBG or gallium-68 DOTATATE or 18F-FDG-PET/CT should be performed. Pheochromocytomas express somatostatin receptors and can be visualized with gallium-68 DOTA-coupled peptides such as DOTATATE. Chang and colleagues[3] showed that gallium-68 DOTATATE PET/CT detected a similar number of lesions with significantly greater lesion-to-background contrast compared with F-18 FDG-PET/CT.

Pheochromocytomas are usually homogeneous; however, they can present as heterogeneous lesions due to intratumoral hemorrhage and necrosis as they get larger, and they can also be cystic. Calcification is an accompanying finding in 10% of cases, and the presence of intracytoplasmic fat can exclude pheochromocytoma.[6] Most pheochromocytomas show intense enhancement in the 70-s phase of contrast enhancement, and they tend to enhance more in the portal venous phase than in the arterial phase. They have washout characteristics similar to malignant lesions with prolonged enhancement (**Fig. 9**); however, approximately one-third of pheochromocytomas show washout values similar to adenomas.[6,83,88] On CT, pheochromocytomas usually have attenuation values higher than those of adenomas and similar to those of muscles. On MR imaging, they have high signal intensity on T2-weighted images, classically described as "light bulb bright"[89]; however, approximately 30% of pheochromocytomas can show intermediate to low signal intensity on T2-weighted images due to cystic degeneration or hemorrhage.[56]

Similar to adrenocortical carcinomas, reliable imaging findings to differentiate malignant from benign pheochromocytomas are distant metastases or local invasion into adjacent organs and vasculature.[90]

Although evaluating imaging studies for pheochromocytoma, special attention should be paid to the findings of potential accompanying syndromes. For instance, the MEN2 syndromes can present with thyroid tumors and parathyroid lesions (MEN2A) or megacolon (MEN2B). Radiologically detectable lesions in von Hippel-Lindau disease include central nervous system hemangioblastomas, renal cysts, renal cell carcinomas, and pancreatic cysts, cystadenomas, and NETs. In patients with neurofibromatosis, neurofibromas, optic nerve gliomas, or other central nervous system lesions or lung lesions can be seen. Tuberous sclerosis can present with subependymal tubers, renal angiomyolipomas, renal cysts, renal cell carcinomas, cardiac rhabdomyomas, and pulmonary lymphangiomatosis. In the familial paraganglioma syndromes, gastrointestinal stromal tumor and renal cell carcinoma can occur. Finally, the Carney complex is associated with extra-adrenal paraganglioma, gastrointestinal stromal tumor and pulmonary chondroma.[91–93]

Hyperandrogenism

The most common etiology of hyperandrogenism is polycystic ovary syndrome (PCOS). Other causes include late-onset 21-hydroxylase deficiency and other steroidogenic enzyme deficiencies; ovarian disorders such as stromal luteoma, ovarian hyperthecosis, and Sertoli-Leydig cell tumor[94]; and adrenocortical tumors. Other endocrine diseases such as ACTH-dependent CS and acromegaly can also cause hyperandrogenism. Common exogenous causes of hyperandrogenism are drugs with androgenic effects, such as testosterone and anabolic steroids.[95] Hyperandrogenism is a difficult diagnosis in men, whereas it can be easier in women who present with acne, increased body/facial hair, deepening of the voice, clitoral enlargement, and menstrual abnormalities.

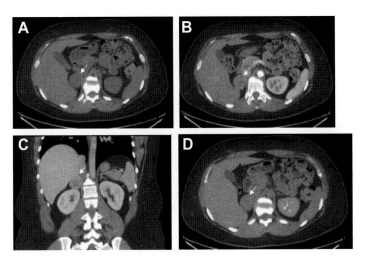

Fig. 9. A 34-year-old woman presented to the endocrinology clinic with an incidental adrenal mass discovered on CT at an outside facility performed after a motor vehicle accident. She reported a history of hypertension and worsening anxiety over the past year. Axial unenhanced CT (*A*) demonstrates a well circumscribed oval mass measuring 4.2 cm in maximal dimension involving the right adrenal gland with a precontrast attenuation of 28 HU. Contrast enhanced CT in arterial phase (*B*) shows a heterogeneously enhancing mass with attenuation of 56 HU, in the context of increased plasma metanephrines, compatible with pheochromocytoma (*arrow*). Coronal reformatted image of CT in the venous phase (*C*) demonstrates attenuation of 91 HU in the mass. Delayed 15-minute axial CT (*D*) shows contrast washout with attenuation of 58 HU, yielding an absolute enhancement washout of 52%. This mass was surgically resected and pathologically proven to represent pheochromocytoma (*arrows* in *A-D*).

To screen for hyperandrogenism, the levels of total testosterone, follicle-stimulating hormone, luteinizing hormone, dehydroepiandrosterone sulfate (DHEAS), androstenedione, and 17-hydroxyprogesterone (17OHP) should be measured. In women, if the total testosterone level is greater than 200 ng/dL and DHEAS is greater than 500 ug/dL, imaging should be done to assess for an adrenal cause; however, if DHEAS is normal or minimally elevated, ovarian causes such as ovarian androgen-secreting tumors or hyperthecosis should be further investigated with pelvic ultrasonography, CT, or MR imaging. DHEAS can be elevated in PCOS, as mentioned in the literature by several studies; for instance, Goodarzi and colleagues[96] reported that 20% to 30% of patients with PCOS have DHEAS excess. Some clinicians use a DHEAS cutoff of 700 ug/dL.[97,98] If the testosterone level is lower than 200 ng/dL, an ACTH stimulation test should be considered. If the stimulated 17OHP is lower than 1000 ng/dL, the etiology is PCOS or functional hyperandrogenism; whereas, for 17OHP levels higher than 1000 ng/dL, the diagnosis is the nonclassic form of 21-hydroxylase deficiency.[97,99–103] Of course, any clinically significant hyperandrogenism should be evaluated regardless of the absolute testosterone level.

Benign or malignant functioning adrenocortical tumors (see **Fig. 8**) typically cause hyperandrogenism but can also present with feminization.[97] Feminizing adrenal tumors are extremely rare, usually seen in men and children, and defined as adrenal neoplasms secreting estrogens with or without other adrenal gland hormones.[104]

SUMMARY

In conclusion, adrenal-related endocrine disorders are commonly encountered pathologies that require a detailed clinical, biochemical, and imaging workup. CT is the standard imaging method for adrenal gland pathologies. Ultrasonography can be considered in neonates and young children. MR imaging and nuclear medicine studies such as MIBG and gallium-68 DOTATATE PET are useful adjuncts to CT when CT is negative or inconclusive. The management of adrenal-related endocrine disorders is one that requires close collaboration and teamwork among endocrinologists, radiologists, and surgeons.

REFERENCES

1. Lumachi F, Marchesi P, Miotto D, et al. CT and MR imaging of the adrenal glands in cortisol-secreting tumors. Anticancer Res 2011;31:2923–6.

2. Choyke PL. ACR appropriateness criteria on incidentally discovered adrenal mass. J Am Coll Radiol 2006;3(7):498–504.

3. Chang CA, Pattison DA, Tothill RW, et al. (68)Ga-DOTATATE and (18)F-FDG PET/CT in Paraganglioma and Pheochromocytoma: utility, patterns and heterogeneity. Cancer Imaging 2016;16:22.

4. Słapa RZ, Jakubowski WS, Dobruch-Sobczak K, et al. Standards of ultrasound imaging of the adrenal gland. J Ultrason 2015;15:377–87.

5. Wagner-Bartak NA, Baiomy A, Habra MA, et al. Cushing syndrome: diagnostic workup and imaging features, with clinical and pathologic correlation. AJR Am J Roentgenol 2017;209:19–32.

6. Schieda N, Alrashed A, Flood TA, et al. Comparison of quantitative MRI and CT washout analysis for differentiation of adrenal pheochromocytoma from adrenal adenoma. AJR Am J Roentgenol 2016;206:1141–8.

7. Laureti S, Vecchi L, Santeusanio F, et al. Is the prevalence of Addison's disease underestimated? J Clin Endocrinol Metab 1999;84:1762.

8. Willis AC, Vince FP. The prevalence of Addison's disease in Coventry, UK. Postgrad Med J 1997; 73:286–8.

9. Bonstein SR. Predisposing factors for adrenal insufficiency. N Engl J Med 2009;360:2328–39.

10. Speckart PF, Nicoloff JT, Bethune JE. Screening for adrenocortical insufficiency with cosyntropin (synthetic ACTH). Arch Intern Med 1971;128:761–3.

11. Bancos I, Hahner S, Tomlinson J, et al. Diagnosis and management of adrenal insufficiency. Lancet Diabetes Endocrinol 2015;3:216–26.

12. Laureti S, Casucci G, Santeusanio F, et al. X-linked adrenoleukodystrophy is a frequent cause of idiopathic Addison's disease in young adult male patients. J Clin Endocrinol Metab 1996;81:470–4.

13. Loes DJ, Fatemi A, Melhem ER. Analysis of MRI patterns aids prediction of progression in X-linked adrenoleukodystrophy. Neurology 2003;61: 369–74.

14. Chambrier ED, Heinrichs C, Avni FE. Sonographic appearance of congenital adrenal hyperplasia in utero. J Ultrasound Med 2002;21:97–100.

15. Rana AI, Kenney PJ, Lockhart ME, et al. Adrenal gland hematomas in trauma patients. Radiology 2004;230:669–75.

16. Morani AC, Jensen CT, Habra MA, et al. Adrenocortical hyperplasia: a review of clinical presentation and imaging. Abdom Radiol (NY) 2020;45(4): 917–27.

17. Wilson DA, Muchmore HG, Tisdal RG, et al. Histoplasmosis of the adrenal glands studied by CT. Radiology 1984;150:779–83.

18. Doppman JL, Gill JR Jr, Nienhuis AW, et al. CT findings in Addison's disease. J Comput Assist Tomogr 1982;6:757–61.

19. Sawczuk IS, Reitelman C, Libby C, et al. CT findings in Addison's disease caused by tuberculosis. Urol Radiol 1986;8:44–5.

20. Jarvis JL, Jenkins D, Sosman MC, et al. Roentgenologic observations in Addison's disease: a review of 120 cases. Radiology 1954;62:16–28.

21. Kawashima A, Sandler CM, Fishman EK, et al. Spectrum of CT findings in nonmalignant disease of the adrenal gland. Radiographics 1998;18: 393–412.

22. Wolverson MK, Kannegiesser H. CT of bilateral adrenal hemorrhage with acute adrenal insufficiency in the adult. AJR Am J Roentgenol 1984; 142:311–4.

23. Rumaneik M, Bosniak AB. Miscellaneous conditions of the adrenals and adrenal pseudotumors. In: Pollack HM, editor. Clinical urography. 1st edition. Philadelphia: Saunders; 1990. p. 2399–412.

24. Elsayes KM, Mukundan G, Narra VR, et al. Adrenal masses: MR imaging features with pathologic correlation. Radiographics 2004;24:73–86.

25. Lee MJ, Mayo-Smith WW, Hahn PF, et al. State-of-the-art MR imaging of the adrenal gland. Radiographics 1994;14:1015–29.

26. Li Y, Sun H, Gao S, et al. Primary bilateral adrenal lymphoma: 2 case reports. J Comput Assist Tomogr 2006;30:791–3.

27. Lee FT Jr, Thornbury JR, Grist TM, et al. MR imaging of adrenal lymphoma. Abdom Imaging 1993; 18:95–6.

28. Song JH, Chaudhry FS, Mayo-Smith WW. The incidental adrenal mass on CT: prevalence of adrenal disease in 1,049 consecutive adrenal masses in patients with no known malignancy. AJR Am J Roentgenol 2008;190:1163–8.

29. Lee JE, Evans DB, Hickey RC, et al. Unknown primary cancer presenting as an adrenal mass: frequency and implications for diagnostic evaluation of adrenal incidentalomas. Surgery 1998;124: 1115–22.

30. Choi YA, Kim CK, Park BK, et al. Evaluation of adrenal metastases from renal cell carcinoma and hepatocellular carcinoma: use of delayed contrast-enhanced CT. Radiology 2013;266: 514–20.

31. Moosavi B, Shabana WM, El-Khodary M, et al. Intracellular lipid in clear cell renal cell carcinoma tumor thrombus and metastases detected by chemical shift (in and opposed phase) MRI: radiologic-pathologic correlation. Acta Radiol 2016;57:241–8.

32. Sydow BD, Rosen MA, Siegelman ES. Intracellular lipid within metastatic hepatocellular carcinoma of the adrenal gland: a potential diagnostic pitfall of chemical shift imaging of the adrenal gland. AJR Am J Roentgenol 2006;187:550–1.

33. Tariq U, Poder L, Carlson D, et al. Multimodality imaging of fat-containing adrenal metastasis from hepatocellular carcinoma. Clin Nucl Med 2012;37:157–9.

34. Young WF Jr. Primary aldosteronism: diagnosis. In: Mansoor GA, editor. Secondary hypertension: clinical presentation, diagnosis, and treatment. Totowa (NJ): Humana Press; 2004. p. 119–37.

35. Montori VM, Young WF Jr. Use of plasma aldosterone concentration-to-plasma renin activity ratio as a screening test for primary aldosteronism. A systematic review of the literature. Endocrinol Metab Clin North Am 2002;31:619–32.

36. Rossi GP. A comprehensive review of the clinical aspects of primary aldosteronism. Nat Rev Endocrinol 2011;7:485–95.

37. Mulatero P, Milan A, Fallo F, et al. Journal of clinical endocrinology and metabolism. Totowa (NJ): Humana Press; 2006. p. 2618–23.

38. Kloos RT, Gross MD, Francis IR, et al. Incidentally discovered adrenal masses. Endocr Rev 1995;16: 460–84.

39. Young WF, Stanson AW, Thompson GB, et al. Role for adrenal venous sampling in primary aldosteronism. Surgery 2004;136:1227–35.

40. Tan YY, Ogilvie JB, Triponez F, et al. Selective use of adrenal venous sampling in the lateralization of aldosterone-producing adenomas. World J Surg 2006;30:879–85.

41. McMahon GT, Dluhy RG. Glucocorticoid-remediable aldosteronism. Cardiol Rev 2004;12:44–8.

42. Dunniek NR, Leight GS Jr, Roubidoux MA, et al. CT in the diagnosis of primary aldosteronism: sensitivity in 29 patients. AJR Am J Roentgenol 1993; 160:321–4.

43. Miyake H, Maeda H, Tashiro M, et al. CT of adrenal tumors: frequency and clinical significance of low-attenuation lesions. AJR Am J Roentgenol 1989; 152:1005–7.

44. Doppman JL, Gill JR Jr. Hyperaldosteronism: sampling the adrenal veins. Radiology 1996;198: 309–12.

45. Lattin GE Jr, Sturgill ED, Tujo CA, et al. From the radiologic pathology archives: adrenal tumors and tumor-like conditions in the adult-radiologic-pathologic correlation. Radiographics 2014;34: 805–29.

46. Wang F, Liu J, Zhang R, et al. CT and MRI of adrenal gland pathologies. Quant Imaging Med Surg 2018;8:853–75.

47. Stratakis CA. Cushing syndrome caused by adrenocortical tumors and hyperplasias (corticotropin-independent Cushing syndrome. Endocr Dev 2008;13:117–32.

48. Guaraldi F, Salvatori R. Cushing syndrome: maybe not so uncommon of an endocrine disease. J Am Board Fam Med 2012;25:199–208.

49. Bansal V, El Asmar N, Selman WR, et al. Pitfalls in the diagnosis and management of Cushing's syndrome. Neurosurg Focus 2015;38:1–11.

50. Castro M, Moreira AC. Screening and diagnosis of Cushing's syndrome. Arq Bras Endocrinol Metabol 2007;51:1191–8.

51. Lad SP, Patil CG, Laws ER Jr, et al. The role of inferior petrosal sinus sampling in the diagnostic localization of Cushing's disease. Neurosurg Focus 2007;23(3):E2.

52. Louiset E, Stratakis CA, Perraudin V, et al. The paradoxical increase in cortisol secretion induced by dexamethasone in primary pigmented nodular adrenocortical disease involves a glucocorticoid receptor-mediated effect of dexamethasone on protein kinase A catalytic subunits. J Clin Endocrinol Metab 2009;4:2406–13.

53. Stratakis CA. Cushing syndrome in pediatrics. Endocrinol Metab Clin North Am 2012;41:793–803.

54. Ueland GÅ, Methlie P, Jøssang DE, et al. Adrenal venous sampling for assessment of autonomous cortisol secretion. J Clin Endocrinol Metab 2018; 103:4553–60.

55. Rockall AG, Babar SA, Sohaib SA, et al. CT and MR imaging of the adrenal glands in ACTH-independent Cushing syndrome. Radiographics 2004;24:435–52.

56. Blake MA, Cronin CG, Boland GW. Adrenal imaging. AJR Am J Roentgenol 2010;194:1450–60.

57. Sebro R, Aslam R, Muglia VF, et al. Low yield of chemical shift MRI for characterization of adrenal lesions with high attenuation density on unenhanced CT. Abdom Imaging 2015;40: 318–26.

58. Seo JM, Park BK, Park SY, et al. Characterization of lipid-poor adrenal adenoma: chemical-shift MRI and washout CT. AJR Am J Roentgenol 2014;202: 1043–50.

59. Sandrasegaran K, Patel AA, Ramaswamy R, et al. Characterization of adrenal masses with diffusion-weighted imaging. AJR Am J Roentgenol 2011; 197:132–8.

60. Boland GW, Lee MJ, Gazelle GS, et al. Characterization of adrenal masses using unenhanced CT: an analysis of the CT literature. AJR Am J Roentgenol 1998;71:201–4.

61. Johnson PT, Horton K, Fishman EK, et al. Adrenal mass imaging with multidetector CT: pathologic conditions, pearls, and pitfalls. Radiographics 2009;29:1333–51.

62. Caoili EM, Korobkin M, Francis IR, et al. Adrenal masses: characterization with combined unenhanced and delayed enhanced CT. Radiology 2002;222:629–33.

63. Siegelman ER. Adrenal MRI: techniques and clinical applications. J Magn Reson Imaging 2012; 36:272–85.

64. Ayala-Ramirez M, Jasim S, Feng L, et al. Adrenocortical carcinoma: clinical outcomes and prognosis of 330 patients at a tertiary care center. Eur J Endocrinol 2013;169:891–9.

65. Icard P, Goudet P, Charpenay C, et al. Adrenocortical carcinomas: surgical trends and results of a 253-patient series from the French Association of Endocrine Surgeons study group. World J Surg 2001;25:891–7.

66. Reznek RH, Narayanan P. Primary adrenal malignancy. Husband & Reznek's imaging in oncology. 3rd edition. London: Informa Healthcare; 2010. p. 280–98.

67. Bharwani N, Rockall AG, Sahdev A, et al. Adrenocortical carcinoma: the range of appearances on CT and MRI. AJR Am J Roentgenol 2011;196: 706–14.

68. Slattery JM, Blake MA, Kalra MK, et al. Adrenocortical carcinoma: contrast washout characteristics on CT. AJR Am J Roentgenol 2006;187:21–4.

69. Outwater EK, Blasbalg R, Siegelman ES, et al. Detection of lipid in abdominal tissues with opposed-phase gradient-echo images at 1.5 T: techniques and diagnostic importance. Radiographics 1998;18:1465–80.

70. Egbert N, Elsayes KM, Azar S, et al. Computed tomography of adrenocortical carcinoma containing macroscopic fat. Cancer Imaging 2010;10: 198–200.

71. Ferrozzi F, Bova D. CT and MR demonstration of fat within an adrenal cortical carcinoma. Abdom Imaging 1995;20:272–4.

72. Heye S, Woestenborghs H, Van Kerkhove F, et al. Adrenocortical carcinoma with fat inclusion: case report. Abdom Imaging 2005;30:641–3.

73. Berland LL, Silverman SG, Gore RM, et al. Managing incidental findings on abdominal CT: white paper of the ACR Incidental Findings Committee. J Am Coll Radiol 2010;7:754–73.

74. Fassnacht M, Arlt W, Bancos I, et al. Management of adrenal incidentalomas: European Society of Endocrinology Clinical Practice Guideline in collaboration with the European Network for the Study of Adrenal Tumors. Eur J Endocrinol 2016; 175:31–4.

75. Ballian N, Adler JT, Sippel RS, et al. Revisiting adrenal mass size as an indication for adrenalectomy. J Surg Res 2009;156:16–20.

76. Courcoutsakis N, Prassopoulos P, Stratakis CA. CT findings of primary pigmented nodular adrenocortical disease: rare cause of ACTH-independent Cushing syndrome. AJR Am J Roentgenol 2010; 94:541.

77. Stratakis CA. Adrenocortical tumors, primary pigmented adrenocortical disease (PPNAD)/Carney complex, and other bilateral hyperplasias: the NIH studies. Horm Metab Res 2007;39:467–73.

78. Doppman JL, Chrousos GP, Papanicolaou DA, et al. Adrenocorticotropin-independent macronodular adrenal hyperplasia: an uncommon cause of primary adrenal hypercortisolism. Radiology 2000;216:797–802.

79. Gimm O. Pheochromocytoma-associated syndromes: genes, proteins and functions of RET, VHL and SDHx. Fam Cancer 2005;4:17–23.

80. Goldifien A. Adrenal medulla. In: Baxter TD, Greenspan FS, editors. Basic endocrinology. 4th edition. Norwalk (CT): Appleton & Lang; 1994. p. 370.

81. Hanafy A, Mujtaba B, Roman-Colon AM, et al. Imaging features of adrenal gland masses in the pediatric population. Abdom Radiol (NY) 2020;45(4):964–81.

82. McDermott S, McCarthy CJ, Blake MA. Images of pheochromocytoma in adrenal glands. Gland Surg 2015;4:350–8.

83. Guller U, Turek J, Eubanks S, et al. Detecting pheochromocytoma: defining the most sensitive test. Ann Surg 2006;243:102–7.

84. Bravo EL, Gifford RW. Current concepts: pheochromocytoma-diagnosis localization and management. N Engl J Med 1984;311:1298–303.

85. Witteles RM, Kaplan EL, Roizen MF. Sensitivity of diagnostic and localization tests for pheochromocytoma in clinical practice. Arch Intern Med 2000;160:2521–4.

86. Bholah R, Bunchman TE. Review of pediatric pheochromocytoma and paraganglioma. Front Pediatr 2017;5:155.

87. Adler JT, Meyer-Rochow GY, Chen H, et al. Pheochromocytoma: current approaches and future directions. Oncologist 2008;13:779–93.

88. Park BK, Kim CK, Kwon GY, et al. Re-evaluation of pheochromocytomas on delayed contrast enhanced CT: washout enhancement and other imaging features. Eur Radiol 2007;17:2804–9.

89. Varghese JC, Hahn PF, Papanicolaou N, et al. MR differentiation of pheochromocytoma from other adrenal lesions based on qualitative analysis of T2 relaxation times. Clin Radiol 1997;52:3–606.

90. Taffel M, Haji-Momenian S, Nikolaidis P, et al. Adrenal imaging: a comprehensive review. Radiol Clin North Am 2012;50:219–43.

91. Scopsi L, Callini P, Muscolino G. A new observation of the Carney's triad, with long follow-up period and additional tumors. Cancer Detect Prev 1999;23:435–43.

92. Opocher G, Schiari F, Conton P, et al. Clinical and genetic aspects of phaeochromocytoma. Horm Res 2003;59:56–61.

93. Ross JH. Pheochromocytoma: special considerations in children. Urol Clin North Am 2000;27:393–402.

94. Udhreja PR, Banerji A, Desai DP, et al. Androgen-secreting steroid cell tumor of the ovary. Indian J Pathol Microbiol 2014;57:94–7.

95. Dolinko AV, Ginsburg ES. Hyperandrogenism in menopause: a case report and literature review. Fertil Res Pract 2015;1:7.

96. Goodarzi MO, Carmina E, Ricardo A. DHEA, DHEAS and PCOS. J Steroid Biochem Mol Biol 2015;145:213–25.

97. Derksen J, Nagesser SK, Meinders AE, et al. Identification of virilizing adrenal tumors in hirsute women. N Engl J Med 1994;331:968–73.

98. Iack MR, Chrousos GP. Neoplasms of the adrenal cortex. Cancer medicine. New York: Lea & Febiger; 1996. p. 1563.

99. d'Alva CB, Abiven-Lepage G, Viallon V, et al. Sex steroids in androgen-secreting adrenocortical tumors: clinical and hormonal features in comparison with nontumoral causes of androgen excess. Eur J Endocrinol 2008;159:641–7.

100. Pascale MM, Pugeat M, Roberts M, et al. Androgen suppressive effect of GnRH agonist in ovarian hyperthecosis and virilizing tumours. Clin Endocrinol (Oxf) 1994;41:571–6.

101. Rivera-Arkoncel ML, Pacquing-Songco D, Lantion-Ang FL. Virilising ovarian tumour in a woman with an adrenal nodule. BMJ Case Rep 2010;2010. bcr0720103139.

102. Auchus RJ, Arlt W. Approach to the patient: the adult with congenital adrenal hyperplasia. J Clin Endocrinol Metab 2013;98:2645–55.

103. Gilchrist VJ, Hecht BR. A practical approach to hirsutism. Am Fam Physician 1995;52:1837–46.

104. Chentli F, Bekkaye I, Azzoug S. Feminizing adrenocortical tumors: literature review. Indian J Endocrinol Metab 2015;19:332–9.

Neuroimaging of the Pituitary Gland
Practical Anatomy and Pathology

Philip R. Chapman, MD*, Aparna Singhal, MD,
Siddhartha Gaddamanugu, MD, Veeranjaneyulu Prattipati, MD

KEYWORDS

- Pituitary adenoma • Macroadenoma • MR imaging • Craniopharyngioma • Meningioma
- Hypophysitis • Apoplexy

KEY POINTS

- MR imaging is the study of choice for evaluating primary tumors and other lesions of the pituitary gland and the central skull base region.
- CT is complimentary in evaluating pituitary and other sellar masses given its ability to detect calcification and assess osseous involvement of skull base.
- The adenoma is the most common lesion of the pituitary gland and can be symptomatic because of its endocrine effects or localized mass effect.
- Macroadenomas can have a variety of imaging appearances based on size, cystic/necrotic change, extent of local invasion, and post-treatment effects.
- There is a broad spectrum of disorders that should be considered in the radiologic evaluation of pituitary, sellar, and suprasellar masses.

INTRODUCTION

The pituitary gland is a small, complex endocrine organ located within the sella of the central skull base. It is anatomically and functionally separated into the anterior lobe (adenohypophysis) and the posterior lobe (neurohypophysis). The anterior lobe produces multiple hormones, including, prolactin, growth hormone (GH), adrenocorticotropic hormone (ACTH), thyroid-stimulating hormone (TSH), follicle-stimulating hormone, and luteinizing hormone. The posterior lobe is an anatomic extension of the hypothalamus and is the site for the secretion of oxytocin and vasopressin. Various pathologic conditions affect the pituitary gland and can produce endocrinologic and neurologic abnormalities. Common lesions include congenital lesions, developmental abnormalities, inflammatory conditions, and a variety of benign and malignant neoplasms. Dedicated MR imaging of the

pituitary is the radiologic modality of choice for evaluating the pituitary gland, central skull base, and parasellar regions. Computed tomography (CT) is complementary and allows for identification of calcification and can evaluate osseous integrity of the central skull base. This review emphasizes basic anatomy, current imaging techniques, and highlights the spectrum of pathologic conditions that affect the pituitary gland and sellar region.

ANATOMY

The pituitary gland is a small endocrine gland located in the sella turcica, a saddle-shaped depression in the central sphenoid bone. It is of critical importance to the body's metabolism because it produces, stores, secretes, and regulates several important hormones. The pituitary gland has an anterior lobe (adenohypophysis) and posterior lobe (neurohypophysis). The

Department of Radiology, School of Medicine, University of Alabama Birmingham, 619 19th Street South, JT N419, Birmingham, AL 35249-6830, USA
* Corresponding author. 2912 Tantallon Drive, Hampton Cove, AL 35763.
E-mail address: pchapman@uabmc.edu

Radiol Clin N Am 58 (2020) 1115–1133
https://doi.org/10.1016/j.rcl.2020.07.009
0033-8389/20/© 2020 Elsevier Inc. All rights reserved.

adenohypophysis constitutes 75% of total pituitary volume and is mainly comprised of the pars distalis. Composed of cords of epithelial cells flanked by vascular sinusoids, the adenohypophysis is where most pituitary hormones are synthesized and stored (GH, prolactin, TSH, ACTH, follicle-stimulating hormone, and luteinizing hormone). The pars intermedia is an endocrinologically inactive narrow zone between the adenohypophysis and neurohypophysis and can contain some microscopic remnants of Rathke cleft (Fig. 1).

Derived from the neural ectoderm, the neurohypophysis extends from the hypothalamus to the sella. Composed of axons arising from hypothalamic neurons of the supraoptic and paraventricular nuclei, it forms the hypothalamohypophyseal tract. Its distal axonal terminals include neurosecretory granules that contain oxytocin or vasopressin. The presence of vasopressin is presumed to be responsible for the hyperintense signal identified on T1-weighted MR images, the so-called pituitary bright spot, a normal finding of the posterior lobe.

The infundibulum (pituitary stalk) is a linear structure extending from the hypothalamus to the pituitary gland. It is comprised of the anterior pars tuberalis and posterior pars infundibularis. The pars tuberalis is considered to be part of the adenohypophysis. It partially surrounds the pars infundibularis, which contains unmyelinated axons of the hypothalamic neurons that extend to the posterior lobe. The normal stalk has a thickness of approximately 2 mm and should be considered abnormal if it measures greater than or equal to 4 mm.

The size of pituitary gland is variable and depends on age and physiologic status. The pituitary size is roughly estimated by its height, and its height is routinely measured from coronal or sagittal MR images. Pituitary dimensions in selected age and gender groups are depicted in Table 1. Note the gradual decrease in size of the pituitary gland in elderly patients.[1]

A thin horizontally oriented dural sheet that stretches across the top of the sella, the diaphragma sellae, separates the sella from suprasellar space. The diaphragma sellae is mildly convex inferiorly and contains a variable-sized central opening or perforation that allows the passage of the pituitary stalk. The diaphragma sellae is attached to the clinoid processes and contiguous with the dural covering of the cavernous sinus roofs bilaterally.

Blood supply to the anterior pituitary is unique and complex. The adenohypophysis lacks a direct blood supply and most of the blood reaches the parenchyma through the hypothalamic hypophyseal portal system. Small branches from superior hypophyseal artery enter the median eminence of the hypothalamus and form a primary capillary plexus. The primary plexus is connected to portal veins that extend through the infundibulum to the adenohypophysis. This portal venous system supplies most of the blood to the adenophyphysis and allows for precise hormonal regulation between the hypothalamus and the pars distalis (Fig. 2). The posterior pituitary has direct blood supply

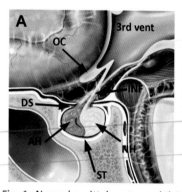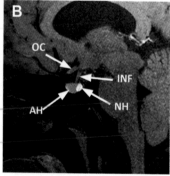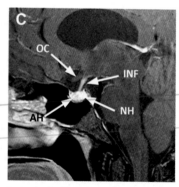

Fig. 1. Normal sagittal anatomy. (A) Sagittal graphic demonstrates key structures including the sella turcica (ST), the anterior pituitary or adenohypophysis (AH), posterior pituitary or neurohypophysis (NH), the pituitary stalk or infundibulum (INF), diaphragma sella (DS), and optic chiasm (OC). (B) Sagittal fat-saturated T1-weighted MR imaging without gadolinium shows hyperintense signal in neurohypophysis, a normal finding referred to as the pituitary bright spot. Note the relationship of the sella turcica to the sphenoid sinus and clivus. (C) Sagittal postgadolinium T1-weighted image shows homogeneous enhancement of the infundibulum and anterior pituitary. ([A] From Osborn AG, Salzman KL, Jhaveri MD, Barkovich AJ. Diagnostic Imaging : Brain. 2015; with permission.)

Table 1
Pituitary gland: age/physiologic status, sex, and size

Age Group/Physiologic Status	Sex	Size (mm)
Prepubertal children	Either	2–6
Prepubertal children	Boys	7–8
	Girls	8–10 (round shape)
Third trimester pregnancy	Women	10
First week postpartum	Women	12
Adult, aged ≥50 y	Men	8
	Women	8

from the inferior hypophyseal artery, which arises from internal carotid artery (ICA). The intrinsic pituitary capillaries are unique in that they are fenestrated and are outside of the blood-brain barrier. Therefore, the pituitary gland homogeneously enhances after administration of intravenous contrast agents.

TECHNIQUE

Dedicated MR imaging of the pituitary gland and sella is the modality of choice for evaluating intrinsic lesions of the pituitary gland, such as adenomas and other lesions localized to the sella. Excellent spatial resolution and multiplanar technique allows for complete evaluation of the lesion

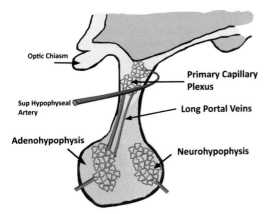

Fig. 2. Schematic diagram depicts the blood supply to the adenohypophysis. Blood enters the hypothalamus at the median eminence by way of branches from superior hypophyseal artery. Within the inferior hypothalamus, there is a primary capillary venous plexus. This is connected to the venous plexus of the pars distalis by way of interconnecting long portal veins that extend through the hypothalamus. The neurohypophysis receives blood primarily through the inferior hypophyseal vessels, and hormones are secreted in this region via terminal axons that originate from the hypothalamus.

and is necessary for treatment or surgical planning. Sagittal and coronal planes are preferred, typically using 2- to 3-mm slice thickness. Routine imaging with a 1.5-T magnet is generally satisfactory. However, the 3-T MR imaging magnet can offer an advantage of increased sensitivity for microadenomas and is recommended if there is strong clinical suspicion of an adenoma and an initial negative scan using 1.5 T.[2,3]

A dedicated pituitary protocol includes precontrast sagittal and coronal T1-weighted images, followed by postgadolinium sequences in same plane. A T2-weighted coronal sequence with fat saturation also is beneficial. The normal adenohyphysis is isointense to brain on routine T1-weighted and T2-weighted images. The posterior pituitary generally contains the pituitary bright spot, if normal. The infundibulum and gland enhance homogeneously after contrast administration. Using such techniques, most adenomas and other sellar pathologies are diagnosed with a high degree of sensitivity. Depending on the circumstances and institutional preferences, optimal evaluation of the whole brain includes performance of axial fluid-attenuated inversion recovery, diffusion-weighted, and whole-brain postgadolinium sequences.

Dynamic MR imaging is a useful technique that is particularly beneficial for identifying microadenomas. Dynamic sequences take advantage of the fact that adenoma tissue enhances more slowly than normal pituitary tissue. If sequential images are obtained in rapid succession during the first-pass arterial phase, a microadenoma is identified as a small focus of nonenhancing tissue against a background of normally enhancing pituitary gland (**Fig. 3**).

Optimization of dynamic sequence with 3-mm thin coronal slices, small field of view (12 × 12 cm), fine matrix size of 256 × 192, and use of spoiled gradient echo techniques instead of spin echo T1 is helpful.[4,5] Dynamic sequences should be acquired every 30 seconds for 3 minutes

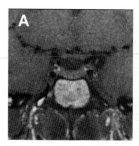 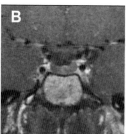 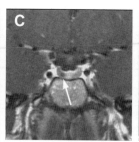 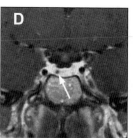

Fig. 3. Sequential same-slice T1-weighted coronal images through anterior pituitary gland during contrast injection of gadolinium. Precontrast and earliest arterial phase contrast images show no obvious abnormality (*A, B*). During contrast infusion, a small hypodense region in right side of the gland (*arrows, C, D*) shows hypoenhancement relative to normal pituitary, consistent with microadenoma.

with five slices/acquisition.[6] The pituitary shows rapid and progressive enhancement usually beginning superiorly and extending inferiorly through the entire gland. Delayed postcontrast images are then obtained in sagittal and coronal planes. On delayed sequences, small adenomas may be isointense to pituitary gland and difficult to see. As new sequences have been developed, some studies have questioned the routine role of dynamic imaging, arguing that other sequences, such as enhanced three-dimensional spoiled gradient echo, may be as sensitive or better.[7]

Diffusion-weighted imaging is not routinely performed for pituitary lesions, but studies are under way to evaluate its utility for sellar and suprasellar lesions. It is challenging because of inhomogeneity at the skull base from air-bone interface from routine echoplanar diffusion imaging. Non–echoplanar diffusion imaging diffusion techniques, such as propeller diffusion-weighted imaging (General Electric, Boston, MA) or BLADE (Siemens, Munich, Germany), are used. Diffusion may help differentiate Rathke cleft cysts from other suprasellar/intrasellar lesions.[8] Some authors suggest that pituitary apoplexy may be detected early using diffusion-weighted MR imaging.[9] Pituitary adenomas with lower apparent diffusion coefficient values correlate with higher collagen content and may have surgical implications.[10] However, perfusion and spectroscopy have limited roles in sellar imaging and are not routinely performed.[11]

High-resolution CT scanning is complementary and may be used primarily if MR imaging is contraindicated. CT allows for identification of any intrinsic calcification/ossification of the lesion, can help in narrowing the differential, and is excellent for evaluating the osseous integrity of the central skull base. CT can be performed with 1-mm axial thin slices with contrast for best spatial resolution. Coronal and sagittal reformats should be obtained.[1,2,4,5,10–14] CT angiography is also complementary, especially in cases where a parasellar vascular lesion, such as aneurysm, is considered.

ADENOMA

The benign adenoma represents the most common pituitary neoplasm and arises from the adenohypophysis. These are benign epithelial lesions and account for about 10% to 15% of all intracranial tumors. Pituitary adenomas occur across a wide age spectrum, from childhood to the elderly. It has been estimated from postmortem and other clinical studies that pituitary adenomas occur in approximately 20% of the normal population, but many are incidental and asymptomatic. Adenomas are most often classified according to hormonal production and size, which predominantly determines the clinical presentation. They can also be classified based on histology and biologic behavior.[14]

Adenomas that are hormone-producing are said to be endocrinologically active or functional, whereas nonfunctional tumors produce no measurable hormone. Prolactinomas are the most common hormone-secreting tumors and account for about 30% of all pituitary adenomas. Nonfunctioning adenomas are the second most common tumors, comprising 25% to 30% of pituitary adenomas.[15]

Microadenoma

Adenomas are unencapsulated tumors, and as they begin to grow they initially infiltrate the parenchyma of pituitary gland itself. Lesions measuring less than 1 cm in size are called microadenomas. These lesions are generally confined to the pituitary gland/sella. In this case, symptoms are not related to the size of the lesions but rather the possible excess production of hormone.

On T1- and T2-weighted images, microadenomas may be isointense to normal pituitary gland. Microadenomas enhance variably with contrast but generally enhance at a slower rate than normal pituitary tissue. Dynamic enhanced images are performed to take advantage of this early differential enhancement and are generally considered to be the most sensitive sequence for microadenoma detection. Using high-resolution techniques, MR imaging can detect adenomas as small as 2 mm. Some institutions perform dynamic imaging routinely as part of pituitary protocol when adenoma is suspected. Others reserve dynamic sequences for cases where adenomas are suspected but conventional imaging is negative, especially in cases of suspected ACTH-secreting tumors, which are typically small, averaging 5 mm in diameter.[6]

Macroadenoma

Macroadenomas are adenomas measuring greater than or equal to 1.0 cm. On unenhanced CT, macroadenomas generally demonstrate a soft tissue mass in the sella that is isodense with gray matter and not clearly discrete from the gland itself. Lesions may show variable attenuation because of cyst formation or necrosis. Occasionally, hemorrhage results in hyperdensity of the lesion. Generally, adenomas do not calcify; however, calcification is seen in 1% to 2%. Postcontrast CT shows moderate, inhomogeneous enhancement.

MR imaging appearance varies according to sequence. T1-weighted images show a lesion isointense to gray matter. T1 hyperintensity seen occasionally in the setting of subacute hemorrhage and intratumoral hemorrhage occurs in up to 10% to 15% of adenomas. The pituitary bright spot is displaced superiorly above the diaphragma sellae in 80% of cases, but may also be absent with larger adenomas. Following contrast, most adenomas demonstrate heterogeneous enhancement. Ultimately, tumors may grow beyond the pituitary capsule and can extend beyond the confines of the sella. In general, macroadenomas can extend superiorly into the suprasellar cistern; laterally into the cavernous sinus; or inferiorly into the sellar floor, clivus, or sphenoid sinus.[16]

Suprasellar Extension

Classically, macroadenomas follow a path of least resistance: tumor growth occurs through the central opening in the diaphragma sellae into the suprasellar cistern. The circumlateral leaflets of the diaphragma sellae are initially displaced upward and can create a horizontal restriction of tumor growth, leading to the typical bilobed appearance in the coronal plane, with the lower sellar component of tumor separated partially from its upper suprasellar component. The classic appearance has been likened to a snowman (**Fig. 4**). As tumor extends superiorly, microscopic invasion of the diaphragma sellae itself often occurs.[17]

As tumor enlarges and extends vertically, it can contact, efface, displace, or compress the optic chiasm. Compression of the optic chiasm can produce a variety of visual deficits, including chiasmal syndrome.[18] Pituitary adenomas are the most common lesions that produce chiasmal syndrome, followed by other lesions that cause extrinsic optic chiasm compression, such as meningiomas or craniopharyngiomas. Although bitemporal hemianopsia, defect of impaired peripheral vision in the temporal (outer) halves of the visual field of each eye, is often suggested as a classic finding associated with pituitary adenoma, actually it is rare. Rather, patients more often present with incomplete bitemporal visual defects or mixed defects.[19]

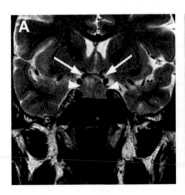 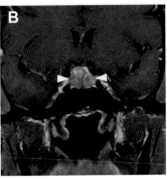

Fig. 4. Nonsecreting pituitary adenoma. This lesion was discovered incidentally in 55-year-old man with no endocrine abnormalities or visual symptoms. (*A*) Coronal T2-weighted image shows a sellar mass (*arrowheads*) extending into the suprasellar region. The lesion minimally splays the proximal cisternal optic nerves (*arrows*). (*B*) Coronal postgadolinium T1-weighted image demonstrates heterogeneous enhancement of the macroadenoma (*arrowheads*). A subtle waist is formed at the level of the diaphragma sellae.

There is no consensus on how best to measure the extent of suprasellar extension or the degree of optic chiasm displacement or compression. However, in general, the larger the tumor and greater the chiasm compression, the more likely the patient is to have more significant visual deficits.

Although no consensus exists, several radiologic reports in the past have used the term "giant macroadenoma" for a mass that exceeds 40 mm in greatest dimension. Symon and colleagues[20] defined giant adenomas as those with an extension of more than 40 mm from the midline of planum sphenoidale in any direction or suprasellar extension to within 6 mm of the foramen of Monro. Other authors have reserved this term for tumors where the superior margin exceeded 20 mm above the planum sphenoidale. Giant macroadenomas are generally regarded as more aggressive, more difficult to resect, and more likely to recur (Fig. 5).[21]

Cavernous Sinus Invasion

Approximately 5% to 10% of all pituitary adenomas extend laterally beyond the margins of the adenohypophysis and sella, invading the adjacent cavernous sinus. Involvement of the cavernous sinus increases surgical procedure complexity, results in higher rates of residual/recurrent tumor,

and is associated with persistent endocrine dysfunction. Definitions of cavernous sinus invasion have been variably based on radiologic, surgical, endoscopic, and microscopic criteria.

The microscopic interface between the pituitary and the cavernous sinus has been evaluated through histologic and microdissection techniques. Songtao and colleagues[22] considered the outer pituitary wall as a two-layered membrane: an inner lamina propria adherent to the pituitary tissue; and a looser, outer pituitary capsule. The outer layer also serves as part of the medial wall of the cavernous sinus. In their description, the medial wall of the cavernous sinus consisted of a fibrous layer in addition to the pituitary capsule. As tumor extends laterally from the sella, it crosses the lamina propria, the pituitary capsule, the fibrous layer of the cavernous sinus, and finally, the endothelial lining of the venous compartment. The authors found that superior margin is thinner, which might explain why adenomas more often extend into the superior compartment of the cavernous sinus.[22]

MR imaging is not reliable at distinguishing these microscopic layers separating the laterally convex pituitary gland from the medial cavernous sinus. MR imaging evaluation of invasion relies on macroscopic findings, such as the relationship of tumor to the cavernous ICA and extent of

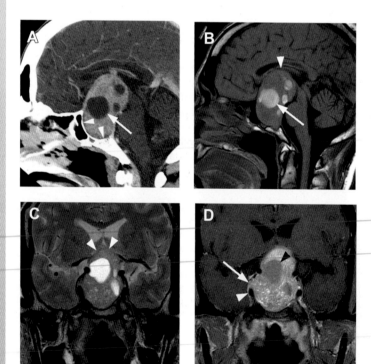

Fig. 5. Giant macroadenoma. A 43-year-old man presents with 2-week history of severe visual loss of left eye. (A) Sagittal reformatted contrast-enhanced CT scan shows a 6.0-cm mass with several cysts (arrowhead) expanding but not destroying the sella (arrowheads) and compressing the anterior third ventricle. (B) Sagittal unenhanced T1-weighted image shows giant macroadenoma with cystic areas (arrow) that contain proteinaceous contents and demonstrate T1 shortening. The lesion compresses the anterior third ventricle superiorly (arrowhead). (C) Coronal T2-weighted image shows a classic snowman appearance of the mass. The optic chiasm is severely compressed and not identified as distinct structure (arrowheads). (D) On coronal contrast-enhanced T1-weighted image, the solid portions of the lesion show moderate enhancement, whereas the cystic areas (black arrowhead) maintain some T1 hyperintensity. The lesion expands the sella and extends into the right cavernous sinus (arrow) passing above the cavernous ICA (white arrowhead).

cavernous sinus involvement. In 1993, Knosp and colleagues[23] introduced an MR imaging–based classification system to predict cavernous sinus invasion. This system was based on lateral tumor extent in relationship to a series of tangential lines drawn between the intracavernous and supracavernous ICAs seen on coronal MR images. This classification system defined five grades of invasion, ranging from 0 to 4 (Fig. 6). The data showed that identification of tumor past the intercarotid line (grade 2 and higher) on coronal MR imaging was highly predictive of cavernous sinus invasion identified at surgery. Conversely, patients with grade 0 or grade 1 were unlikely to have definitive invasion. Their results also showed that the degree of cavernous invasion was directly related to tumor size.

The Knosp-Steiner classification of potential cavernous sinus invasion by macroadenoma (see Fig. 6) involves using coronal MR imaging to determine extent of lateral tumor growth in relationship to tangential lines drawn between the cavernous ICA and supraclinoid ICA.

Others have evaluated the Knosp-Steiner macroadenoma classification and other MR imaging findings that might predict the presence of cavernous sinus invasion. Cottier and colleagues[24] found the most specific sign of cavernous sinus invasion to be partial tumor encasement of the intracavernous ICA, defined as involvement of 67% of its circumference (positive predictive value of 100%). Macroadenomas with Knosp-Steiner grade of 3 had a positive predictive value of 85%. Invasion is highly probable (positive predictive value of 95%) if the carotid sulcus venous compartment (medial venous compartment inferior to the cavernous ICA on coronal MR imaging) is obliterated. Cavernous sinus invasion could be ruled out with a negative predictive value of 100% if the percentage of encasement of the perimeter of intracavernous ICA was lower than 25% or with Knosp-Steiner grade of 0 or 1 (Fig. 7).

Skull Base Invasion

Adenomas that originate in or involve the inferior aspect of the gland and sella can involve the underlying dura and bone of the central skull base. Selman and colleagues[25] performed transphenoidal surgery for pituitary adenoma in 65 patients and reported that 51 (85%) demonstrated microscopic dural invasion of the sellar floor. These authors demonstrated a direct correlation between overall tumor size and the presence of dural invasion. Dural invasion was present in 95% of cases of macroadenoma (>10 mm). The authors also noted that microscopic dural invasion occurred even in some microadenomas. Meij and colleagues,[26] in a larger study of 354 patients, found dural invasion in 45% of all cases and confirmed a correlation between tumor size and dural invasion.

As the macroadenoma infiltrates the gland, generalized expansion of the sella can occur, often with preservation of smooth cortical margins of the bony sella. With progressive enlargement, cortical thinning of the underlying bone can occur and is most often identified along the roof of the sphenoid sinus. Focal dehiscence of the sphenoid roof can occur, and the tumor can protrude directly into the sphenoid sinus (Fig. 8). The tumor can also infiltrate into the

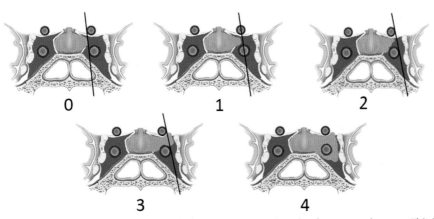

Fig. 6. The Knosp-Steiner classification of potential cavernous sinus invasion by macroadenoma. This involves using coronal MR imaging to determine extent of lateral tumor growth in relationship to tangential lines drawn between the cavernous ICA and supraclinoid ICA. The classification ranges from 0 to 4 and expresses likelihood of cavernous sinus invasion that would be encountered at surgery. Stage 0 is unlikely to correlate with tumor invasion. Stage 4 demonstrates encasement of the cavernous ICA, a definitive finding for tumor invasion.

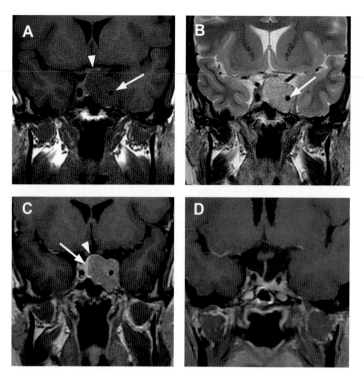

Fig. 7. ACTH-secreting macroadenoma. A 33-year-old woman presented with clinical findings and biochemical evidence of Cushing disease. (*A*) Unenhanced coronal T1-weighted MR imaging shows large left-sided sellar mass with suprasellar extension and left cavernous sinus invasion. There is mild compression of the optic chiasm (*arrowhead*) and encasement of the cavernous ICA (*arrow*). (*B*) Coronal T2-weighted image shows heterogeneously hyperintense mass with left cavernous ICA encasement (*arrow*). (*C*) Coronal postcontrast T1-weighted MR image shows solid heterogeneously enhancing sellar mass that measures 3.0 × 2.7 × 2.5 cm. The mass displaces the normal pituitary (*arrow*) and infundibulum (*arrowhead*) to the right. (*D*) Postoperative coronal image shows satisfactory resection of the large lesion despite the cavernous sinus invasion.

trabecular bone and marrow space of the clivus. In rare instances, the inferior growth pattern can dominate (**Fig. 9**). The bony change of the clivus can include focal irregularity, permeative change, mixed sclerotic-permeative change, or frank lysis. Large tumors can expand and destroy the clivus, mimicking chordoma, myeloma, or metastatic disease. Most reports of infrasellar invasion are small case series or case reports. Luo and colleagues[27] reported 28% incidence of infrasellar extension with involvement of the floor of the sella and sphenoid sinus.

Chen and colleagues[28] recently evaluated clival invasion of pituitary macroadenomas using CT in 390 patients. Thirty-two patients (8.21%) had clival

invasion detected by CT and confirmed at surgery. In this study, the authors found female sex to be the strongest risk factor for clival invasion. This finding contradicted previous studies that suggested a greater propensity of clival invasion in men. As with cavernous sinus invasion, larger tumor volume was found to be a strong risk factor for clival invasion. In this report, clival invasion was more frequent in null-cell adenomas even after correction for larger average tumor volume. Some macroadenomas have a preferential invasion for the central skull base. The tumor is mistaken for a primary sphenoid bone lesion encroaching on the floor of the sella. In these cases, identification of tumor contiguity with the

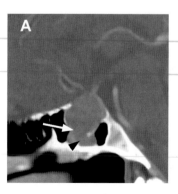
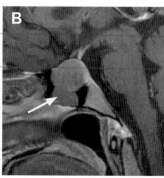

Fig. 8. Macroadenoma invasive to sphenoid sinus. (*A*) Sagittal postcontrast CT reformation with bone windows shows an expansile mass of the sella with dehiscence of the sellar floor (*arrow*) and soft tissue mass in the ventral sphenoid sinus (*arrowhead*). (*B*) Sagittal postcontrast T1-weighted MR imaging shows that there is significant inferior vector of tumor growth (*arrow*). The pituitary gland is not identified as a separate structure from the main mass.

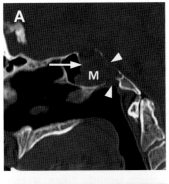
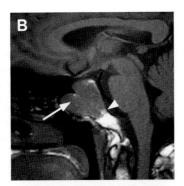
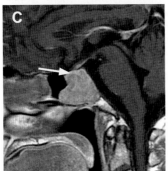
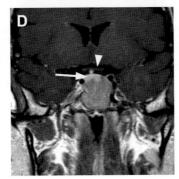

Fig. 9. Nonsecreting macroadenoma invasive to the clivus. (A) Sagittal reformation CT scan with bone windows reveals a large invasive soft tissue mass (M) that involves the sella, sphenoid sinus, and clivus. There is dehiscence of the sellar floor (arrow) and cortical erosions of the clivus (arrowheads). (B) Sagittal unenhanced T1-weighted image shows the ventral extension to the sphenoid sinus (arrow), and there is demarcation of the inferior margin (arrowhead) from normal residual fatty marrow of the clivus. (C) Sagittal postcontrast T1-weighted image shows homogeneous enhancement of the tumor that blends with residual normal pituitary superiorly (arrow). (D) Although there is some suprasellar extension, the major vector is inferiorly, and the chiasm (arrowhead) is not compressed. Some residual normal pituitary tissue is seen along upper edge of pituitary (arrow).

inferior pituitary gland is the best clue to its pituitary origin.

Pituitary Tumor Apoplexy

Pituitary tumor apoplexy is a clinical syndrome that occurs when an existing pituitary adenoma undergoes an acute hemorrhage or infarction, or both.[29] Most cases occur in males during the fifth or sixth decade of life, and most often occur in previously undiagnosed nonfunctioning pituitary adenomas or prolactinomas.[30] Patients typically present with an abrupt onset of severe headache, variable visual disturbance (including vision loss, field defects, and ophthalmoplegia), and acute hypopituitarism. Radiologic studies are performed as an adjunct to clinical findings to exclude other etiologies and to confirm the presence of a hemorrhagic pituitary lesion. Unenhanced CT is often the first study performed in an acute setting and may demonstrate a variably hyperdense mass of the sella and suprasellar region. With sensitivity greater than 90%, MR imaging is the preferred study of choice and can identify the adenoma, the intrinsic hemorrhage, and necrosis, and evaluate effects on adjacent structures.[31,32]

MR imaging generally demonstrates a sellar mass with variable and complex signals on T1- and T2-weighted images. Imaging findings depend on several factors, including size of the underlying tumor, extent of hemorrhage or necrosis, and timing of the examination. Like hemorrhage elsewhere in the brain, MR imaging appearance varies depending on the sequence and stage of the hemorrhage (hemoglobin degradation). Typically, a sellar and suprasellar mass shows significant regions of T1 hyperintensity, T2 hypointensity, and nonenhancing necrotic tissue centrally (**Fig. 10**). Some peripheral nodular enhancing tissue is identified to confirm presence of underlying adenoma.[33]

PITUITARY CARCINOMA

Pituitary adenomas are benign tumors but can demonstrate aggressive or invasive features. Tumors are considered aggressive if the growth rate is greater than usual or if the tumor progresses despite satisfactory treatment.[34] Pituitary carcinomas are rare, accounting for 0.1% of pituitary tumors.[27] Unlike many other situations, the term carcinoma in this case is applied when adenomas demonstrate aggressive biologic behavior and evidence of metastatic disease. The distinction is not based on histologic criteria. Rather, a tumor of pituitary origin is classified as a carcinoma when there is evidence of noncontiguous leptomeningeal spread to the intracranial compartment or

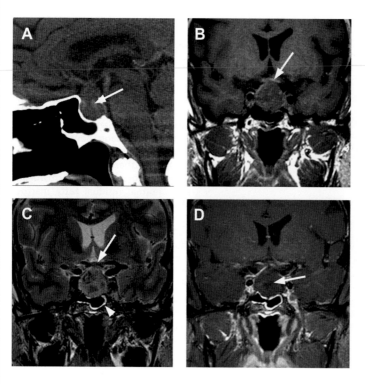

Fig. 10. Pituitary tumor apoplexy in nonfunctioning adenoma. A 65-year-old woman presents with acute onset of headache, nausea, and vomiting, and pituitary insufficiency was detected by laboratory evaluation. (A) Sagittal unenhanced CT scan demonstrates an expansile sellar and suprasellar mass (arrow). (B) Coronal T1-weighted MR image shows that the mass contacts the optic chiasm (arrow). (C) Coronal T2-weighted image shows that the mass contacts the optic chiasm (arrow). There is mild mucosal edema in sphenoid sinus (arrowhead). There are areas of intrinsic T2 hypointensity within the mass, consistent with hemorrhage. (D) Coronal postcontrast image shows large zone of centrally necrotic tissue (arrow), consistent with hemorrhage and/or infarction.

spine, or there is evidence of distant metastases via hematogenous or lymphatic spread (Fig. 11).[35,36] Such lesions are found during initial work-up of the primary lesion or are observed as progression or recurrence following treatment of the original lesion.[37]

METASTATIC LESIONS TO THE PITUITARY

Metastasis to the pituitary gland is a rare finding in a typical neuroradiologic practice. The incidence of metastatic lesions to the pituitary gland may be as low as 1% in some surgical series.[37] Autopsy series in the setting of widely metastatic disease have suggested higher incidence, ranging from 3% to 27%.[38] The rich vascularity of the pituitary gland presumably facilitates hematogenous transport, implantation, and growth of micrometastases. Breast and lung cancers are the most common primary malignancies associated with pituitary metastases, accounting for 37% and 25%, respectively.[39] Although most metastases to pituitary gland are asymptomatic, they can present with clinical symptoms, most commonly panhypopituitarism or diabetes insipidus.[38] Occasionally, metastasis to the pituitary gland may occur as the initial manifestation of metastatic disease. In one report, pituitary metastasis was the presenting lesion in more than half the patients, with a variety of symptoms, including diabetes insipidus, visual field defects, cranial nerve abnormalities, or headache.[40]

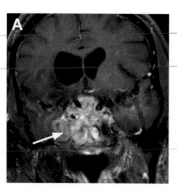
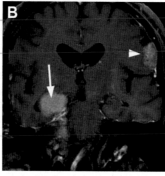

Fig. 11. Pituitary carcinoma. A 69-year-old patient with persistent pituitary adenoma despite surgical and radiation treatments. (A) Coronal postcontrast T1-weighted MR image shows persistent tumor invading the skull base and cavernous sinuses (arrow). (B) Coronal postcontrast T1-weighted image shows invasion of mass into right temporal lobe (arrow) and a new left frontal convexity mass (arrowhead), consistent with leptomeningeal spread.

The MR imaging and CT features of metastatic disease to the pituitary gland are largely nonspecific. Often, metastatic disease may appear similar to macroadenomas, creating a diagnostic dilemma.[41] Clues that suggest metastasis to pituitary include a new pituitary mass that develops during metastatic surveillance, presence of additional metastatic foci, or if a suspected incidental adenoma in a patients with cancer undergoes rapid growth and becomes symptomatic. CT may demonstrate a sellar mass that is isodense or hyperdense, and associated with heterogeneous enhancement. The clinoid processes or bony sellar floor may be eroded.[39] Also, the tumor can extend into the suprasellar space or laterally into the cavernous sinus. MR imaging can have an appearance indistinguishable from adenoma (Fig. 12). The lesion can show heterogeneous signal related to intrinsic necrosis or hemorrhage, variable enhancement, and the margins of the lesion may be slightly more irregular than macroadenoma.[42]

PITUITARY HYPERPLASIA

Pituitary hyperplasia is simply defined as the nonneoplastic increase in the number of pituitary cells. If this hyperplasia is significant, the gland can demonstrate an increase in overall size. This can be a normal physiologic response and does not

necessarily indicate pathology. For example, the pituitary gland normally increases in size during pregnancy because of hyperplasia of prolactin cells. Hyperplasia can also occur in pathologic conditions. With primary hypothyroidism, there is a lack of circulating thyroxine. With decreased thyroxine, the hypothalamus produces excess thyrotropin-releasing hormone, which stimulates the thyrotrophs of the anterior pituitary and produces pituitary enlargement. The associated diffuse enlargement of the anterior lobe of pituitary gland can mimic the appearance of pituitary macroadenoma, with an enhancing sellar and suprasellar mass.[43] With adequate hormone replacement, follow-up studies show normalization of the pituitary gland (Fig. 13).

RATHKE CLEFT CYST

Rathke cleft cyst is a nonneoplastic lesion arising from remnants of the embryologic Rathke pouch and generally presents as an asymptomatic cyst in the sella with or without suprasellar extension. Famini and colleagues[35] examined brain MR imaging findings in 2598 patients and found an incidence of 3.4%. Rarely, such cysts are symptomatic with the most common complaint being headache, followed by visual disturbance and pituitary dysfunction. The cyst wall is a delicate epithelial wall made of simple or

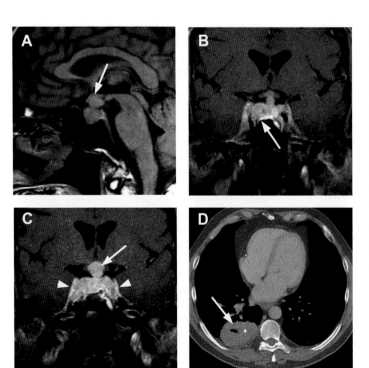

Fig. 12. Metastatic non–small cell lung cancer. A 60-year-old man with no prior history presented with severe headache for 1 month, found to have diabetes insipidus and panhypopituitarism. (A) Sagittal T1-weighted MR imaging shows sellar and suprasellar mass effacing optic chiasm (arrow). (B) Coronal postcontrast T1-weighted image shows asymmetric enlargement of the pituitary gland (arrow). (C) Coronal postcontrast T1-weighted image slightly more posterior shows marked enlargement of infundibulum (arrow) and bilateral cavernous sinus infiltration (arrowheads). (D) Contrast-enhanced chest CT demonstrated primary lung cancer right lower lobe (arrow).

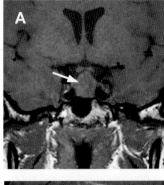
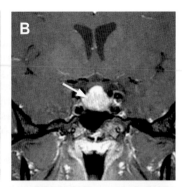
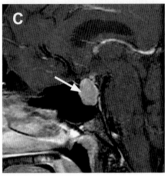
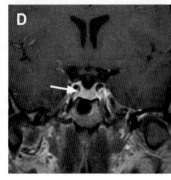

Fig. 13. Pituitary hyperplasia secondary to hypothyroidism. A 32-year-old woman with history of obesity and hypothyroidism was treated with thyroid-replacement therapy, and presented with vague symptoms of headache, nausea, and blurred vision. She had stopped her thyroid-replacement therapy 4 months earlier. (*A*) Coronal unenhanced T1-weighted MR image demonstrates mass-like enlargement of pituitary gland (*arrow*) contacting optic chiasm. (*B, C*) Coronal and sagittal postcontrast T1-weighted images show homogeneous enhancement of enlarged pituitary gland (*arrow*), similar to appearance of a macroadenoma. (*D*) Follow-up study after resumption of thyroid hormone replacement shows marked decrease in size of pituitary gland (*arrow*).

pseudostratified cuboidal or columnar cells and may contain cilia and goblet cells. The cyst generally contains mucoid or gelatinous material and can have fluid of variable consistency. CT demonstrates homogenous masses of variable density relative to brain, with 10% to 15% containing peripheral calcification. MR imaging demonstrates a nonenhancing cystic lesion that is variable in signal depending on contents of the cyst. On T1-weighted images, approximately 50% are hyperintense and the other 50% hypointense (**Fig. 14**). On T2-weighted images, 70% are hyperintense and 30% isointense/hypointense. Some lesions contain a small intracystic nodule that is typically hyperintense on T1, hypointense on T2, and shows enhancement.[44]

CRANIOPHARYNGIOMA

Craniopharyngiomas are rare epithelial tumors that arise from the Rathke pouch and occur along the path of the craniopharyngeal duct. These lesions typically occur in a suprasellar location (75%–90%) and involve the infundibulum. However, 20% of craniopharyngiomas show suprasellar and sellar components and 5% are intrasellar in location.[45] Although the lesions are histologically benign, they can be locally aggressive and cause significant morbidity. Symptoms in childhood cases are dominated by nonspecific manifestations of intracranial pressure (headache, nausea,

and vomiting). Visual impairment (62%–84%) and endocrine deficits, such as GH deficiency (52%–87%), are also common. In adult cases, patients also present with visual field deficits and headache. The hormonal deficits in adults are more pronounced when compared with childhood-onset cases. At the time of diagnosis, 40% to 87% of patients present with at least one hormonal deficit. Endocrine deficits are found with GH secretion (75%), gonadotropins (40%), ACTH (25%), and TSH (25%). Diabetes insipidus is found in 17% to 27%.[46]

There are two broad types of craniopharyngiomas. Adamantinomatous lesions are more common in childhood, generally present as heterogeneous solid and cystic lesions, and are associated with calcifications identified on CT in 90% of cases. The solid components generally enhance, whereas the cystic components do not enhance and show heterogeneous, often complex signal (**Fig. 15**). The papillary type is more typically solid, enhance, rarely show calcification, and are the most common type found in adulthood (**Fig. 16**). When evaluating craniopharyngiomas on MR imaging, it is important to identify the full extent of the tumor preoperatively, establishing the relationship of the tumor to the surrounding structures including the optic chiasm, the chiasmatic cistern, the third ventricle, the stalk, and the hypothalamus.[47]

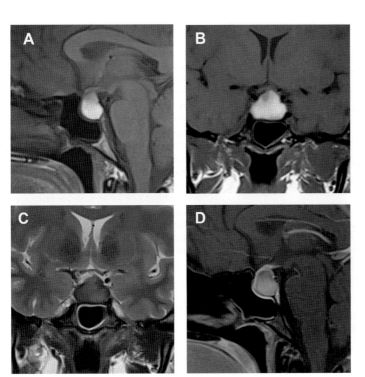

Fig. 14. Rathke cleft cyst. A 39-year-old woman with incidentally discovered sellar mass. (*A, B*) Sagittal and coronal T1-weighted unenhanced MR imaging demonstrates large cystic sellar and suprasellar lesion that is T1 hyperintense, secondary to proteinaceous contents. (*C*) Coronal T2-weighted image demonstrates diffuse hypointensity of the lesion. (*D*) Sagittal postcontrast T1-weighted image shows no nodular enhancing tissue.

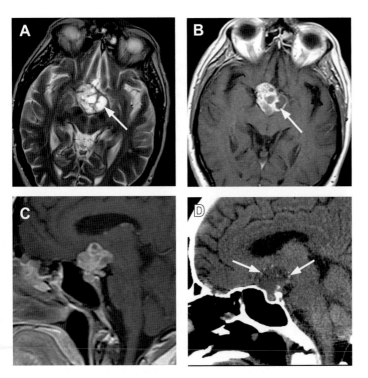

Fig. 15. Craniopharyngioma, adamantinomatous type. A 68-year-old man presented with bitemporal vison loss. (*A*) Axial T2-weighted MR imaging shows suprasellar lesion with multiple cystic areas (*arrow*). (*B*) Axial enhanced T1-weighted MR imaging demonstrates complex sellar and suprasellar lesion with enhancing solid and cystic components (*arrow*). (*C*) Sagittal enhanced T1-weighted MR imaging demonstrates multilobular appearance. (*D*) Sagittal CT identifies punctate calcifications around the margin of the lesion (*arrows*), characteristic of craniopharyngioma.

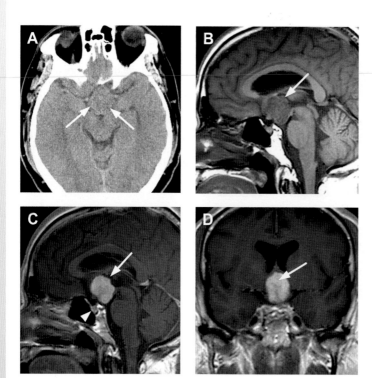

Fig. 16. Craniopharyngioma, papillary type. A 57-year-old man presented acutely with transient episode of tunnel vison and diplopia. (*A*) Axial CT demonstrates 3.0-cm isodense suprasellar mass (*arrows*) without calcifications. (*B*) Sagittal T1-weighted MR demonstrates large suprasellar mass that obscures the pituitary stalk, pushes the chiasm anteriorly, and extends into the anterior third ventricle (*arrow*). (*C, D*) Sagittal and coronal postcontrast T1-weighted MR images show homogeneously enhancing suprasellar mass (*arrows*). Note the normal appearing enhancing pituitary tissue in sella (*arrowhead* in *C*).

GERMINOMA/GERM CELL TUMORS

Germinoma is the most common (67%) of intracranial germ cell tumors. Most tumors occur in children and adolescents, and most occur before age 20.[48] Although germinomas are most commonly located in the pineal region and affect males, 20% to 40% arise in the suprasellar region and more commonly occur in females.[49] Tumors that involve both regions at presentation are termed "bifocal," and the incidence of bifocal germinoma ranges from 2% to 41%.[50] Suprasellar lesions are locally invasive and can invade the infundibulum, the chiasm, and hypothalamus. Distinction from other nongerminomatous germ cell tumors is determined histologically and through evaluation of protein markers in cerebrospinal fluid. Suprasellar germinomas often present with diabetes insipidus and other endocrine deficiencies. Visual disturbance and obstructive hydrocephalus can occur. Germinomas can spread easily through cerebrospinal fluid dissemination, and imaging of the entire neuroaxis is warranted for staging. On CT, lesions are isodense to hyperdense to brain parenchyma and rarely demonstrate calcification or osseous invasion. MR imaging typically shows an ill-defined enhancing mass in the region of the infundibulum that invades and compresses the chiasm and third ventricle (**Fig. 17**).[49]

PITUICYTOMA

Pituicytoma is a rare World Health Organization grade I sellar and/or suprasellar neoplasm presumably derived from neurohypophyseal pituicytes.[51] These lesions are similar to adenomas on conventional MR imaging, demonstrating T1 isointensity, heterogeneous hyperintensity on T2-weighted images, and heterogeneous enhancement. No distinctive imaging features can confidently allow preoperative diagnosis. These lesions represent a unique surgical subgroup, and resection is associated with significant morbidity including increased intraoperative hemorrhage, diabetes insipidus, and panhypopituitarism (**Fig. 18**).[52]

MENINGIOMA

Meningiomas arise from arachnoid cap cells and can occur anywhere that meninges are found; 10% to 15% involve the sella and parasellar regions.[53] Most meningiomas are benign, World Health Organization grade I lesions based on histologic subtype and lack of anaplastic features. Grade II meningiomas are atypical, and grade III meningiomas are considered anaplastic or malignant. Midline meningiomas of the skull base are challenging in terms of diagnosis and management given their proximity to the pituitary gland,

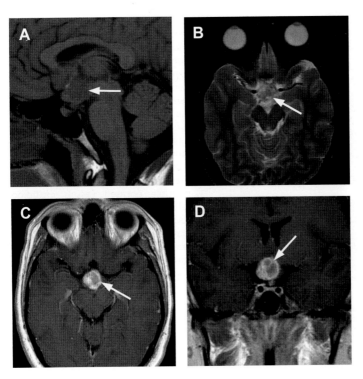

Fig. 17. Suprasellar germ cell tumor. A 20 year old with panhypopituitarism presents with recent worsening in peripheral vision. (A) Sagittal T1-weighted MR imaging shows large isointense suprasellar mass (arrow). (B) Axial T2-weighted image shows lobular T2 hyperintense suprasellar lesion (arrow). (C, D) Axial and coronal enhanced T1-weighted images show the rounded mass is heterogeneously enhancing (arrows). Elevated cerebrospinal a-fetoprotein and human chorionic gonadotropin (HCG) were noted, indicating that the lesion is not pure germinoma.

cavernous sinus, carotid vessels, and cranial nerves. Meningiomas can have a variety of growth patterns ranging from pedunculated focal mass to en plaque dural infiltration.

High-resolution CT or MR imaging is often necessary to separate an enhancing tumor from adjacent enhancing structures including the cavernous sinus or pituitary gland. Fat-saturation sequences are also invaluable in distinguishing an enhancing tumor from skull base fat on T1-weighted images. The dural tail sign is a common finding but is not pathognomonic. Meningiomas can encase the ICA and result in narrowing. In contrast, pituitary adenomas that surround the ICA usually do not significantly constrict or occlude the vessel.

The effect of meningioma growth on underlying skull base is variable. Most meningiomas do not cause obvious changes in the underlying bone, but some meningiomas cause hyperostosis. Pieper and colleagues[54] suggested that hyperostosis associated with meningiomas of the skull base demonstrates histologic tumor invasion. Osseous invasion can have a range of appearances, ranging from sclerosis to permeative to lytic.

Meningiomas are variably classified in the literature according to the anatomic site of origin or involvement. Lesions involving the skull base

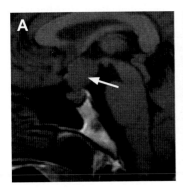
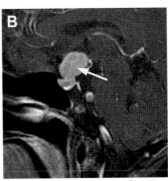

Fig. 18. Pituicytoma. A 60-year-old man presented with trauma. CT showed an incidental sellar and suprasellar mass. (A) Sagittal MR imaging shows T1-isointense predominantly suprasellar mass (arrow) that displaces optic chiasm and compresses the anterior third ventricle. (B) Sagittal postcontrast T1-weighted image demonstrates homogeneous enhancement of the mass (arrow).

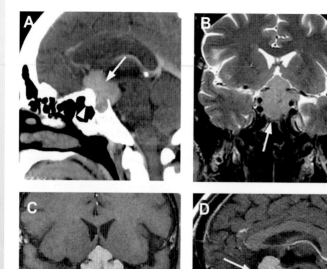

Fig. 19. Meningioma. (*A*) Sagittal reformation of enhanced CT scan shows large sellar and suprasellar enhancing mass (*arrow*). There is expansion of the sella and focal hyperostosis of the tuberculum sella (*arrowhead*). (*B*) Coronal T2-weighted MR imaging shows multilobulated mass. Compressed pituitary tissue is identified along floor of sella (*arrow*). (*C*) Coronal postcontrast T1-weighted image shows avid enhancement of the meningioma. There are multiple encased vessels including left supraclinoid carotid artery (*arrow*). (*D*) Sagittal postcontrast T1-weighted image shows large lobulated lesion with subtle dural tail (*arrow*) along planum sphenoidale.

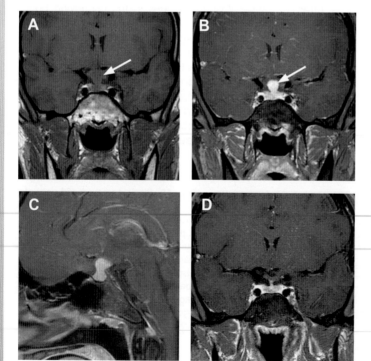

Fig. 20. Primary hypophysitis. A 20 year old presented with headache, blurred vision, and 6 months of multiple symptoms related to panhypopituitarism. (*A*) Coronal T1-weighted unenhanced MR image shows marked enlargement of infundibulum (*arrow*). (*B*) Coronal enhanced T1-weighted image shows marked enhancement of the enlarged infundibulum (*arrow*). (*C*) Sagittal enhanced T1-weighted image shows the process involves the pituitary and the infundibulum. (*D*) After temporary treatment with steroids, the 1-year follow-up coronal enhanced T1-weighted image shows normalization of the infundibulum.

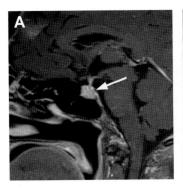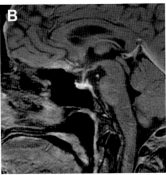

Fig. 21. Ipilumimab-related hypophysitis. A 55 year old with metastatic melanoma was treated with four doses of combination ipilumimab and nivolumab and developed progressive fatigue and adrenal insufficiency. (*A*) Sagittal enhanced T1-weighted MR imaging shows global enlargement of the pituitary gland (*arrow*) and mild enlargement of the stalk. (*B*) Three weeks after steroid therapy, repeat MR imaging showed normalization of the gland.

may be localized to the planum sphenoidale, the sella, cavernous sinus, or clinoid processes. Planum meningiomas can directly arise from the superior surface of the planum. Planum meningiomas, like tuberculum sella meningiomas, can extend laterally to involve the optic nerve canal or superiorly to involve the suprasellar region, resulting in unilateral or bilateral vision loss. Meningiomas primarily involving or largely involving the sella can present with mild elevation of prolactin levels, but most do not have significant endocrine dysfunction preoperatively.[55] Sellar meningiomas is difficult to differentiate from a large macroadenoma. An enhancing dural tail, lesion calcification, or adjacent skull base hyperostosis may suggest meningioma (**Fig. 19**).

HYPOPHYSITIS

Hypophysitis is a broad nonspecific term that includes a diverse group of conditions that result in localized inflammation of the pituitary gland and/or stalk. The associated pituitary gland inflammation can lead to abnormal enlargement of the infundibulum and the gland itself. Hypophysitis has been classified according to etiology, anatomic location, and histologic variants, and elucidation of this classification is beyond the scope of this article.[56] In general, MR imaging of these lesions demonstrates enlargement and intense homogeneous enhancement of the infundibulum and/or gland on dedicated postgadolinium MR imaging sequences, without deviation of the stalk. These lesions are difficult to differentiate radiologically from adenomas or germinomas. Clinically, patients can present with headache, anterior and posterior pituitary deficiencies, and visual defects.

Primary hypophysitis is considered idiopathic, possibly autoimmune in cause; secondary forms are caused by known associated etiologies (medication or systemic disease). The most common primary form is lymphocytic hypophysitis. It is probably autoimmune in nature and typically occurs in females during last month of pregnancy or in early postpartum period. Other forms of primary hypophysitis show similar imaging features and symptoms but are not associated with pregnancy (**Fig. 20**).

One unique form of secondary hypophysitis occurs after therapy with immune checkpoint inhibitors, such as ipilumimab, an established therapy for metastatic melanoma. Patients generally present after three or four infusions, with an incidence that may be 17%.[57] Symptoms are not specific but may include lethargy, headaches, myalgia, or nausea and vomiting. Patients may also have eye pain, diplopia, or other visual defects. Gadolinium-enhanced MR imaging shows diffuse enlargement of the pituitary gland and/or stalk (**Fig. 21**). Treatment with corticosteroids usually results in normalization of the pituitary findings.

SUMMARY

The most common primary lesion of the pituitary gland, sella, and suprasellar region is the adenoma. However, the spectrum of nonadenomatous abnormalities is broad, and a reasonable differential should be considered for each lesion. The pituitary gland is best evaluated with dedicated MR imaging, with CT performing a complementary role in evaluation. For any lesion, it is important to consider location, point of origin, relationship to adjacent structures, and clinical scenario to propose the most appropriate diagnosis.

DISCLOSURE

The authors have nothing to disclose.

REFERENCES

1. Elster AD. Imaging of the sella: anatomy and pathology. Semin Ultrasound CT MR 1993;14(3):182–94.

2. Stobo DB, Lindsay RS, Connell JM, et al. Initial experience of 3 Tesla versus conventional field strength magnetic resonance imaging of small functioning pituitary tumours. Clin Endocrinol (Oxf) 2011;75(5): 673–7.

3. Erickson D, Erickson B, Watson R, et al. 3 Tesla magnetic resonance imaging with and without corticotropin releasing hormone stimulation for the detection of microadenomas in Cushing's syndrome. Clin Endocrinol (Oxf) 2010;72(6):793–9.

4. Bladowska J, Sasiadek M. Diagnostic imaging of the pituitary and parasellar region. In: Rahimi-Movaghar PV, editor. Pituitary adenomas. InTech; 2012.

5. Chowdhury IN, Sinaii N, Oldfield EH, et al. A change in pituitary magnetic resonance imaging protocol detects ACTH-secreting tumours in patients with previously negative results. Clin Endocrinol (Oxf) 2010;72(4):502–6.

6. Friedman TC, Zuckerbraun E, Lee ML, et al. Dynamic pituitary MRI has high sensitivity and specificity for the diagnosis of mild Cushing's syndrome and should be part of the initial workup. Horm Metab Res 2007;39(6):451–6.

7. Grober Y, Grober H, Wintermark M, et al. Comparison of MRI techniques for detecting microadenomas in Cushing's disease. J Neurosurg 2018;128(4): 1051–7.

8. Kunii N, Abe T, Kawamo M, et al. Rathke's cleft cysts: differentiation from other cystic lesions in the pituitary fossa by use of single-shot fast spin-echo diffusion-weighted MR imaging. Acta Neurochir (Wien) 2007;149(8):759–69 [discussion: 769].

9. Rogg JM, Tung GA, Anderson G, et al. Pituitary apoplexy: early detection with diffusion-weighted MR imaging. AJNR Am J Neuroradiol 2002;23(7): 1240–5.

10. Yiping L, Ji X, Daoying G, et al. Prediction of the consistency of pituitary adenoma: a comparative study on diffusion-weighted imaging and pathological results. J Neuroradiol 2016;43(3):186–94.

11. Bou-Ayache JM, Delman BN. Advances in imaging of the pediatric pituitary gland. Endocrinol Metab Clin North Am 2016;45(2):443–52.

12. Chaudhary V, Bano S. Imaging of the pituitary: recent advances. Indian J Endocrinol Metab 2011; 15(Suppl 3):S216–23.

13. Di Iorgi N, Allegri AE, Napoli F, et al. The use of neuroimaging for assessing disorders of pituitary development. Clin Endocrinol (Oxf) 2012;76(2):161–76.

14. Zamora C, Castillo M. Sellar and parasellar imaging. Neurosurgery 2017;80(1):17–38.

15. Go JL, Rajamohan AG. Imaging of the sella and parasellar region. Radiol Clin North Am 2017;55(1): 83–101.

16. Rennert J, Doerfler A. Imaging of sellar and parasellar lesions. Clin Neurol Neurosurg 2007;109(2): 111–24.

17. Shaffi OM, Wrightson P. Dural invasion by pituitary tumours. N Z Med J 1975;81(538):386–90.

18. Trevino R. Chiasmal syndrome. J Am Optom Assoc 1995;66(9):559–75.

19. Lee IH, Miller NR, Zan E, et al. Visual defects in patients with pituitary adenomas: the myth of bitemporal hemianopsia. AJR Am J Roentgenol 2015;205(5): W512–8.

20. Symon L, Jakubowski J, Kendall B. Surgical treatment of giant pituitary adenomas. J Neurol Neurosurg Psychiatry 1979;42(11):973–82.

21. Mohr G, Hardy J, Comtois R, et al. Surgical management of giant pituitary adenomas. Can J Neurol Sci 1990;17(1):62–6.

22. Songtao Q, Yuntao L, Jun P, et al. Membranous layers of the pituitary gland: histological anatomic study and related clinical issues. Neurosurgery 2009;64(3 Suppl):ons1–9 [discussion: ons9–10].

23. Knosp E, Steiner E, Kitz K, et al. Pituitary adenomas with invasion of the cavernous sinus space: a magnetic resonance imaging classification compared with surgical findings. Neurosurgery 1993;33(4): 610–7 [discussion: 617–18].

24. Cottier JP, Destrieux C, Brunereau L, et al. Cavernous sinus invasion by pituitary adenoma: MR imaging. Radiology 2000;215(2):463–9.

25. Selman WR, Laws ER Jr, Scheithauer BW, et al. The occurrence of dural invasion in pituitary adenomas. J Neurosurg 1986;64(3):402–7.

26. Meij BP, Lopes MB, Ellegala DB, et al. The long-term significance of microscopic dural invasion in 354 patients with pituitary adenomas treated with transsphenoidal surgery. J Neurosurg 2002;96(2): 195–208.

27. Luo CB, Teng MM, Chen SS, et al. Imaging of invasiveness of pituitary adenomas. Kaohsiung J Med Sci 2000;16(1):26–31.

28. Chen X, Dai J, Ai L, et al. Clival invasion on multidetector CT in 390 pituitary macroadenomas: correlation with sex, subtype and rates of operative complication and recurrence. AJNR Am J Neuroradiol 2011;32(4):785–9.

29. Barkhoudarian G, Kelly DF. Pituitary apoplexy. Neurosurg Clin N Am 2019;30(4):457–63.

30. Wildemberg LE, Glezer A, Bronstein MD, et al. Apoplexy in nonfunctioning pituitary adenomas. Pituitary 2018;21(2):138–44.

31. Semple PL, Jane JA, Lopes MB, et al. Pituitary apoplexy: correlation between magnetic resonance imaging and histopathological results. J Neurosurg 2008;108(5):909–15.

32. Burns J, Policeni B, Bykowski J, et al. ACR Appropriateness Criteria Neuroendocrine Imaging. Expert panel on neurologic imaging. J Am Coll Radiol 2019;16(5S):S161–73.

33. Dubuisson AS, Beckers A, Stevenaert A. Classical pituitary tumour apoplexy: clinical features,

management and outcomes in a series of 24 patients. Clin Neurol Neurosurg 2007;109(1):63–70.

34. Kasuki L, Raverot G. Definition and diagnosis of aggressive pituitary tumors. Rev Endocr Metab Disord 2020;21(2):203–8.

35. Famini P, Maya MM, Melmed S. Pituitary magnetic resonance imaging for sellar and parasellar masses: ten-year experience in 2598 patients. J Clin Endocrinol Metab 2011;96(6):1633–41.

36. Ragel BT, Couldwell WT. Pituitary carcinoma: a review of the literature. Neurosurg Focus 2004; 16(4):E7.

37. Sansur CA, Oldfield EH. Pituitary carcinoma. Semin Oncol 2010;37(6):591–3.

38. Di Nunno V, Mollica V, Corcioni B, et al. Clinical management of a pituitary gland metastasis from clear cell renal cell carcinoma. Anticancer Drugs 2018; 29(7):710–5.

39. Angelousi A, Alexandraki KI, Kyriakopoulos G, et al. Neoplastic metastases to the endocrine glands. Endocr Relat Cancer 2020;27(1):R1–20.

40. Morita A, Meyer FB, Laws ER Jr. Symptomatic pituitary metastases. J Neurosurg 1998;89(1):69–73.

41. Spinelli GP, Lo Russo G, Miele E, et al. Breast cancer metastatic to the pituitary gland: a case report. World J Surg Oncol 2012;10:137.

42. He W, Chen F, Dalm B, et al. Metastatic involvement of the pituitary gland: a systematic review with pooled individual patient data analysis. Pituitary 2015;18(1):159–68.

43. Al-Gahtany M, Horvath E, Kovacs K. Pituitary hyperplasia. Hormones (Athens) 2003;2(3):149–58.

44. Larkin S, Karavitaki N, Ansorge O. Rathke's cleft cyst. Handb Clin Neurol 2014;124:255–69.

45. Zada G, Lin N, Ojerholm E, et al. Craniopharyngioma and other cystic epithelial lesions of the sellar region: a review of clinical, imaging, and histopathological relationships. Neurosurg Focus 2010;28(4):E4.

46. Muller HL. Craniopharyngioma. Endocr Rev 2014; 35(3):513–43.

47. Prieto R, Pascual JM, Barrios L. Topographic diagnosis of craniopharyngiomas: the accuracy of MRI findings observed on conventional T1 and T2 images. AJNR Am J Neuroradiol 2017;38(11):2073–80.

48. Osorio DS, Allen JC. Management of CNS germinoma. CNS Oncol 2015;4(4):273–9.

49. Chung EM, Biko DM, Schroeder JW, et al. From the radiologic pathology archives: precocious puberty: radiologic-pathologic correlation. Radiographics 2012;32(7):2071–99.

50. Lee L, Saran F, Hargrave D, et al. Germinoma with synchronous lesions in the pineal and suprasellar regions. Childs Nerv Syst 2006;22(12):1513–8.

51. Viaene AN, Lee EB, Rosenbaum JN, et al. Histologic, immunohistochemical, and molecular features of pituicytomas and atypical pituicytomas. Acta Neuropathol Commun 2019;7(1):69.

52. Guerrero-Perez F, Marengo AP, Vidal N, et al. Primary tumors of the posterior pituitary: a systematic review. Rev Endocr Metab Disord 2019;20(2): 219–38.

53. FitzPatrick M, Tartaglino LM, Hollander MD, et al. Imaging of sellar and parasellar pathology. Radiol Clin North Am 1999;37(1):101–21, x.

54. Pieper DR, Al-Mefty O, Hanada Y, et al. Hyperostosis associated with meningioma of the cranial base: secondary changes or tumor invasion. Neurosurgery 1999;44(4):742–6 [discussion: 746–7].

55. Sathananthan M, Sathananthan A, Scheithauer BW, et al. Sellar meningiomas: an endocrinologic perspective. Pituitary 2013;16(2):182–8.

56. Faje A. Hypophysitis: evaluation and management. Clin Diabetes Endocrinol 2016;2:15.

57. Dillard T, Yedinak CG, Alumkal J, et al. Anti-CTLA-4 antibody therapy associated autoimmune hypophysitis: serious immune related adverse events across a spectrum of cancer subtypes. Pituitary 2010;13(1): 29–38.

Molecular Imaging in the Head and Neck
Diagnosis and Therapy

Brandon A. Howard, MD, PhD

KEYWORDS

- Head and neck • Nuclear medicine • PET • SPECT • Radionuclide therapy • Dosimetry

KEY POINTS

- I-131 sodium iodide continues to be invaluable for remnant ablation and adjuvant therapy of well-differentiated thyroid cancer.
- Recent studies of patients after I-131 radioablative therapy have shown a small increased rate of solid cancer mortality and development of secondary cancers; further studies are needed.
- Tc99m-sestamibi remains a workhorse for workup of hyperparathyroidism, with F-18 fluorocholine PET/computed tomography scans showing promise in detection of parathyroid adenomas and multigland disease.
- Ga-68 DOTATATE is highly sensitive and specific for staging of somatostatin receptor-positive neuroendocrine tumors of the head and neck, having supplanted In-111 Octreoscan and playing a complementary role to I-123 meta-iodo-benzyl-guanidine.

INTRODUCTION

From the first production of radioactive iodine in 1936 by Enrico Fermi to the subsequent application of [130]I-sodium iodide (later ^{131}I) to treat hyperthyroid patients in 1946 by Drs Saul Hertz and others, molecular imaging and therapy of the head and neck was born.[1]

THYROID-BENIGN DISEASE

The thyroid gland descends during development from the foramen cecum at the base of the tongue to its location anterior to the trachea and inferior to the thyroid cartilage, weighs approximately 25 g, and measures 4 to 5 cm tall and 1 to 2 cm wide. Ectopic thyroid can occur anywhere along this descent, including at the base of tongue (lingual thyroid), hyoid bone (thyroglossal duct cyst), superior to either lobe or isthmus (pyramidal lobe), or in the mediastinum (substernal goiter).[2] Symptoms of the hyperthyroid patient can be due to Graves

disease (caused by autoantibodies to the thyroid-stimulating hormone [TSH] receptor), toxic multinodular goiter (caused by hyperplasia of follicular cells which become autonomous of TSH, and TSH receptor mutations),[3] toxic adenoma, or thyroiditis.[4] Unusual causes of thyrotoxicosis, including struma ovarii, lithium, and the Jod–Basdow effect (from iodinated contrast), and of hypothyroidism (lingual thyroid) have been previously reviewed.[5] Nuclear techniques can differentiate between these entities and provide definitive treatment.

Imaging of the thyroid is performed with a thyroid uptake and scan, either with I-123 sodium iodide, or I-131 sodium iodide for the uptake and Tc99m-pertechnetate for the scan (Table 1). On a thyroid scan in a patient with Graves' disease, the thyroid gland seems to be homogeneous with convex contours, with a 24-hour iodine uptake of typically 60% to 80%. A mildly elevated or high-normal 24-hour uptake can sometimes be observed with rapid turnover Graves' disease,

No funding for this article.

Division of Nuclear Medicine, Department of Radiology, Duke University School of Medicine, DUMC Box 3949, 2301 Erwin Road, Durham, NC 27710, USA

E-mail address: brandon.howard@duke.edu

Radiol Clin N Am 58 (2020) 1135–1146
https://doi.org/10.1016/j.rcl.2020.08.001

Table 1
-Technical details of molecular imaging of the thyroid and parathyroid glands

Imaging Protocol	Notes
Thyroid uptake and scan - pediatric/mediastinal mass characterization Off PTU or methimazole >3 d	400 µCi I-123 sodium iodide via capsule or oral solution; pediatric 5.7 µC/kg; Uptake and scan: 4 h post images: anterior /anterior 10 cm/RAO, LAO, 5 min Uptake: 24 h Pinhole collimator, 159 keV 20% window Captus uptake probe
Thyroid uptake and scan - routine Off PTU or methimazole >3 d	5–12 µCi sodium iodide I-131 capsule by mouth Adult dose: 6 mCi Tc-99m pertechnetate IV Returns 24 h after post I-131 for uptake measurement and then scan 20 min after injection Give crackers and water after injection Views: anterior, anterior −10 cm, RAO, LAO, 5 min/view Pinhole collimator, 140 keV, 20% window
Total body iodine scan No CT contrast within 4 wks Preparation options: 1) Discontinue levothyroxine for 4 wks 2) At 4 wks, switch from levothyroxine to liothyronine, then cease liothyronine at 2 wks prior to scan 3) Thyrogen™	Adult dose: 2 mCi sodium I-123 oral solution Pediatric dose: 28.6 µCi/kg Patients on Thyrogen™: dosed at least 4 h after second Thyrogen™ shot Uptake w/Captus probe Images: whole body - anterior and post 8 cm/min; neck statics, neck statics w/sternal notch marker
Parathyroid scan	Adult dose: 25 mCi Tc99m-sestamibi Pediatric dose: 0.28 mCi/kg Images: immediate, anterior (10 min) Images: 2 h, anterior (10 min)
Parathyroid SPECT/CT	2 h SPECT/CT 128 × 128 matrix, 1.5 zoom, dual head 30 sec/stop, step and shoot with body contour If unable to tolerate SPECT/CT, may acquire RAO and LAO views

Abbreviations: LAO, left anterior oblique; PTU, propylthiouracil; RAO, right anterior oblique.

when a 4-hour uptake (typically only obtained with I-123) would have been elevated. Although patients are often first treated medically with methimazole, radioablative therapy is ultimately pursued owing to the unfavorable side effect profile of thionamides. Radioablation for Graves' disease with ^{131}I-sodium iodide typically uses a calculated method, with the dose proportional to the weight of the gland (in grams) and a constant (100–200 µCi/g), and inversely related to the uptake fraction; typically 10–15 mCi is the resulting dose. This method is selected to avoid radiation thyroiditis and ensure ablation success, but studies have shown that the risk of thyroid storm is very low and does not correlate with untreated hyperthyroidism before radioiodine ablation[1]; an empiric, fixed-dose method is similarly efficacious.[6] Side effects include sialadenitis with possible xerostomia, sore throat, neck discomfort, and dysgeusia. Graves' ophthalmopathy can be worsened by I-131 therapy, which is thought to result from deposition of antigen–antibody complexes. Compared with methimazole, radioiodine was associated with a lower recurrence but a higher incidence of ophthalmopathy in a large meta-analysis.[7,8]

Toxic multinodular goiter exhibits patchy uptake on scintigraphy, with a 24-hour radioiodine uptake of 30% to 60%. Although photopenic regions may represent degenerating adenomas or suppressed normal thyroid tissue, the "cold nodule" carries a 10% risk of malignancy and warrants ultrasound examination and potential biopsy.[9] Thyroid malignancy is more common in patients with underlying thyroid disease and prior head and neck radiation. In cases of large nontoxic multinodular goiter when the patient is not a surgical candidate, recombinant human thyroid stimulating hormone (rhTSH: Thyrogen™, Genzyme Corporation, Cambridge, MA) can be used.[10] In a hyperthyroid patient with a solitary tracer-avid focus and absent uptake elsewhere in the gland, this entity is likely a toxic adenoma. Toxic adenomas larger than 4 cm are usually surgically excised, but smaller nodules may be ablated successfully with 20 to 30 mCi I-131 sodium iodide (more activity is needed owing to suppressed gland and lower uptake). Toxic multinodular goiter is treated with a similar dose. After radioablative therapy, the failure rate is 10%, with underestimation of a large gland size representing the most common reason. A recent retrospective cohort study of 18,805 patients by Kitahara and colleagues[11] showed a modest association between greater absorbed organ doses of radioactive iodine and increased risk of death from solid cancers, including breast cancer (5%–10% increase per 100-mGy dose).

Scintigraphic evaluation is occasionally performed for workup of neonatal hypothyroidism, which is usually secondary to thyroid dysgenesis or aplasia, or organification defect. For the latter, a perchlorate washout test may be performed using Tc99m pertechnetate and I-123; in this procedure, trapping of iodide is demonstrated on a Tc99m pertechnetate scan; however, a relative washout of more than 10% is observed on I-123 scans after administration of perchlorate, an inhibitor of iodide trapping (i.e., a sodium–iodine symporter), thereby confirming lack of organification.[12] Additional use of I-123 sodium iodide scanning includes verification of the thyroid origin of indeterminate mediastinal masses.

THYROID-MALIGNANT DISEASE

Thyroid cancer has increased in incidence, likely owing to increased detection, with more than 60,000 new cases in 2013, and is now the fifth most common cancer in women.[13] Follicular epithelial-derived cancers (papillary, follicular, some poorly differentiated) concentrate iodine, enabling adjuvant treatment with I-131 sodium iodide, and express thyroglobulin, which may be used as a marker for tumor recurrence after ablation of remnant tissue after thyroidectomy. Follicular cancer is more aggressive and more likely to present with distant metastases than papillary histology (Fig. 1). Hurthle cell carcinoma and anaplastic thyroid cancer are typically not iodine avid. Staging is either based on disease-specific mortality (American Joint Committee on Cancer) or the risk of recurrence (American Thyroid Association [ATA]). In the American Joint Committee on

Cancer system, stages I to IV are based on T-, N-, and M parameters, with age less than 55 years being a positive factor and extrathyroidal extension, age greater than 55 years, and distant metastases being negative prognostic factors. In the 2009 ATA guidelines, high-risk patients may have distant metastases, gross extrathyroidal extension, or incomplete resection; intermediate-risk patients have nodal metastasis, advanced age, and adverse histology (e.g. tall cell); and low-risk patients have tumors confined to the thyroid, favorable histology, and no nodal or distant metastatic disease. After the issuance of the 2015 ATA guidelines, microscopic nodal metastases were placed into the low-risk category along with other changes.[14] The 5-year survival of patients with localized tumor is 100%, nodal metastasis is 97%, and distant metastasis is 57%.

Factors associated with higher recurrence or mortality include advanced age, extrathyroidal extension, multiple and enlarged nodal metastases in the lateral neck, and distant metastatic disease (to the lungs or bones), and I-131 treatment is unquestionably the standard of practice for such patients. Its benefit in low-risk patients has not consistently been shown and radioablative therapy is now tending to be reserved for intermediate- or high-risk patients. Moreover, a recent large study demonstrated a slightly increased risk of salivary gland malignancies and leukemia with radioiodine therapy, which is dose dependent and inversely correlated with age.[14–16]

Total body iodine scanning plays an integral role in the patient's initial staging evaluation (see Table 1). After thyroidectomy, the patient is typically prepared by thyroid hormone withdrawal for 4 weeks, or Thyrogen™ 0.9 mg IM × 2 days (plus 1 week of a low-iodine diet) to achieve TSH stimulation, then administered 2 mCi I-123 sodium iodide, followed by a total body scan and uptake the following day.

Diagnostic I-131 sodium iodide total body scan is less preferred, owing to concern of "stunning" the thyroid cancer cells and making them more resistant to subsequent radioiodine therapy. The total body scan may reveal unanticipated distant metastatic disease, prominent residual thyroid tissue that may warrant further surgery, or a burden of pulmonary metastases that may require dosimetry. A pretherapy scan is advocated by Van Nostrand and colleagues[17] who, in a study of 355 scans, found that 53% of the patients had findings on preradioablation whole body scan that might have altered the management. Alternatively, the nuclear radiologist can treat empirically based on clinicopathologic data, and obtain a post-therapy scan 5 to 7 days later to complete the diagnostic

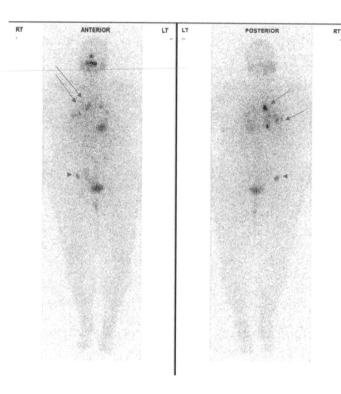

Fig. 1. A 67-year-old woman with follicular thyroid carcinoma metastatic to lungs (*arrows*) and right ilium (*arrowhead*) on I-123 total body scan.

evaluation; in the event of unanticipated metastatic disease, additional I-131 could still be given at a later time. Chen and colleagues[18] also reported that I-123 preablation whole body scan was able to provide additional critical information in 25% of the patients, requiring significant changes in the I-131 therapy strategy. I-123 single photon emission computed tomography/computed tomography (SPECT/CT) scan can change management, most often on post-therapy scan, with a less clear benefit for the pretherapy scan.[19] A SPECT scan is helpful for evaluating unexpected distant sites of iodine uptake (Fig. 2).

Thyrogen™ is approved by the US Food and Drug Administration for remnant ablation, but is increasingly used off-label in patients with metastatic disease owing to increased convenience and patient comfort relative to thyroid hormone withdrawal. It has been demonstrated that renal clearance is lower with thyroid hormone withdrawal, suggesting that dose to tumor would be higher than with Thyrogen™.[20] This finding is supported by studies of 124 I-PET/CT, which have showed a lower radiation dose to metastases with recombinant human TSH stimulation compared with thyroid hormone withdrawal[21] and decreased detection of metastases compared with thyroid hormone withdrawal.[1,22]

Other methods of treatment for thyroid cancer include thyroid hormone suppression, radiation, tyrosine kinase inhibition, and restoration of iodine avidity in iodine-negative cancers via the mitogen-activated protein kinase pathway (under investigation).[23] I-124 PET/CT imaging has been used to quantitate difference in sodium-iodine symporter expression before and after such redifferentiation therapy in patients with radioiodine-refractory metastatic thyroid cancer.[24]

State-of-the-art radioiodine therapy offers the opportunity to provide personalized dosimetry. In patients with renal impairment or diffuse pulmonary metastases (Fig. 3), a pre-dosing and post-dosing I-123 total body scan can be used to compute the effective renal clearance half-time, and using a modified Benua–Leeper approach, calculate maximum tolerated doses of I-131 sodium iodide to avoid bone marrow and lung toxicity, respectively.[25] Sgouros and colleagues[26] have suggested that the 80 mCi at 48-hour Benua threshold for lung toxicity may overestimate the risk of pulmonary complications. Lesion-specific dosimetry is possible using OLINDA software, but its use is not widespread.[27]

Although the selection of I-131 dose for thyroid cancer treatment is controversial, and ranges from 30 to 200 mCi, there are certain consistent themes, such as 100 to 200 mCi for therapy of

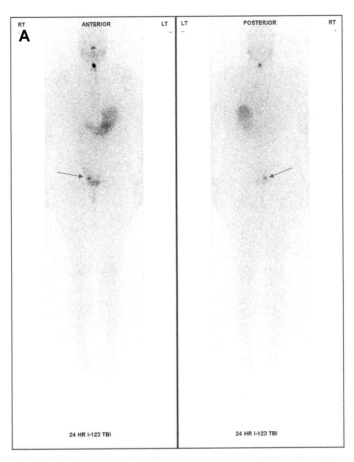

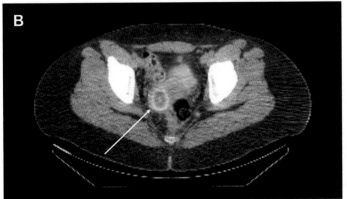

Fig. 2. A 27-year-old woman with thyroid cancer status post thyroidectomy. (*A*) I-123 total body scan shows remnant thyroid activity and unexpected focal activity in the right pelvis (*arrow*). (*B*) On SPECT/CT scanning, this activity localized to the right uterus (*arrow*). Given a normal follow-up pelvic ultrasound examination, this result was favored to represent physiologic uterine activity.

distant metastatic disease and 30 mCi for remnant ablation. The recommendations of the ATA and Society of Nuclear Medicine and Molecular Imaging are summarized by Ylli and colleagues.[28] Similar to hyperthyroid therapy, side effects of I-131 therapy for thyroid cancer include sialadenitis, lacrimal gland dysfunction, and xerostomia, the risk of which can likely be mitigated by lemon juice at 24 hours after therapy.

A PET/CT scan fludeoxyglucose (FDG) is useful in the detection of iodine-negative thyroid carcinoma that has become dedifferentiated and for initial staging and follow-up of invasive and metastatic Hurthle cell and anaplastic thyroid carcinoma. Medullary thyroid cancer can be evaluated by a FDG PET/CT scan after surgery, if the patient has persistently elevated calcitonin.[29] Incidental thyroid uptake on FDG PET scans is

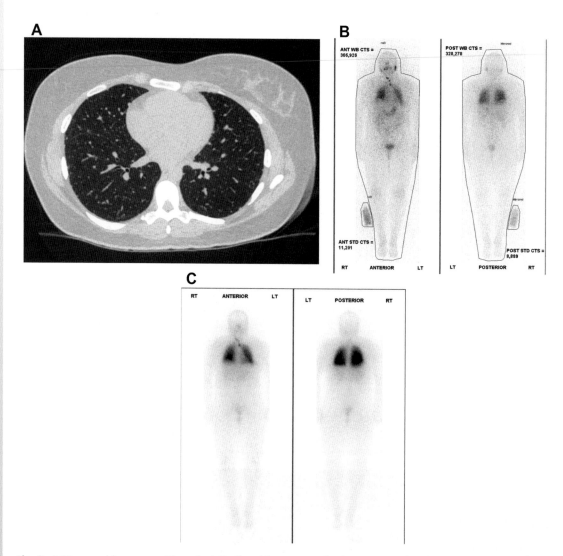

Fig. 3. A 21-year-old woman with metastatic thyroid cancer to the lungs, treated with 100 mCi I-131 6 months previously at an outside hospital. (*A*) A CT scan demonstrates persistence of innumerable small pulmonary nodules. (*B*) On I-123 total body scan performed before repeat I-131 therapy, the pulmonary metastases were diffusely iodine avid; a scan was performed using regions of interest about the whole body and I-123 standard bottle, as part of dosimetry to avoid pulmonary toxicity. (*C*) Total body iodine scan performed 7 days after dosimetrically determined therapy with 125 mC I-131, showing intense uptake in pulmonary metastases.

usually benign, such as follicular adenoma or Hurthle cell lesions; however, Nayan and colleagues[30] showed that 20% are primary thyroid cancers; 15% of those are papillary, and further evaluation is warranted with ultrasound examination.

PARATHYROID DISEASE

Patients with hyperparathyroidism present with hypercalcemia. The underlying cause is a solitary parathyroid adenoma in 85%, multigland hyperplasia (or double adenoma) in 15%, and carcinoma in 1% of instances. Complete resection of

the hyperfunctioning tissue is necessary to resolve the patient's symptoms. The parathyroid glands can range from 2 to 6 in number (usually 4) and are located adjacent to the upper and lower thyroid poles. Ectopic glands can occur in the thymus, carotid sheath, and mediastinum; they can also be retroesophageal or intrathyroid in location. Preoperative scintigraphy can obviate the need for bilateral neck exploration.[31,32]

Tc99m sestamibi (2-methoxy-isobutyl-isonitrile) is delivered to the hypervascular parathyroid adenoma, passively diffuses into the cell, and is believed to bind electrostatically to the mitochondrial membrane. Adenomas have a high proportion of the mitochondria-rich oxyphil cells, which results in retention on dual phase parathyroid scan with SPECT scanning. Other protocols include dual isotope Tc99m sestamibi/Tc99m pertechnetate and Tc99m sestamibi/I-123-iodide, both with subtraction; in the latter, I-123 is given first with imaging at 4 hours, followed by Tc99m-sestamibi imaging (see Table 1). Subtraction imaging can be affected by patient motion. The characteristic appearance of parathyroid adenoma is a focal tracer-avid area on immediate image, which remains avid on delays, whereas the thyroid activity washes out. False negatives can occur with a rapid washout adenoma, small adenoma less than 500 mg, parathyroid hyperplasia (which contain more chief cells than oxyphil cells and are usually smaller than adenomas), and expression of P-glycoprotein/multidrug resistance protein.[33] False positives include thyroid adenoma or multinodular goiter, nodal or thyroid metastatic disease (i.e., breast or lung cancer), chronic lymphocytic thyroiditis, or Hurthle cell lesions. A 4-dimensional CT scan may be helpful for imaging after discordant ultrasound examination and scintigraphy, persistent or recurrent hyperparathyroidism, or multiglandular disease.[34–38] In a large meta-analysis of 1236 patients, the detection rate of sestamibi was 88%.[39] An advantage of SPECT scanning is the ability to differentiate ectopic superior glands in the tracheoesophageal groove (the most common site of missed ectopic adenoma) from inferior glands.[40] It is also highly

sensitive for recurrent or persistent disease after surgery for primary hyperparathyroidism or 4-gland parathyroidectomy and autotransplantation.[41,42] Using an intraoperative gamma probe, a count ratio of 1.5 times the background thyroid is suggestive of an adenoma; an ex vivo count of more than 20% greater than thyroid background and/or intraoperative parathyroid hormone assay is confirmatory.[43–45]

After several investigators imaging prostate cancer with C-11 and F-18-choline PET/CT scans incidentally noted uptake in a parathyroid adenoma, this was more systematically investigated. Lezaic and colleagues[46] compared F-18 fluorocholine-PET/CT scans and conventional parathyroid scintigraphic imaging consisting of Tc99m-sestamibi SPECT/CT scans, Tc99m-sestamibi dual-phase imaging, and Tc99m-sestamibi/pertechnetate subtraction imaging in 24 patients and compared against histology, postoperative serum calcium, and intact parathyroid hormone values. The sensitivity and specificity of F-18 fluorocholine-PET/CT scans were 92% and 100%, respectively, in contrast with 49% and 100%, 46% and 100%, and 44% and 100% for Tc99m-sestamibi SPECT/CT scans, Tc99m-sestamibi dual-phase imaging, and Tc99m-sestamibi/pertechnetate subtraction imaging, respectively. The performance of (18)F-fluorocholine PET/CT scans was found to be superior in patients with multiple lesions or hyperplasia. Michaud and colleagues[47,48] found that in 12

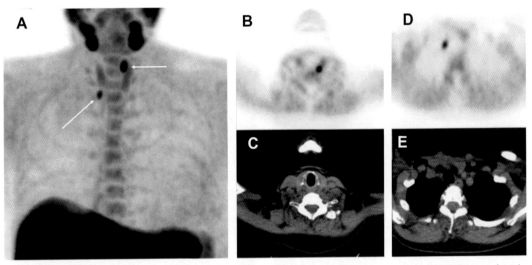

Fig. 4. Patient with hypercalcemia and hyperparathyroidism underwent F-18-fluorocholine PET/CT scan showing a double parathyroid adenoma. (A) On a coronal PET image, 2 foci of intense choline uptake are noted in the neck (arrows), with physiologic uptake in the salivary glands, thyroid gland, liver, spleen, and marrow. Axial PET (B) and CT (C) images show foci of uptake posterior and superior to the left thyroid lobe measuring 7 × 5 mm and maximum standardized uptake value of 8.7. Axial PET (D) and CT (E) images show uptake inferior to the right thyroid lobe measuring 6 × 4 mm and maximum standardized uptake value of 5.6. (Courtesy of Dr. Wouter Broos.)

patients with discordant ultrasound examinations and sestamibi scintigraphy results, F-18 fluoro-choline detected hyperfunctioning parathyroid tissue in 11 of 12 patients, and 7 adenomas and 10 hyperplasias, with surgical pathology correlation (**Fig. 4**).

Secondary hyperparathyroidism is a complication of end-stage renal disease, where diffuse hyperplasia in response to hypophosphatemia and other factors gives way to asymmetric nodular growth; patients are then treated with subtotal parathyroidectomy or total parathyroidectomy with autotransplantation. Scintigraphy can identify supernumerary or ectopic glands, which may change the operative approach. The sensitivity of Tc99m-sestamibi in this situation is reported to be significantly higher using a Tc99m-sestamibi/I-123 subtraction protocol (75%) compared with 56% to 63% for dual phase Tc99m-sestamibi and 52% to 63% for Tc99m-sestamib/pertechnetate subtraction protocols.[49]

SALIVARY GLANDS

The most common primary tumors of the salivary glands are the Warthin tumor and pleomorphic adenoma, which appear as enhancing, circumscribed FDG-avid nodules on PET/CT scans and most commonly occupy the parotid gland (**Fig. 5**). Tumors in the submandibular and sublingual glands are less common, and in the minor salivary glands in the oral cavity, tongue, and larynx even rarer, although they are more likely to be malignant; adenoid cystic and mucoepidermoid carcinoma, and adenocarcinoma are examples. Adenoid cystic and mucoepidermoid carcinomas have a propensity for perineural invasion.[50,51]

NEUROENDOCRINE TUMORS OF THE HEAD AND NECK

The major neuroendocrine tumors in the head and neck are paragangliomas. These slow-growing hypervascular tumors may involve the carotid bifurcation (carotid body), jugular bulb (glomus jugulare), or cochlear promontory (glomus tympanicum) and are associated with germline or sporadic succinate dehydrogenase mutations. These tumors express somatostatin receptors (SSTRs), decarboxylate amino acid precursors, and in 30% of cases have an active catecholamine pathway. Given these physiologic characteristics, they can be imaged with the radiopharmaceuticals I-123 meta-iodo-benzyl-guanidine (MIBG)—a norepinephrine analog, and the SSTR-targeting agents In-111 DTPA-octreotide (Octreoscan) and Ga-68 DOTATATE (targeting SSTR type 2 and approved by the US Food and Drug Administration in 2016).[52]

SSTR imaging is superior to I-123/I-131 MIBG for paragangliomas in the head and neck. In a study of 29 patients with head and neck paragangliomas, Koopmans and colleagues[53] found a sensitivity of 93% versus 44% and 89% versus 42% for Octreoscan versus MIBG on a per-patient and per-lesion basis, respectively. Data are limited for Ga-68 DOTATATE PET/CT in head and neck paragangliomas, but it does visualize them and has been shown to be superior to CT scans, MR imaging, F-18 DOPA PET/CT scans, and F-18 FDG PET/CT scans (38/38 lesions for

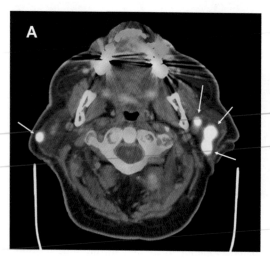
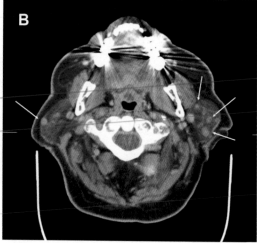

Fig. 5. A 77-year-old man with metastatic melanoma and stable hypermetabolic parotid nodules compatible with Warthin tumors. (*A*) FDG PET/CT fusion imaging showing multiple hypermetabolic parotid nodules (*arrows*). (*B*) CT imaging showing multiple parotid soft tissue nodules (*arrows*).

DOTATATE, 37/38 for DOPA, 27/38 for FDG, and 23/38 for CT/MR imaging).[54,55]

Patients who are germline mutation carriers of succinate dehydrogenase (SDHx) are at risk for later development of paraganglioma and pheochromocytoma. Kong and colleagues[56] retrospectively reviewed 20 SDHx carriers with these tumors who underwent Ga-68 DOTATATE PET/CT scans, and found the modality to have a sensitivity and specificity of 100% and 100%, compared with 85% and 50% for MR imaging/CT scans on a per-patient basis, and 100% and 75% compared with 80% and 25% on a per-lesion basis, as well as resulting in a management change in 40% of patients.

Lu-177 DOTATATE therapy showed strong efficacy in patients with gastroenteropancreatic carcinoid in the NETTER-1 trial, and was approved in 2018 by the US Food and Drug Administration. Several small series have reported on the use of this therapy for head and neck paragangliomas, after confirming expression of SSTR by Ga-68 DOTA PET. Estevao and colleagues reviewed 14 patients treated with 3 cycles of Lu-177 DOTATATE. Ten of the 14 patients showed decreased uptake after treatment; 90% of patients with jugulotympanic paragangliomas had symptomatic improvement or stabilization, and patients with carotid body paragangliomas had a worse response to the treatment.[57,58]

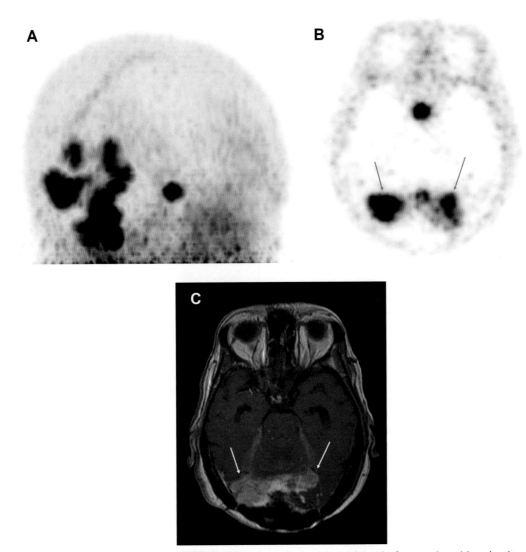

Fig. 6. An 80-year-old woman with grade II occipital meningioma complained of worsening vision despite surgery and radiotherapy. (*A*) Three-dimensional and (*B*) axial Ga-68 DOTATATE PET (*arrows*) and (*C*) post-contrast MRI (*arrows*) showed tracer-avid enhancing dural-based masses, consistent with somatostatin receptor-positive meningioma. Based on these findings, she started octreotide therapy and improved clinically.

Meningiomas are the most common intracranial tumor and usually are treated with surgery and radiotherapy if high grade. Although meningiomas are not commonly thought of as neuroendocrine tumors, they highly express SSTR type 2 and may be imaged with somatostatin scintigraphy. Compared with standard MR imaging, SSTR PET scans may add valuable additional diagnostic information in these patients, particularly in the differential diagnosis of newly diagnosed brain lesions suspicious for meningiomas, delineation of meningioma extent for resection or radiotherapy planning, and the differentiation of tumor progression from a post-treatment change.

Ivanidze and colleagues[59] reported on 20 patients with biopsy-confirmed meningioma who had undergone surgery or radiation. Ga-68 DOTA-TATE PET/MR imaging was able to identify 49 meningiomas and differentiate them from post-treatment change based on a higher maximum standardized uptake value (17 vs 1.7; $P<.0001$) (Fig. 6).

SUMMARY

I-131 ablative therapy remains a critical tool in the treatment of benign and malignant thyroid disease, and there is a trend to decreasing dose for certain subsets of patients, although recent data have shown an increased rate of secondary cancers with this therapy. This risk needs to be weighed against the benefit of treating potentially fatal hyperthyroid symptoms and adequately addressing thyroid cancer, which may become iodine negative and refractory if not treated fully. Parathyroid scintigraphy remains a valuable adjunct to a multimodality preoperative workup, with superior performance promised by radiolabeled choline tracers. SSTR-targeted diagnostic imaging and therapy (i.e., "Theranostics") is an exciting recent development. With a much higher binding affinity to SSTR type 2 than In-111 Octreoscan, Ga-68 DOTATATE PET/CT scans have a high sensitivity and specificity. Along with Lu-177 DOTATATE, its beta-emitting cousin, a new era in diagnosis and therapy of neuroendocrine tumors in the head and neck has arrived.

DISCLOSURE

None.

REFERENCES

1. Bonnema SJ, Hegedus L. Radioiodine therapy in benign thyroid diseases: effects, side effects, and factors affecting therapeutic outcome. Endocr Rev 2012;33:920–80.
2. Nilsson M, Fagman H. Development of the thyroid gland. Development 2017;144:2123–40.
3. Siegel RD, Lee SL. Toxic nodular goiter. Toxic adenoma and toxic multinodular goiter. Endocrinol Metab Clin North Am 1998;27:151–68.
4. Sarkar SD. Benign thyroid disease: what is the role of nuclear medicine? Semin Nucl Med 2006;36:185–93.
5. Mittra ES, Niederkohr RD, Rodriguez C, et al. Uncommon causes of thyrotoxicosis. J Nucl Med 2008;49:265–78.
6. de Rooij A, Vandenbroucke JP, Smit JW, et al. Clinical outcomes after estimated versus calculated activity of radioiodine for the treatment of hyperthyroidism: systematic review and meta-analysis. Eur J Endocrinol 2009;161:771–7.
7. Ma C, Xie J, Wang H, et al. Radioiodine therapy versus antithyroid medications for graves' disease. Cochrane Database Syst Rev 2016;(2):CD010094.
8. Thou S, Vinjamuri S. The relationship between thyroid eye disease and radioiodine treatment. Nucl Med Commun 2019;40:194–8.
9. Achong DM. Clinical significance of a solitary cold thyroid nodule in the setting of graves disease. Clin Nucl Med 2018;43:e27–8.
10. Fast S, Nielsen VE, Bonnema SJ, et al. Time to reconsider nonsurgical therapy of benign non-toxic multinodular goitre: focus on recombinant human TSH augmented radioiodine therapy. Eur J Endocrinol 2009;160:517–28.
11. Kitahara CM, Berrington de Gonzalez A, Bouville A, et al. Association of radioactive iodine treatment with cancer mortality in patients with hyperthyroidism. JAMA Intern Med 2019;179(8):1034–42.
12. Cone L, Oates E, Vazquez R. Congenital hypothyroidism: diagnostic scintigraphic evaluation of an organification defect. Clin Nucl Med 1988;13:419–20.
13. Mayson SE, Yoo DC, Gopalakrishnan G. The evolving use of radioiodine therapy in differentiated thyroid cancer. Oncology 2015;88:247–56.
14. Haugen BR, Alexander EK, Bible KC, et al. 2015 American Thyroid Association management guidelines for adult patients with thyroid nodules and differentiated thyroid cancer: the American Thyroid Association guidelines task force on thyroid nodules and differentiated thyroid cancer. Thyroid 2016;26:1–133.
15. Iyer NG, Morris LG, Tuttle RM, et al. Rising incidence of second cancers in patients with low-risk (T1N0) thyroid cancer who receive radioactive iodine therapy. Cancer 2011;117:4439–46.
16. Tuttle RM, Ahuja S, Avram AM, et al. Controversies, consensus, and collaboration in the use of (131)I therapy in differentiated thyroid cancer: a joint statement from the American Thyroid Association, the European Association of Nuclear Medicine, the Society of Nuclear Medicine and Molecular Imaging, and the

European Thyroid Association. Thyroid 2019;29: 461–70.

17. Van Nostrand D, Aiken M, Atkins F, et al. The utility of radioiodine scans prior to iodine 131 ablation in patients with well-differentiated thyroid cancer. Thyroid 2009;19:849–55.

18. Chen MK, Yasrebi M, Samii J, et al. The utility of I-123 pretherapy scan in I-131 radioiodine therapy for thyroid cancer. Thyroid 2012;22:304–9.

19. Lee SW. SPECT/CT in the treatment of differentiated thyroid cancer. Nucl Med Mol Imaging 2017;51: 297–303.

20. Menzel C, Kranert WT, Dobert N, et al. RhTSH stimulation before radioiodine therapy in thyroid cancer reduces the effective half-life of (131)I. J Nucl Med 2003;44:1065–8.

21. Freudenberg LS, Jentzen W, Petrich T, et al. Lesion dose in differentiated thyroid carcinoma metastases after rhTSH or thyroid hormone withdrawal: 124I PET/CT dosimetric comparisons. Eur J Nucl Med Mol Imaging 2010;37:2267–76.

22. Van Nostrand D, Khorjekar GR, O'Neil J, et al. Recombinant human thyroid-stimulating hormone versus thyroid hormone withdrawal in the identification of metastasis in differentiated thyroid cancer with 131I planar whole-body imaging and 124I PET. J Nucl Med 2012;53:359–62.

23. Kreissl MC, Janssen MJR, Nagarajah J. Current treatment strategies in metastasized differentiated thyroid cancer. J Nucl Med 2019;60:9–15.

24. Nagarajah J, Janssen M, Hetkamp P, et al. Iodine symporter targeting with (124)I/(131)I theranostics. J Nucl Med 2017;58:34S–8S.

25. Howard BA, James OG, Perkins JM, et al. A practical method of i-131 thyroid cancer therapy dose optimization using estimated effective renal clearance. SAGE Open Med Case Rep 2017;5. 2050313X17745203.

26. Sgouros G, Song H, Ladenson PW, et al. Lung toxicity in radioiodine therapy of thyroid carcinoma: development of a dose-rate method and dosimetric implications of the 80-mCi rule. J Nucl Med 2006;47: 1977–84.

27. Stabin MG, Sparks RB, Crowe E. Olinda/exm: the second-generation personal computer software for internal dose assessment in nuclear medicine. J Nucl Med 2005;46:1023–7.

28. Ylli D, Van Nostrand D, Wartofsky L. Conventional radioiodine therapy for differentiated thyroid cancer. Endocrinol Metab Clin North Am 2019;48: 181–97.

29. Lauridsen JK, Rohde M, Thomassen A. 18F–fluorodeoxyglucose-positron emission tomography/ computed tomography in malignancies of the thyroid and in head and neck squamous cell carcinoma: a review of the literature. PET Clin 2015;10: 75–88.

30. Nayan S, Ramakrishna J, Gupta MK. The proportion of malignancy in incidental thyroid lesions on 18-FDG PET study: a systematic review and meta-analysis. Otolaryngol Head Neck Surg 2014;151: 190–200.

31. Liddy S, Worsley D, Torreggiani W, et al. Preoperative imaging in primary hyperparathyroidism: Literature review and recommendations. Can Assoc Radiol J 2017;68:47–55.

32. Kettle AG, O'Doherty MJ. Parathyroid imaging: how good is it and how should it be done? Semin Nucl Med 2006;36:206–11.

33. Agrawal K, Esmail AA, Gnanasegaran G, et al. Pitfalls and limitations of radionuclide imaging in endocrinology. Semin Nucl Med 2015;45:440–57.

34. Lee JH, Anzai Y. Imaging of thyroid and parathyroid glands. Semin Roentgenol 2013;48:87–104.

35. Greenspan BS, Dillehay G, Intenzo C, et al. SNM practice guideline for parathyroid scintigraphy 4.0. J Nucl Med Technol 2012;40:111–8.

36. Bunch PM, Kelly HR. Preoperative imaging techniques in primary hyperparathyroidism: a review. JAMA Otolaryngol Head Neck Surg 2018;144: 929–37.

37. Smith JR, Oates ME. Radionuclide imaging of the parathyroid glands: patterns, pearls, and pitfalls. Radiographics 2004;24:1101–15.

38. Eslamy HK, Ziessman HA. Parathyroid scintigraphy in patients with primary hyperparathyroidism: 99mTc sestamibi SPECT and SPECT/CT. Radiographics 2008;28:1461–76.

39. Treglia G, Sadeghi R, Schalin-Jantti C, et al. Detection rate of (99m) Tc-mibi single photon emission computed tomography (SPECT)/CT in preoperative planning for patients with primary hyperparathyroidism: a meta-analysis. Head Neck 2016;38(Suppl 1): E2159–72.

40. Lavely WC, Goetze S, Friedman KP, et al. Comparison of SPECT/CT, SPECT, and planar imaging with single- and dual-phase (99m)Tc-sestamibi parathyroid scintigraphy. J Nucl Med 2007;48:1084–9.

41. Chien D, Jacene H. Imaging of parathyroid glands. Otolaryngol Clin North Am 2010;43:399–415, x.

42. Wein RO, Weber RS. Parathyroid surgery: what the radiologists need to know. Neuroimaging Clin N Am 2008;18:551–8, ix.

43. Mariani G, Gulec SA, Rubello D, et al. Preoperative localization and radioguided parathyroid surgery. J Nucl Med 2003;44:1443–58.

44. Ikeda Y, Takayama J, Takami H. Minimally invasive radioguided parathyroidectomy for hyperparathyroidism. Ann Nucl Med 2010;24:233–40.

45. Judson BL, Shaha AR. Nuclear imaging and minimally invasive surgery in the management of hyperparathyroidism. J Nucl Med 2008;49:1813–8.

46. Lezaic L, Rep S, Sever MJ, et al. 18F-fluorocholine PET/CT for localization of hyperfunctioning

parathyroid tissue in primary hyperparathyroidism: a
pilot study. Eur J Nucl Med Mol Imaging 2014;41:
2083–9.

47. Michaud L, Burgess A, Huchet V, et al. Is 18F-fluoro-
choline-positron emission tomography/computer-
ized tomography a new imaging tool for detecting
hyperfunctioning parathyroid glands in primary or
secondary hyperparathyroidism? J Clin Endocrinol
Metab 2014;99:4531–6.

48. Michaud L, Balogova S, Burgess A, et al. A pilot
comparison of 18F-fluorocholine PET/CT, ultrasonography and 123I/99mTc-sestamibi dual-phase
dual-isotope scintigraphy in the preoperative localization of hyperfunctioning parathyroid glands in primary or secondary hyperparathyroidism: influence
of thyroid anomalies. Medicine (Baltimore) 2015;
94:e1701.

49. Taieb D, Urena-Torres P, Zanotti-Fregonara P, et al.
Parathyroid scintigraphy in renal hyperparathyroid-
ism: the added diagnostic value of SPECT and
SPECT/CT. Clin Nucl Med 2013;38:630–5.

50. Guzzo M, Locati LD, Prott FJ, et al. Major and minor
salivary gland tumors. Crit Rev Oncol Hematol 2010;
74:134–48.

51. Hadiprodjo D, Ryan T, Truong MT, et al. Parotid
gland tumors: preliminary data for the value of
FDG PET/CT diagnostic parameters. AJR Am J
Roentgenol 2012;198:W185–90.

52. Woolen S, Gemmete JJ. Paragangliomas of the head
and neck. Neuroimaging Clin N Am 2016;26:259–78.

53. Koopmans KP, Jager PL, Kema IP, et al. 111In-oc-
treotide is superior to 123i-metaiodobenzylguani-
dine for scintigraphic detection of head and neck
paragangliomas. J Nucl Med 2008;49:1232–7.

54. Quah RC. Imaging of bilateral neck paragangliomas
with 68Ga-DOTATATE positron-emission tomogra-
phy/CT. AJNR Am J Neuroradiol 2011;32:E71–2.

55. Janssen I, Chen CC, Taieb D, et al. 68Ga-DOTATATE
PET/CT in the localization of head and neck paragangliomas compared with other functional imaging
modalities and CT/MRI. J Nucl Med 2016;57:
186–91.

56. Kong G, Schenberg T, Yates CJ, et al. The role of
68Ga-DOTA–octreotate PET/CT in follow-up of sdh-
associated pheochromocytoma and paraganglioma. J Clin Endocrinol Metab 2019;104:5091–9.

57. Puranik AD, Kulkarni HR, Singh A, et al. Peptide receptor radionuclide therapy with (90)Y/(177)Lu-
labelled peptides for inoperable head and neck paragangliomas (glomus tumours). Eur J Nucl Med Mol
Imaging 2015;42:1223–30.

58. Estevao R, Duarte H, Lopes F, et al. Peptide receptor
radionuclide therapy in head and neck paragangliomas - report of 14 cases. Rev Laryngol Otol Rhinol
(Bord) 2015;136:155–8.

59. Ivanidze J, Roytman M, Lin E, et al. Gallium-68 dotatate PET in the evaluation of intracranial meningiomas. J Neuroimaging 2019;29:650–6.

Multimodality Imaging of Neuroendocrine Tumors

Samuel J. Galgano, MD[a,b,*], Kedar Sharbidre, MD[a], Desiree E. Morgan, MD[a]

KEYWORDS

- Neuroendocrine tumor • DOTATATE • PET • CT • MR imaging • Carcinoid

KEY POINTS

- Neuroendocrine tumors are a heterogeneous group of tumors and knowledge of pathology is essential to selecting the appropriate imaging modality.
- DOTATATE-PET/computed tomography scans offer substantial improvement for systemic staging of well-differentiated neuroendocrine tumors compared with computed tomography scans and MR imaging and offer potential value for theranostic applications.
- Neuroendocrine tumors can occur as part of systemic syndromes, such as multiple endocrine neoplasia, and detection of 1 neoplasm may prompt additional screening for other neuroendocrine neoplasms.

INTRODUCTION

Neuroendocrine tumors (NET) are a rare type of solid tumor with an estimated 12,000 people in the United States diagnosed with a NET each year and approximately 170,000 people living with a NET.[1] In the past several decades, the incidence rate of NETs has continued to increase, with a 6.4-fold increase between 1973 and 2012.[1] This increase is thought to be in part owing to an increased awareness of NETs, but largely attributed to improvements medical imaging and endoscopy (including endoscopic ultrasound). There is a wide spectrum of disease in NETs, ranging from slow-growing and indolent tumors that are incidentally found on imaging for unrelated clinical indications to highly aggressive malignancies with a poor prognosis. Despite the increase in the prevalence and detection of NETs, significant improvements in overall survival have been observed since 2000. In 2018, the US Food and Drug Administration approved a targeted systemic therapy to somatostatin receptor (SSTR)-expressing gastroenteropancreatic NETs (GEP-NETs).[1] The focus of this article is on the evaluation, detection, and staging of the most common types of NETs with multiple imaging modalities, because the information gained with a multimodality approach is often complementary and leads to image-guided treatment decision making at a patient-specific level. Additionally, given the spectrum of pathology in NETs, the article briefly addresses key pathologic issues that guide imaging evaluation in patients with NETs.

IMAGING PROTOCOLS

Computed Tomography Scans and MR Imaging

The current American College of Radiology Appropriateness Criteria for neuroendocrine imaging focuses only on pituitary imaging, which are covered in a different chapter of this book.[2] However, no American College of Radiology Appropriateness Criteria exist to describe appropriate imaging of NETs in the chest, abdomen, and pelvis.

[a] Department of Radiology, Section of Abdominal Imaging, University of Alabama at Birmingham, 619 19th Street South, JT N325, Birmingham, AL 35249, USA; [b] Department of Radiology, Section of Molecular Imaging & Therapeutics, University of Alabama at Birmingham, 619 19th Street South, JT N325, Birmingham, AL 35249, USA
* Corresponding author. Department of Radiology, Section of Abdominal Imaging, University of Alabama at Birmingham, 619 19th Street South, JT N325, Birmingham, AL 35249.
E-mail address: samuelgalgano@uabmc.edu

Radiol Clin N Am 58 (2020) 1147–1159
https://doi.org/10.1016/j.rcl.2020.07.008

Multidetector computed tomography (CT) scanning is widely used in the assessment of pancreatic NETs with detection rates of up to 69% to 94%.[3] On dual phase pancreatic CT protocols used to evaluated suspected pancreatic masses, NETs are typically hypervascular and demonstrate avid enhancement in the arterial phase. This factor is especially important in the diagnosis of liver metastases from NET. Some studies have shown that the contrast enhancement pattern of NETs can correlate with the tumor grade. Cappelli and colleagues[4] showed that tumors with venous and delayed phase enhancement are likely to be high grade compared with tumors with arterial enhancement and venous phase washout. Other findings, such as tumor size, ill-defined tumor margins, pancreatic duct dilation, and vascular invasion, have also been found to be significant in predicting grading of tumors. Dual energy CT scans can help to improve the detection of small pancreatic NETs, particularly using low-energy monochromatic and iodine density images.[5] For assessment of small bowel NETs, CT scans and MR enterography protocols are used with unenhanced images, followed by arterial and venous phase acquisitions after distension of the bowel by neutral contrast. Recent studies have shown that CT scans and MR enterography have higher sensitivity (100% and 86%–94%, respectively) and specificity (96.2% and 95%–98%, respectively) for the detection of small bowel neoplasms, including NETs.[6,7]

Owing to its superior soft tissue characterization, MR imaging has an improved detection rate compared with CT, particularly for the characterization of previously indeterminate pancreatic lesions.[8] Additional sequences such as diffusion-weighted imaging and apparent diffusion coefficient mapping can help to localize and potentially grade the tumors.[9–11] MR cholangiopancreatography is useful to evaluate the status of pancreatic duct and biliary system and should be performed for surgical planning.[12] Other focal pancreatic lesions like hypervascular metastasis, intrapancreatic accessory splenule, or serous cystadenoma can be sometimes be confused with NETs, and MR imaging can aid with problem solving in such cases.[13,14]

[68Ga]DOTATATE PET/Computed Tomography Scans and PET/MR Imaging

[68Ga]DOTATATE was approved in 2016 for the localization of SSTR-positive NETs in adult and pediatric patients.[15] Once injected, DOTATATE binds to SSTRs on the cell surface, with highest affinity for the SSTR2 receptor.[16] Clinically, [68Ga]

DOTATATE-PET/CT is rapidly becoming the standard of care in the evaluation of NET, owing to its superior sensitivity and specificity for detection of metastatic disease when compared with [111In] pentetreotide scintigraphy.[17] Frequently, the findings from a [68Ga]DOTATATE-PET/CT are complementary to CT and MR imaging, which offer higher spatial resolution and aid in surgical planning and decision-making. As peptide receptor radionuclide therapy (PRRT) with [177Lu]DOTATATE becomes increasingly available and offered to patients, [68Ga]DOTATATE-PET/CT is essential to assess patient eligibility before PRRT. Finally, as the emerging hybrid imaging modality PET/MR imaging becomes increasingly available, [68Ga] DOTATATE-PET/MR imaging allows for synchronous acquisition of both PET and MR imaging data with excellent anatomic co-registration and may allow for simultaneous assessment of metastatic disease using both [68Ga]DOTATATE-PET and diagnostic contrast-enhanced MR imaging of the abdomen (**Fig. 1**).

[68Ga]DOTATATE-PET scans require preparation of the radiopharmaceutical before injection into the patient. The radionuclide [68Ga] is eluted from a [68Ge] generator and has a half-life of 68 minutes, which somewhat limits its ability to be commercially distributed compared with [18F], which has a half-life of 110 minutes. The recommended dose of [68Ga]DOTATATE is 2 MBq/kg (0.054 mCi/kg) up to 200 MBq (5.4 mCi). Patients are instructed to be well-hydrated before performance of the PET scan and are advised to void frequently after injection of radiotracer to decrease radiation exposure. Approximately 40 to 90 minutes following injection of [68Ga]DOTATATE, patients can be scanned with a typical field-of-view from skull base to the mid thigh.

[111In]Pentetreotide Scintigraphy

Before the approval of [68Ga]DOTATATE for imaging of NETs, [111In]pentetreotide (Octreoscan; Covidien Inc., Dublin, Ireland) was the standard of care for molecular imaging of NETs.[18] The mechanism of action of pentetreotide is the binding of SSTRs at the cell surface, albeit with a lower affinity than [68Ga]DOTATATE. Additionally, owing to the gamma emission of 171 keV and 245 keV photons from [111In] during its decay, imaging is limited to planar and single photon emission CT (SPECT) or SPECT/CT images on a gamma camera. The half-life of [111In] is 2.8 days, and images obtained during [111In]pentetreotide scintigraphy are routinely acquired at 24 hours after injection, with optional imaging at 4 and 48 hours after injection. This nature leads to patients having to return

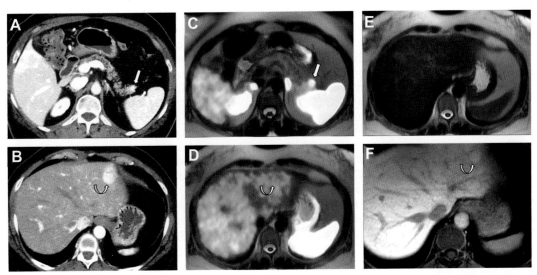

Fig. 1. Patient with suspected pancreatic tail NET on contrast-enhanced portal venous phase CT scan (A) and possible hepatic metastasis on contrast-enhanced arterial-phase CT scan (B). Subsequent [68Ga]DOTATATE-PET/MR imaging shows focal activity (arrow) in the pancreatic tail NET (C) and no activity in the suspected liver metastasis (curved arrow) (D). Corresponding T2-weighted (E) and hepatobiliary phase T1-weighted postcontrast MR images (F) demonstrate no increased T2 signal in the liver lesion, which demonstrates hepatobiliary phase contrast retention (curved arrow), consistent with focal nodular hyperplasia.

to the nuclear medicine department multiple times, which is a significant drawback when compared with [68Ga]DOTATATE-PET/CT. Although an important historical radiotracer that provided key diagnostic information about NETs, current use of [111In]pentetreotide is limited to practice settings with limited or no access to [68Ga]DOTATATE and has been shown to be an inferior molecular imaging agent.[17]

PATHOLOGY AND IMAGING CONSIDERATIONS
Variable Somatostatin Receptor Expression Among Neuroendocrine Tumors

It is well-known that NETs are a heterogeneous group of tumors and that certain NETs overexpress different SSTR subtypes at the cell surface.[19–21] Historically, [111In]pentetreotide scintigraphy preferentially localized to the SSTR2 and SSTR5 receptors, which are upregulated in pheochromocytomas, gastrinomas, glucagonomas, and nonfunctional GEP-NETs. However, both insulinomas and medullary thyroid cancer demonstrate variable levels of SSTR expression, particularly the SSTR2 receptor.[22,23] As a result, studies of [111In]pentetreotide scintigraphy demonstrated low sensitivity for the detection of medullary thyroid cancer and insulinomas.[24–26] [68Ga]DOTATATE-PET/CT scanning has demonstrated significant improvement in detection of insulinomas owing to the higher cell receptor

binding and spatial resolution of the PET radiotracer.[27] Thus, when performing a molecular imaging study to evaluate for either primary or metastatic NET, it is essential that the interpreting physician know the suspected pathology of the tumor and the potential limitations of the examination, particularly if performing [111In]pentetreotide scintigraphy. Additionally, certain NETs (such as gastrinoma) occur in characteristic anatomic locations (eg, the gastrinoma triangle), and providing this information to the interpreting physician can allow for greater scrutiny of the scan in the areas of concern.

Neuroendocrine Tumor Differentiation and Choice of Molecular Imaging Agent

Another key pathologic consideration in molecular imaging of NETs is the degree of pathologic differentiation, because it may influence the choice of molecular imaging agent. NETs are classified by the 2017 World Health Organization into 3 pathologic grades (G1–G3) on the basis of the number of mitoses seen on high-powered microscopy, the Ki-67 index, and the presence or absence of tumor necrosis and apoptosis.[28] As an example, G1 NETs are well-differentiated with extremely low Ki-67 (<3%), low number of mitoses, and rare tumor necrosis. The 2017 World Health Organization criteria also introduced a separate subtype of poorly differentiated neuroendocrine carcinoma, which also has large cell and small cell variants, and renamed mixed neuroendocrine or non-neuroendocrine neoplasms.[29] In regard to the selection of PET radiotracers, knowledge of the pathology is paramount, because more aggressive tumors may be better imaged with PET scanning with [^{18}F]fluorodeoxyglucose (FDG-PET)/CT scanning rather than [^{68}Ga]DOTA-TATE-PET/CT, owing to their more aggressive cellular behavior and poor differentiation, which together result in decreased expression of SSTRs at the cell surface. In cases of G2 NETs, both [^{18}F]FDG-PET/CT scans and [^{68}Ga]DOTATATE-PET/CT scans may be performed before therapeutic intervention, as differential uptake on these 2 examinations may influence therapeutic management between PRRT, systemic chemotherapy, and/or surgery. Thus, interpreting physicians should take caution when interpreting [^{68}Ga]DOTATATE-PET/CT without pathologic data, because low expression in a known NET or suspected metastasis could represent a poorly differentiated NET and may require a [^{18}F]FDG-PET/CT for adequate staging (**Fig. 2**).

GASTROENTEROPANCREATIC NEUROENDOCRINE TUMORS

The gastrointestinal tract and pancreas are the most common locations (about 70%) for NETs.[30] GEP-NETs account for about 1.5% to 2.0% of all primary gastrointestinal and pancreatic neoplasms, and their incidence in the United States is estimated at 3.56 per 100,000 population.[1] The majority of these cases are sporadic, and a small percentage occur in patients with genetic syndromes such as multiple endocrine neoplasia type 1 (MEN-1), neurofibromatosis type 1, Von Hippel-Lindau disease, and tuberous sclerosis complex.

Pancreatic NETs account for about 1% to 2% of all pancreatic neoplasms with an incidence of less than 1%, al though increasing over the last 20 to 30 years.[31] Functioning pancreatic NETs are diagnosed earlier because of the symptoms, but are less common (10%–30%) than nonfunctioning tumors. Among functional NETs, insulinomas are the most common tumors, followed by gastrinomas.[32] The nonfunctioning tumors produce nonspecific symptoms. Because of slow growth and late detection, these tumors can have an advanced stage when diagnosed.[33,34] In patients with functioning NETs, laboratory analyses of the specific hormone levels are often diagnostic and can be tested in urine or serum. Chromogranin A is the most commonly used serum marker for diagnosis and is found to be elevated in 60% to 80% patients.[13,35]

The gastrointestinal tract is the most common site of NETs (67%); the distal part of the ileum being the most common location.[36] The majority of ileal NETs are hormonally inactive and can present as vague abdominal pain, gastrointestinal bleeding, or bowel obstruction. Classic carcinoid syndrome (diarrhea, tachycardia, hot flushes, and skin reddening) is seen in 6% to 30% of patients and more commonly occurs (about 95% of cases) with hepatic metastasis.[35] Gastric NETs are rare and account for approximately 0.3% of gastric tumors. Three distinct types of gastric NETs have been described, of which type I and II are asymptomatic and generally manifest as multiple small polyps in gastric fundus and body, incidentally diagnosed on endoscopy[37] (**Fig. 3**). Type III gastric NETs demonstrate marked enhancement and can have an infiltrative appearance on imaging. Duodenal NETs are most commonly gastrinomas, and one-third of these tumors develop Zollinger-Ellison syndrome owing to excess gastrin

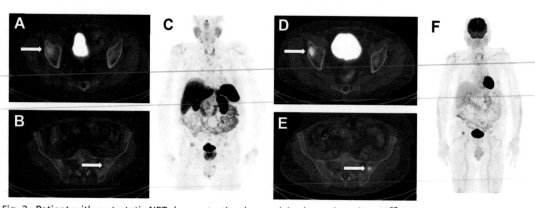

Fig. 2. Patient with metastatic NET demonstrating low activity (*arrow*) on fused [^{68}Ga]DOTATATE-PET/CT images (*A, B*) and maximum intensity projection image (*C*). Subsequent [^{18}F]FDG-PET/CT images (*D–F*) demonstrate substantially higher FDG activity (*arrow*) than [^{68}Ga]DOTATATE-PET/CT, indicating poorly differentiated histology.

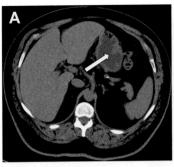
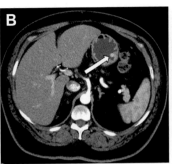
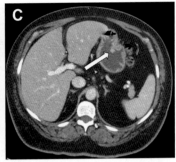

Fig. 3. CT images in noncontrast (A), arterial (B), and portal venous (C) phases demonstrate a small enhancing polyp in the stomach (arrow), subsequently biopsied and found to represent gastric NET.

secretion. Multiple gastrinomas are more commonly seen in patients with MEN-1 syndrome.

Functioning NETs are usually smaller in size (1–2 cm), well-defined, and hypervascular (Fig. 4). Insulinomas are typically solitary and smaller compared with other functioning NETs. Gastrinomas are located in the gastrinoma triangle, which is bounded by the cystic duct junction with the common bile duct, the pancreatic neck, and the junction of the second and third portions of the duodenum; 60% tumors found in pancreas, and remainder are seen in duodenum or peripancreatic lymph nodes. Those within the duodenum are usually multiple, subcentimeter in size, and better detected by endoscopic ultrasound imaging rather than CT scans or MR imaging.

Nonfunctioning NETs are usually larger in size, may be symptomatic owing to the mass effect, have encapsulated margins, and show heterogeneous enhancement, often characterized by areas of cystic degeneration, necrosis, or sometimes fibrosis (Fig. 5). Cystic degenerated NETs are seen in up to 17% of cases, and more commonly in patients with MEN-1 syndrome. The presence of a hypervascular rim on CT scanning or MR imaging can help to suggest the diagnosis compared with other cystic pancreatic masses.[38] Both functioning and nonfunctioning NETs very rarely involve the main pancreatic duct to cause duct

dilation, a finding commonly seen in patients with pancreatic adenocarcinoma. Pancreatic NETs usually metastasize to liver and regional lymph nodes, whereas locally invasive tumors can extend into the retroperitoneum.

On CT scans and MR imaging, small bowel NETs may present as polypoid hypervascular masses or focal concentric bowel wall thickening. More often, NETs are diagnosed by detection of a mesenteric mass with a surrounding desmoplastic reaction owing to local effects of serotonin. Smaller NETs of the small bowel are difficult to diagnose and may present with only metastatic disease. Appendiceal NETs are incidentally discovered during appendicectomy in 70% cases, have a favorable prognosis compared with other NETs, and metastasize less frequently. As with other GEP-NETs, appendiceal NETs are seen as small arterial hyperenhancing lesions on CT scans and MR imaging and are typically located in the appendiceal tip. Uncommonly, NETs may arise in the colon and rectum, accounting for about 11% of all GEP-NETs.[36] The majority of these tumors are incidentally detected on colonoscopy, but occasionally patients may present with gastrointestinal bleeding and pain.

Nodal staging of NETs is usually performed by CT scan, MR imaging, or PET imaging. Like the primary lesions, nodal metastases are also typically

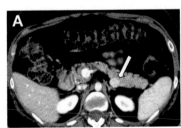
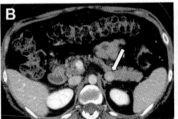
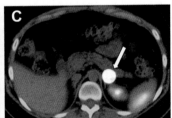

Fig. 4. CT images in arterial (A) and portal venous (B) phases demonstrate a small well-circumscribed avidly enhancing mass in the pancreatic tail (arrow), likely a NET. Fused image from subsequent [68Ga]DOTATATE-PET/CT (C) demonstrates avid tracer activity in the lesion, consistent with pancreatic NETs.

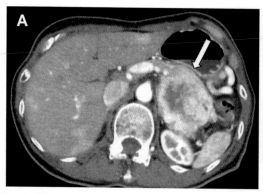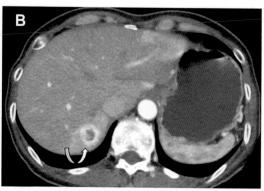

Fig. 5. CT images in the arterial phase demonstrate a large heterogeneous enhancing mass (*arrow*) arising from the pancreatic tail (*A*) with a similar appearing metastatic lesion (*curved arrow*) in the liver (*B*). Subsequent biopsy confirmed nonfunctional metastatic pancreatic NETs.

hypervascular and more conspicuous on arterial phase. Liver metastases are also typically hypervascular in arterial phase; lesions with hypoenhancement in all phases suggest a poor prognosis.[39] MR imaging is a more sensitive modality compared with CT scans for the detection of NET liver metastases. Dynamic contrast-enhanced MR imaging, in particular using gadoxetic acid and diffusion-weighted imaging, is helpful in increasing diagnostic confidence for liver metastasis detection.

Somatostatin receptor imaging has long been a part of the diagnosis and staging for GEP-NETs. The initial experience with [111In]pentetreotide demonstrated a similar sensitivity, specificity, and accuracy between helical CT scans and somatostatin receptor scintigraphy.[40] The performance of [111In]pentetreotide somatostatin receptor scintigraphy is increased when performed as an SPECT/CT scans compared with SPECT scans or planar scintigraphy alone.[41] However, given advances in CT scans and MR imaging technology and acquisition techniques, CT scanning and MR imaging now perform better than [111In]pentetreotide, and the use of somatostatin receptor scintigraphy should be limited to cases in which disease is occult on CT or MR imaging.[42] More recently, US Food and Drug Administration approval of [68Ga]DOTATATE and [177Lu]DOTATATE has substantially altered the imaging diagnosis, management, and treatment of GEP-NETs. Multiple studies have shown superior performance of [68Ga]DOTATATE-PET/CT scans compared with [111In]pentetreotide somatostatin receptor scintigraphy, resulting in changes in treatment plans in up to 36% of patients who underwent both scans.[17,43,44] Given the superior performance of [68Ga]DOTATATE-PET/CT scans among molecular imaging agents and the potential for targeted

molecular therapy with [177Lu]DOTATATE PRRT, this approach is the current favored method of systemic staging for patients with NETs before treatment.

LUNG AND THYMIC CARCINOID TUMORS

Lung carcinoid tumors account for approximately 1% to 2% of all lung cancers, with approximately 2000 to 4500 newly diagnosed cases in the United States each year.[45] Lung carcinoid tumors are classified as typical or atypical, with typical lung carcinoid tumors arising in slightly younger patients (the average age at diagnosis is 45 years).[45] Lung carcinoid tumors are generally classified as well-differentiated NETs and are often slow growing with a benign clinical courses.[45–47] Frequently, lung carcinoid tumors are endobronchial lesions that present with symptoms of cough, hemoptysis, or pneumonia secondary to bronchial obstruction from the lesion.[46] Thymic carcinoid tumors (also referred to as NETs of the thymus) are rare tumors, accounting for only 2% to 5% of thymic tumors and 0.4% of all carcinoid tumors, with an estimated incidence of 0.2 per million in the United States.[48,49] Thymic NETs are associated with the genetic syndrome MEN-1. Thymic carcinoid tumors have heterogeneous clinical behaviors and pathologic appearances, ranging from asymptomatic and nonaggressive to symptomatic and highly aggressive.[50] If symptomatic, patients often present secondary to symptoms of mass effect or invasion of the mediastinal structures; carcinoid syndrome is an uncommon clinical presentation.[46,51] Interestingly, up to 50% of patients with thymic carcinoid tumors have hormonal abnormalities, the most frequent being Cushing syndrome secondary to primary tumoral secretion of adenocorticotropic hormone.[52] Up to 30% of patients with thymic carcinoid present with advanced-stage disease, much higher than lung carcinoid tumors.

Given the general benign course of many lung carcinoid tumors, these lesions are frequently incidentally detected on CT scans of the chest performed for other reasons. Approximately 60% to 70% of lung carcinoids arise in the central airways and involve the main, lobar, or segmental bronchi.[46] These centrally located tumors are more frequently typical carcinoid tumors, but the imaging features of both typical and atypical lung carcinoid tumors overlap and are too similar for confident differentiation on CT scan. Chest radiography often shows a well-defined hilar or perihilar mass with or without the presence of distal airspace disease. When carcinoid tumors arise distal to the segmental bronchi in the lung, these are termed peripheral carcinoids and are more frequently atypical on histology.[46] These carcinoid tumors are typically appear as a well-circumscribed slightly lobulated spherical or ovoid nodule or mass with the long axis parallel to adjacent bronchi or pulmonary artery branches. On CT scans, up to 30% of lung carcinoid tumors demonstrate punctate or diffuse calcifications and may demonstrate avid vascularity and internal enhancement. For endobronchial carcinoid tumors, evaluation with thin section CT chest scanning is useful to establish the relationship between the lesion and the bronchi, and can aid in directing bronchoscopic evaluation and biopsy (Fig. 6). Mediastinal and hilar adenopathy is a common finding on CT scans and may be reactive secondary to recurrent pneumonia versus lymph node metastases, the latter being more common with atypical carcinoids.[53,54] Thymic carcinoids arise in the anterior mediastinum and on CT scanning may mimic a thymoma.[55] The appearance of thymic carcinoid is overall nonspecific, but these masses tend to be large, ranging from 6 to 20 cm, and demonstrate heterogeneous enhancement and locally aggressive features.[56] Scattered calcifications may be present within thymic carcinoids.[57] MR imaging is seldom used for the evaluation of pulmonary nodules and masses, but may

be used in the evaluation of mediastinal or thymic lesions to assist in the characterization of the internal components. Small case series report that primary thymic NETs are isointense to mildly hyperintense to skeletal muscle on T1-weighted images and heterogeneously T2 hyperintense.[57]

Historically, carcinoid tumors of the lung have been evaluated with several types of radiotracers, including [^{111}In]pentetreotide, [^{18}F]FDG, and most recently [^{68}Ga]DOTATATE. A study comparing the performance of [^{111}In]pentetreotide SPECT/CT scans with contrast-enhanced CT scans demonstrated increased sensitivity (96.0% vs 87.5%, respectively) with slightly less specificity (92% vs 97%, respectively) for detection of the primary lesion or recurrent disease.[58] As with other radiotracers imaged with SPECT/CT scans, a known limitation of the imaging modality is decreased spatial resolution when compared with a standard diagnostic contrast-enhanced CT scan. [^{111}In]Pentetreotide has been studied in evaluation of thymic tumors, many of which demonstrate increased SSTR expression. Although [^{111}In]pentetreotide is able to accurately exclude a diagnosis of thymic hyperplasia, it is unable to differentiate between other thymic tumors owing to overexpression of SSTRs.[59] An [^{18}F] FDG-PET/CT scan is a frequently performed examination during the initial evaluation of solid pulmonary nodules and for staging of known lung cancer. Given the difficulty differentiating lung carcinoid tumors from other etiologies of pulmonary nodules, there are frequently initially evaluated with [^{18}F]FDG-PET/CT. Although typical lung carcinoid tumors have less FDG uptake than other lung malignancies, atypical lung carcinoid tumors frequently demonstrate marked FDG uptake and seem to be similar to other primary lung malignancies[60–62] (Fig. 7). Neuroendocrine neoplasms, including lung carcinoids, which demonstrate high metabolic tumor volume on [^{18}F]FDG-PET/CT scans are associated with poor survival given their more aggressive histologic features.[63] [^{68}Ga]DOTATATE-PET/CT scans (and other DOTA-peptide PET/CT imaging) has shown promising results for lung carcinoid tumors, particularly

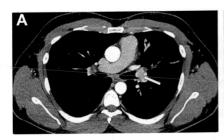
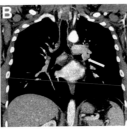

Fig. 6. Axial (A) and coronal (B) contrast-enhanced CT images of the chest demonstrate an avidly enhancing endobronchial lesion in the left mainstem bronchus (arrow), consistent with a lung carcinoid.

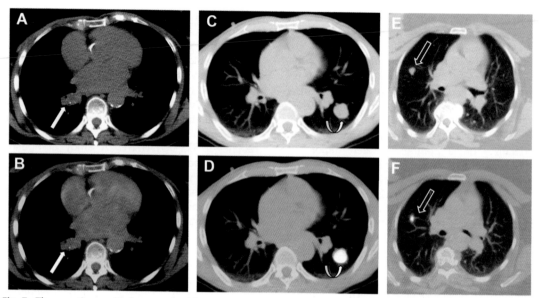

Fig. 7. Three patients with lung carcinoid tumors. Axial CT (*A*) and fused [^{18}F]FDG-PET/CT (*B*) images demonstrate a right-sided endobronchial lesion (*arrow*) with calcifications and low FDG uptake, biopsy-proven to represent a typical lung carcinoid. Axial CT (*C*) and fused [^{68}Ga]DOTATATE-PET/CT (*D*) images from a different patient demonstrate a well-circumscribed left nodule (*curved arrow*) with very high tracer activity, consistent with a typical lung carcinoid. Axial CT (*E*) and fused [^{18}F]FDG-PET/CT (*F*) images from a third patient demonstrate increased tracer activity in a peripheral right lung nodule (*open arrow*), which was subsequently biopsied and found to represent an atypical lung carcinoid.

typical carcinoids[17] (see **Fig. 7**). [^{68}Ga]DOTATATE-PET/CT scanning has been shown to have superior diagnostic performance when compared with [^{18}F]FDG-PET/CT scans in the evaluation of typical pulmonary carcinoid, while an [^{18}F]FDG-PET/CT scan is superior in the evaluation of atypical pulmonary carcinoid.[60,64] Thus, in the initial molecular imaging evaluation of patients with lung carcinoid tumors of unknown histology, both [^{18}F]FDG and [^{68}Ga]DOTATATE imaging can be performed for a comprehensive initial evaluation; knowledge of pathologic findings is key to determining which radiotracer is more suitable for both initial staging and follow-up PET/CT examinations.

PHEOCHROMOCYTOMA AND PARAGANGLIOMA

Paragangliomas and pheochromocytomas are rare neuroendocrine neoplasms with a combined estimated annual incidence of approximately 0.8 per 100,000 person-years; between 500 and 1600 cases are diagnosed in the United States each year.[65,66] However, given the nonfunctional behavior of many paragangliomas, autopsy series suggest that the prevalence may be higher than reported owing to undiagnosed tumors.[67] Many paragangliomas are diagnosed in the third to fifth decades with a mean age of diagnosis of

47 years.[68] Paragangliomas are associated with the genetic syndromes MEN 2A and 2B, neurofibromatosis type, hereditary paraganglioma-pheochromocytoma syndrome, and von Hippel Lindau disease (**Fig. 8**). In these patients with a genetic predisposition to develop paragangliomas and pheochromocytomas, the mean age of diagnosis is younger than those diagnosed with sporadic paragangliomas. These tumors may arise from either the sympathetic or parasympathetic paraganglia in the head, neck, skull base, adrenal gland, or along the abdominopelvic sympathetic chain. These lesions may be nonsecretory or secrete catecholamines (commonly referred to as pheochromocytomas), and they are classified by the World Health Organization (2004) by anatomic site of origin, regardless of secretory status. When secretory, catecholamine-secreting paragangliomas present with severe hypertension and other symptoms related to excess catecholamine. However, the vast majority of paragangliomas are nonsecretory and are either incidentally discovered or produce symptoms secondary to local mass effect, particularly in the head, neck, and skull base. Approximately 26% of paragangliomas are multiple (more common in hereditary cases), 15% to 20% are extra-adrenal, and 33% to 50% are associated with a hereditary syndrome.[69] Rates of malignant paragangliomas vary by

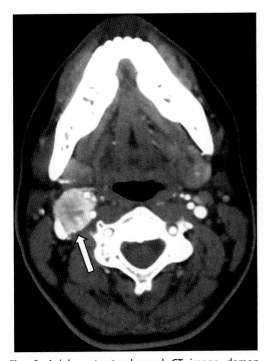

Fig. 8. Axial contrast-enhanced CT image demonstrating an avidly enhancing mass (*arrow*) in the right carotid space with splaying of the internal and external carotid arteries, characteristic of a carotid body paraganglioma. The patient subsequently underwent genetic testing and was found to have hereditary paraganglioma–pheochromocytoma syndrome secondary to a *SDHB* mutation.

anatomic location, with approximately 20% of extra-adrenal secretory paragangliomas being malignant and most skull base and neck paragangliomas being benign.[70,71]

The initial imaging evaluation of pheochromocytomas and paragangliomas may differ based on patient presentation (eg, secretory vs nonsecretory). For patients with nonsecretory paragangliomas, these lesions are often incidentally discovered on CT scans or MR imaging of the abdomen and pelvis performed for alternate reasons. On CT scanning, paragangliomas and pheochromocytomas demonstrate avid contrast enhancement with delayed washout. On MR imaging, paragangliomas and pheochromocytomas demonstrate T1 hypointensity when compared with the liver and adrenal gland and have a characteristic high signal on T2-weighted images. Additionally, MR imaging may also demonstrate the so-called salt and pepper appearance of paragangliomas and pheochromocytomas owing to flow voids within the lesion from high vascularity, superimposed on the avid contrast enhancement[72] (**Fig. 9**). Although CT scans and MR imaging offer superb sensitivity and spatial resolution compared with molecular imaging modalities, they frequently are unable to definitively characterize a mass as a paraganglioma and/or a pheochromocytoma.[73] In such cases, a noninvasive molecular imaging evaluation is often preferred to an invasive percutaneous biopsy of these lesions secondary to concerns of precipitating a hypertensive crisis secondary to catecholamine

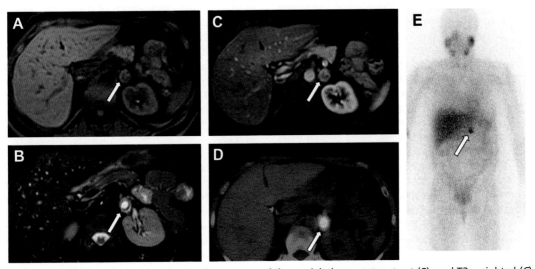

Fig. 9. Axial MR imaging with T1-weighted precontrast (*A*), arterial phase postcontrast (*B*), and T2-weighted (*C*) images demonstrate a T2 hyperintense enhancing left adrenal mass (*arrows*), which demonstrated marked activity of both SPECT/CT (*D*) and planar (*E*) images from subsequent [^{123}I]MIBG scan, confirming the diagnosis of pheochromocytoma.

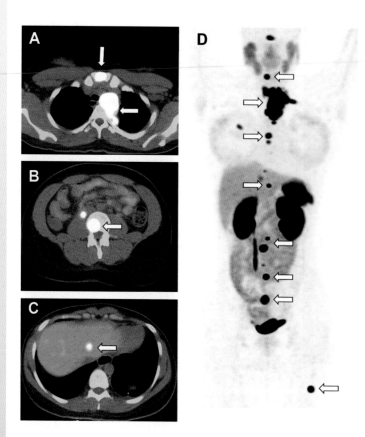

Fig. 10. Axial fused [⁶⁸Ga]DOTATATE-PET/CT (*A–C*) and maximum intensity projection image (*D*) in a patient with metastatic paraganglioma. Metastases (*arrows*) are present in the sternum, upper mediastinal and cervical lymph nodes, spine, liver, right, and left femur.

release during biopsy in a patient with pheochromocytoma who has not undergone periprocedural alpha-blockade.

Molecular imaging has long been the mainstay of noninvasive definitive diagnosis of paragangliomas and pheochromocytomas. For secretory pheochromocytomas, [¹²³I] or [¹³¹I]meta-iodobenzylguanidine (MIBG) is a molecular imaging analog of norepinephrine that targets the presynaptic norepinephrine transporter.[74] This mechanism results in the accumulation of radiotracer in patients with hyperfunctioning lesions. After administration, patients are imaged with both planar gamma cameras and SPECT/CT scans to localize the lesion and any possible metastases. Early clinical trials are evaluating the potential use of therapeutic [¹³¹I]MIBG for the treatment of metastatic and/or recurrent pheochromocytoma or paraganglioma.[75] This theranostic approach could expand utilization of MIBG scans, particularly given that currently [¹⁷⁷Lu]DOTATATE is only approved for use in GEP-NETs. However, for tumors that are nonsecretory, MIBG scans may be limited in their ability to detect and characterize lesions. Alternately, [⁶⁸Ga]DOTATATE-PET/CT scans can be used for imaging owing to overexpression of SSTRs at the cell surface of both

pheochromocytomas and paragangliomas (**Fig. 10**). Although few studies have directly compared MIBG scans with [⁶⁸Ga]DOTATATE-PET/CT, early studies suggest that [⁶⁸Ga]DOTATATE-PET/CT scanning performs similarly in the evaluation and identification of the primary lesion, but superior to [¹³¹I]MIBG and [¹⁸F]FDG-PET/CT scan in the mapping of metastatic lesions.[76–78] [¹⁸F]FDG-PET/CT scanning may also play a role for malignant paragangliomas and the information may be synergistic with findings on [⁶⁸Ga]DOTATATE-PET/CT scans for comprehensive staging and evaluation of patients.

SUMMARY

NETs are a wide spectrum of disease that affect a broad range of organ systems throughout the body. Although varied in location, NETs tend to share common imaging features such as avid contrast enhancement and overexpression of SSTRs. However, malignant NETs may express only some or none of these features, and knowledge of NET pathology before imaging modality selection is important. Thus, imaging of NETs requires both standard anatomic and functional molecular imaging modalities to comprehensively stage patients and make informed treatment decisions. As the roles of PRRT and theranostics expand, other NETs beyond GEP-NETs may be treated in a theranostic approach with both [^{177}Lu]DOTATATE and [^{131}I]MIBG.

DISCLOSURE

The authors have nothing to disclose.

REFERENCES

1. Dasari A, Shen C, Halperin D, et al. Trends in the incidence, prevalence, and survival outcomes in patients with neuroendocrine tumors in the United States. JAMA Oncol 2017;3(10):1335–42.

2. Expert Panel on Neurologic I, Burns J, Policeni B, et al. ACR appropriateness criteria((R)) neuroendocrine imaging. J Am Coll Radiol 2019;16(5S): S161–73.

3. Sundin A, Vullierme MP, Kaltsas G, et al, Mallorca Consensus Conference Participants European Neuroendocrine Tumor Society. ENETS Consensus guidelines for the standards of care in neuroendocrine tumors: radiological examinations. Neuroendocrinology 2009;90(2):167–83.

4. Cappelli C, Boggi U, Mazzeo S, et al. Contrast enhancement pattern on multidetector CT predicts malignancy in pancreatic endocrine tumours. Eur Radiol 2015;25(3):751–9.

5. George E, Wortman JR, Fulwadhva UP, et al. Dual energy CT applications in pancreatic pathologies. Br J Radiol 2017;90(1080):20170411.

6. Kamaoui I, De-Luca V, Ficarelli S, et al. Value of CT enteroclysis in suspected small-bowel carcinoid tumors. AJR Am J Roentgenol 2010;194(3):629–33.

7. Van Weyenberg SJ, Meijerink MR, Jacobs MA, et al. MR enteroclysis in the diagnosis of small-bowel neoplasms. Radiology 2010;254(3):765–73.

8. Thoeni RF, Mueller-Lisse UG, Chan R, et al. Detection of small, functional islet cell tumors in the pancreas: selection of MR imaging sequences for optimal sensitivity. Radiology 2000;214(2):483–90.

9. Anaye A, Mathieu A, Closset J, et al. Successful preoperative localization of a small pancreatic insulinoma by diffusion-weighted MRI. JOP 2009;10(5): 528–31.

10. Kang BK, Kim JH, Byun JH, et al. Diffusion-weighted MRI: usefulness for differentiating intrapancreatic accessory spleen and small hypervascular neuroendocrine tumor of the pancreas. Acta Radiol 2014; 55(10):1157–65.

11. Jang KM, Kim SH, Lee SJ, et al. The value of gadoxetic acid-enhanced and diffusion-weighted MRI for prediction of grading of pancreatic neuroendocrine tumors. Acta Radiol 2014;55(2):140–8.

12. Caramella C, Dromain C, De Baere T, et al. Endocrine pancreatic tumours: which are the most useful MRI sequences? Eur Radiol 2010;20(11):2618–27.

13. Sahani DV, Bonaffini PA, Fernandez-Del Castillo C, et al. Gastroenteropancreatic neuroendocrine tumors: role of imaging in diagnosis and management. Radiology 2013;266(1):38–61.

14. Tamm EP, Kim EE, Ng CS. Imaging of neuroendocrine tumors. Hematol Oncol Clin North Am 2007; 21(3):409–32, vii.

15. Subramaniam RM, Bradshaw ML, Lewis K, et al. ACR Practice Parameter for the Performance of Gallium-68 DOTATATE PET/CT for Neuroendocrine Tumors. Clin Nucl Med 2018;43(12):899–908.

16. Poeppel TD, Binse I, Petersenn S, et al. 68Ga-DOTATOC versus 68Ga-DOTATATE PET/CT in functional imaging of neuroendocrine tumors. J Nucl Med 2011;52(12):1864–70.

17. Deppen SA, Liu E, Blume JD, et al. Safety and Efficacy of 68Ga-DOTATATE PET/CT for diagnosis, staging, and treatment management of neuroendocrine tumors. J Nucl Med 2016;57(5):708–14.

18. Balon HR, Brown TL, Goldsmith SJ, et al. The SNM practice guideline for somatostatin receptor scintigraphy 2.0. J Nucl Med Technol 2011;39(4):317–24.

19. Portela-Gomes GM, Stridsberg M, Grimelius L, et al. Differential expression of the five somatostatin receptor subtypes in human benign and malignant insulinomas - predominance of receptor subtype 4. Endocr Pathol 2007;18(2):79–85.

20. Herrera-Martinez AD, Gahete MD, Pedraza-Arevalo S, et al. Clinical and functional implication of the components of somatostatin system in gastroenteropancreatic neuroendocrine tumors. Endocrine 2018;59(2):426–37.

21. Leijon H, Remes S, Hagstrom J, et al. Variable somatostatin receptor subtype expression in 151 primary pheochromocytomas and paragangliomas. Hum Pathol 2019;86:66–75.

22. Papotti M, Bongiovanni M, Volante M, et al. Expression of somatostatin receptor types 1-5 in 81 cases of gastrointestinal and pancreatic endocrine tumors. A correlative immunohistochemical and reverse-transcriptase polymerase chain reaction analysis. Virchows Arch 2002;440(5):461–75.

23. Mato E, Matias-Guiu X, Chico A, et al. Somatostatin and somatostatin receptor subtype gene expression in medullary thyroid carcinoma. J Clin Endocrinol Metab 1998;83(7):2417–20.

24. Schillaci O, Massa R, Scopinaro F. 111In-pentetreotide scintigraphy in the detection of insulinomas: importance of SPECT imaging. J Nucl Med 2000; 41(3):459–62.

25. Adams S, Baum RP, Hertel A, et al. Comparison of metabolic and receptor imaging in recurrent medullary thyroid carcinoma with histopathological findings. Eur J Nucl Med 1998;25(9):1277–83.

26. Whiteman ML, Serafini AN, Telischi FF, et al. 111In octreotide scintigraphy in the evaluation of head and neck lesions. AJNR Am J Neuroradiol 1997; 18(6):1073–80.

27. Nockel P, Babic B, Millo C, et al. Localization of insulinoma using 68Ga-DOTATATE PET/CT Scan. J Clin Endocrinol Metab 2017;102(1):195–9.

28. Rindi G, Klimstra DS, Abedi-Ardekani B, et al. A common classification framework for neuroendocrine neoplasms: an International Agency for Research on Cancer (IARC) and World Health Organization (WHO) expert consensus proposal. Mod Pathol 2018;31(12):1770–86.

29. Inzani F, Petrone G, Rindi G. The new world health organization classification for pancreatic neuroendocrine neoplasia. Endocrinol Metab Clin North Am 2018;47(3):463–70.

30. Walczyk J, Sowa-Staszczak A. Diagnostic imaging of gastrointestinal neuroendocrine neoplasms with a focus on ultrasound. J Ultrason 2019;19(78): 228–35.

31. McKenna LR, Edil BH. Update on pancreatic neuroendocrine tumors. Gland Surg 2014;3(4):258–75.

32. Tan EH, Tan CH. Imaging of gastroenteropancreatic neuroendocrine tumors. World J Clin Oncol 2011; 2(1):28–43.

33. Hill JS, McPhee JT, McDade TP, et al. Pancreatic neuroendocrine tumors: the impact of surgical resection on survival. Cancer 2009;115(4):741–51.

34. Wu J, Sun C, Li E, et al. Non-functional pancreatic neuroendocrine tumours: emerging trends in incidence and mortality. BMC Cancer 2019;19(1):334.

35. Modlin IM, Oberg K, Chung DC, et al. Gastroenteropancreatic neuroendocrine tumours. Lancet Oncol 2008;9(1):61–72.

36. Chang S, Choi D, Lee SJ, et al. Neuroendocrine neoplasms of the gastrointestinal tract: classification, pathologic basis, and imaging features. Radiographics 2007;27(6):1667–79.

37. Baxi AJ, Chintapalli K, Katkar A, et al. Multimodality imaging findings in carcinoid tumors: a head-to-toe spectrum. Radiographics 2017;37(2):516–36.

38. Lewis RB, Lattin GE Jr, Paal E. Pancreatic endocrine tumors: radiologic-clinicopathologic correlation. Radiographics 2010;30(6):1445–64.

39. Denecke T, Baur AD, Ihm C, et al. Evaluation of radiological prognostic factors of hepatic metastases in patients with non-functional pancreatic neuroendocrine tumors. Eur J Radiol 2013;82(10): e550–5.

40. Kumbasar B, Kamel IR, Tekes A, et al. Imaging of neuroendocrine tumors: accuracy of helical CT versus SRS. Abdom Imaging 2004;29(6):696–702.

41. Wong KK, Cahill JM, Frey KA, et al. Incremental value of 111-in pentetreotide SPECT/CT fusion imaging of neuroendocrine tumors. Acad Radiol 2010; 17(3):291–7.

42. Shaverdian N, Pinchot SN, Zarebczan B, et al. Utility of (1)(1)(1)indium-pentetreotide scintigraphy in patients with neuroendocrine tumors. Ann Surg Oncol 2013;20(2):640–5.

43. Sadowski SM, Neychev V, Millo C, et al. Prospective Study of 68Ga-DOTATATE positron emission tomography/computed tomography for detecting gastro-entero-pancreatic neuroendocrine tumors and unknown primary sites. J Clin Oncol 2016;34(6): 588–96.

44. Van Binnebeek S, Vanbilloen B, Baete K, et al. Comparison of diagnostic accuracy of (111)In-pentetreotide SPECT and (68)Ga-DOTATOC PET/CT: a lesion-by-lesion analysis in patients with metastatic neuroendocrine tumours. Eur Radiol 2016;26(3): 900–9.

45. Hilal T. Current understanding and approach to well differentiated lung neuroendocrine tumors: an update on classification and management. Ther Adv Med Oncol 2017;9(3):189–99.

46. Rosado de Christenson ML, Abbott GF, Kirejczyk WM, et al. Thoracic carcinoids: radiologic-pathologic correlation. Radiographics 1999;19(3):707–36.

47. Chong S, Lee KS, Chung MJ, et al. Neuroendocrine tumors of the lung: clinical, pathologic, and imaging findings. Radiographics 2006;26(1):41–57 [discussion: 57–8].

48. Chaer R, Massad MG, Evans A, et al. Primary neuroendocrine tumors of the thymus. Ann Thorac Surg 2002;74(5):1733–40.

49. Gaur P, Leary C, Yao JC. Thymic neuroendocrine tumors: a SEER database analysis of 160 patients. Ann Surg 2010;251(6):1117–21.

50. Moran CA, Suster S. Neuroendocrine carcinomas (carcinoid tumor) of the thymus. A clinicopathologic analysis of 80 cases. Am J Clin Pathol 2000;114(1): 100–10.

51. Nishino M, Ashiku SK, Kocher ON, et al. The thymus: a comprehensive review. Radiographics 2006;26(2): 335–48.

52. Walts AE, Frye J, Engman DM, et al. Carcinoid tumors of the thymus and Cushing's syndrome: clinicopathologic features and current best evidence regarding the cell of origin of these unusual neoplasms. Ann Diagn Pathol 2019;38:71–9.

53. Jeung MY, Gasser B, Gangi A, et al. Bronchial carcinoid tumors of the thorax: spectrum of radiologic findings. Radiographics 2002;22(2):351–65.

54. Gould PM, Bonner JA, Sawyer TE, et al. Bronchial carcinoid tumors: importance of prognostic factors that influence patterns of recurrence and overall survival. Radiology 1998;208(1):181–5.

55. Scarsbrook AF, Ganeshan A, Statham J, et al. Anatomic and functional imaging of metastatic carcinoid tumors. Radiographics 2007;27(2): 455–77.

56. Brown LR, Aughenbaugh GL. Masses of the anterior mediastinum: CT and MR imaging. AJR Am J Roentgenol 1991;157(6):1171–80.

57. Araki T, Sholl LM, Hatabu H, et al. Radiological features and metastatic patterns of thymic neuroendocrine tumours. Clin Radiol 2018;73(5):479–84.

58. Chiaravalloti A, Spanu A, Danieli R, et al. 111In-pentetreotide SPECT/CT in pulmonary carcinoid. Anticancer Res 2015;35(7):4265–70.

59. Guidoccio F, Grosso M, Maccauro M, et al. Current role of 111In-DTPA-octreotide scintigraphy in diagnosis of thymic masses. Tumori 2011;97(2):191–5.

60. Jindal T, Kumar A, Venkitaraman B, et al. Evaluation of the role of [18F]FDG-PET/CT and [68Ga] DOTATOC-PET/CT in differentiating typical and atypical pulmonary carcinoids. Cancer Imaging 2011;11:70–5.

61. Moore W, Freiberg E, Bishawi M, et al. FDG-PET imaging in patients with pulmonary carcinoid tumor. Clin Nucl Med 2013;38(7):501–5.

62. Erasmus JJ, McAdams HP, Patz EF Jr, et al. Evaluation of primary pulmonary carcinoid tumors using FDG PET. AJR Am J Roentgenol 1998;170(5): 1369–73.

63. Chan DL, Bernard E, Schembri G, et al. High metabolic tumour volume on FDG PET predicts poor survival from neuroendocrine neoplasms. Neuroendocrinology 2019. https://doi.org/10.1159/000504673.

64. Lococo F, Perotti G, Cardillo G, et al. Multicenter comparison of 18F-FDG and 68Ga-DOTA-peptide PET/CT for pulmonary carcinoid. Clin Nucl Med 2015;40(3):e183–9.

65. Chen H, Sippel RS, O'Dorisio MS, et al. The North American Neuroendocrine Tumor Society consensus guideline for the diagnosis and management of neuroendocrine tumors: pheochromocytoma, paraganglioma, and medullary thyroid cancer. Pancreas 2010;39(6):775–83.

66. Beard CM, Sheps SG, Kurland LT, et al. Occurrence of pheochromocytoma in Rochester, Minnesota, 1950 through 1979. Mayo Clin Proc 1983;58(12): 802–4.

67. Sutton MG, Sheps SG, Lie JT. Prevalence of clinically unsuspected pheochromocytoma. Review of a 50-year autopsy series. Mayo Clin Proc 1981; 56(6):354–60.

68. Erickson D, Kudva YC, Ebersold MJ, et al. Benign paragangliomas: clinical presentation and treatment outcomes in 236 patients. J Clin Endocrinol Metab 2001;86(11):5210–6.

69. Parenti G, Zampetti B, Rapizzi E, et al. Updated and new perspectives on diagnosis, prognosis, and therapy of malignant pheochromocytoma/paraganglioma. J Oncol 2012;2012:872713.

70. Lee JH, Barich F, Karnell LH, et al. National Cancer Data Base report on malignant paragangliomas of the head and neck. Cancer 2002;94(3):730–7.

71. Chrisoulidou A, Kaltsas G, Ilias I, et al. The diagnosis and management of malignant phaeochromocytoma and paraganglioma. Endocr Relat Cancer 2007;14(3):569–85.

72. Blake MA, Kalra MK, Maher MM, et al. Pheochromocytoma: an imaging chameleon. Radiographics 2004;24(Suppl 1):S87–99.

73. Baez JC, Jagannathan JP, Krajewski K, et al. Pheochromocytoma and paraganglioma: imaging characteristics. Cancer Imaging 2012;12:153–62.

74. Vallabhajosula S, Nikolopoulou A. Radioiodinated metaiodobenzylguanidine (MIBG): radiochemistry, biology, and pharmacology. Semin Nucl Med 2011; 41(5):324–33.

75. Noto RB, Pryma DA, Jensen J, et al. Phase 1 study of high-specific-activity I-131 MIBG for Metastatic and/or recurrent pheochromocytoma or paraganglioma. J Clin Endocrinol Metab 2018;103(1): 213–20.

76. Tan TH, Hussein Z, Saad FF, et al. Diagnostic performance of (68)Ga-DOTATATE PET/CT, (18)F-FDG PET/CT and (131)I-MIBG scintigraphy in mapping metastatic pheochromocytoma and paraganglioma. Nucl Med Mol Imaging 2015;49(2):143–51.

77. Jing H, Li F, Wang L, et al. Comparison of the 68Ga-DOTATATA PET/CT, FDG PET/CT, and MIBG SPECT/CT in the evaluation of suspected primary pheochromocytomas and paragangliomas. Clin Nucl Med 2017;42(7):525–9.

78. Han S, Suh CH, Woo S, et al. Performance of (68) Ga-DOTA-Conjugated somatostatin receptor-targeting peptide PET in detection of pheochromocytoma and paraganglioma: a systematic review and metaanalysis. J Nucl Med 2019;60(3):369–76.

Neuroendocrine Tumors
Imaging of Treatment and Follow-up

Agata E. Migut, MD[a], Harmeet Kaur, MD[b], Rony Avritscher, MD[a,c],*

KEYWORDS

- Neuroendocrine tumor • Carcinoid • Therapy • Imaging • Embolization

KEY POINTS

- Accurate neuroendocrine tumor (NET) imaging assessment and follow-up require familiarity with the entire range of disease sites, morphologic manifestations, as well as the impact of the various therapeutic options on clinical course.
- The variable conspicuity of NETs requires multiple phases of contrast enhancement to detect both tumor recurrence and metastasis. Although these tumors are typically hypervascular, they may exhibit little or no enhancement on the arterial phase and be optimally identified only on the porto-venous phase.
- ^{68}Ga-DOTA-SSTR imaging is indicated for initial staging, detection of occult disease, diagnosis of recurrence, patient selection before peptide receptor radionuclide therapy, and disease confirmation in sites not amenable to biopsy.
- Transcatheter arterial embolization strategies show similar response outcomes, but differ importantly on their toxicity with reports of increased risk for biliary injury in patients with NET after chemoembolization using drug-eluting beads (DEB-TACE).
- Objective measurements used in RECIST 1.1 do not always offer the most accurate evaluation for targeted therapy response. Alternative response criteria using lesion attenuation and morphology offer promising results and seem better suited to assess response to target agents.

INTRODUCTION

Neuroendocrine neoplasms are a heterogeneous group of tumors that arise from cells that are distributed throughout the body, including central nervous system, thyroid, parathyroid glands, larynx, breast, as well as the respiratory, gastrointestinal, and urogenital tracts. The lungs (22%–27%) and gastrointestinal tract (62%–67%) are the most common primary sites.[1] Given the wide variety of disease sites and clinical behavior, the treatment of neuroendocrine tumors (NETs) requires a multidisciplinary approach. Endocrine surgeons offer curative treatment for patients with locoregional tumors, endocrinologists and gastrointestinal medical oncologists offer a gamut of systemic therapeutic options, whereas radiologists aid in the diagnosis, treatment, and palliation of unresectable metastatic disease.

NETs account for approximately 0.5% of all newly diagnosed malignancies. The incidence is approximately 6.98/100,000 per year.[2,3] These tumors can arise in association with multiple endocrine neoplasia syndrome, von Hippel-Lindau syndrome, neurofibromatosis, tuberous sclerosis, but are in the great majority sporadic in nature. The management of NETs is predicated on histologic classification of NETs, which separates tumors into well-differentiated (G1) characterized

[a] Department of Interventional Radiology, The University of Texas MD Anderson Cancer Center, 1515 Holcombe Boulevard, Houston, TX 77030, USA; [b] Department of Diagnostic Radiology, The University of Texas MD Anderson Cancer Center, 1515 Holcombe Boulevard, Houston, TX 77030, USA; [c] Department of Interventional Radiology, 1400 Pressler Street, Unit 1471, Houston, TX 77030, USA
* Corresponding author. Department of Interventional Radiology, 1400 Pressler Street, Unit 1471, Houston, TX 77030.
E-mail address: rony.avritscher@mdanderson.org

Radiol Clin N Am 58 (2020) 1161–1171
https://doi.org/10.1016/j.rcl.2020.08.002
0033-8389/20/© 2020 Elsevier Inc. All rights reserved.

by slow growth; moderately differentiated (G2) with heterogeneous differentiation; (G3) displaying poor-differentiation; and undifferentiated or anaplastic (G4).[3] Imaging plays a central role in the diagnosis, workup, and monitoring of patients with NET. Establishing the site of the primary tumor has critical prognostic implications, as a combination of NET site, grade, and stage (local, regional, or distant) are the determinants of management and clinical outcome. Patients with primary rectal NETs have the best prognosis, followed by small intestine, lung/bronchus, stomach, and colon. Patients with pancreatic NET have the highest mortality risk.[4]

Local and regional disease is typically managed with surgical resection, whenever possible. However, the treatment of patients with NET with higher grade, unresectable or metastatic disease can be complex involving a combination of systemic targeted agents, as well as transarterial embolization and peptide receptor targeted therapies and will be discussed in detail. The most important concept in modern NET workup is that an optimal diagnostic strategy requires combination of both anatomic and functional imaging modalities. This combined approach enables a more accurate identification of the primary disease site and disease staging. Because of their unique symptomatology, NETs often present with unknown primary site of disease, despite adequate cross-sectional imaging workup, and ^{68}Ga-DOTA-TATE PET can now diagnose these lesions with great sensitivity.[5] Finally, functional imaging is essential to select ideal candidates for peptide receptor radionuclide therapy (PRRT).

TREATMENT CONSIDERATIONS AND EXPECTED OUTCOMES

In cases with limited metastases, surgical resection of the primary tumor and metastases is possible. Overall survival rate was 50.4% at 10 years after resection in one study, and systematic review estimates overall survival to be 41% to 100% at 5 years after resection.[6] Surgical resection of gastrointestinal NETs showed overall survival rates to be 84%, 67%, and 31% at 5 years, 10 years, and 20 years after resection, respectively, with overall median survival at 161 months. Recurrence after resection is expected, but decreasing tumor burden has been shown to improve symptoms and quality of life in patients.[7]

Imaging is an integral part of the management and follow-up of patients with advanced locoregional or distant disease. Approximately 40% to 50% of patients with NET present with metastatic disease at initial diagnosis.[8] Treatment for these patients encompasses long established approaches, such as somatostatin analogs to reduce both tumor growth and symptomatology and liver-directed therapies, reserved for patients with metastatic liver disease, particularly those with poorly controlled carcinoid syndrome. Modern approaches using precision medicine targeted therapies are used as systemic antitumor agents, and finally, peptide receptor radionuclides therapies are typically indicated for metastatic tumors expressing somatostatin receptors. Familiarity with the expected objective response and time to progression of each of these therapeutic approaches is required to establish optimal treatment surveillance strategies.

SOMATOSTATIN ANALOGS

Somatostatin analogs (SSAs), namely octreotide and lanreotide, were originally used to modulate hormonal effects and growth of NET tumor cells by binding somatostatin receptors. These agents remain as the first-line management and therapy for NETs and have a remarkably successful history over decades.[9] These therapies take advantage of somatostatin receptor overexpression characteristic of NETs. Initially, these agents were used mainly to regulate symptoms of hormone excess from carcinoid syndrome; they are now increasingly used also to control tumor growth. Octreotide was shown to increase median times to tumor progression to 14.3 months as compared with 6 months in the placebo group (PROMID trial, $P = .000072$).[10] Stable disease was maintained in 66.7% of the octreotide group and 37.2% of the placebo group after 6 months of treatment. Lanreotide treatment for 2 years was shown to increase progression-free survival (PFS) in patients with locally advanced or metastatic nonfunctioning pancreatic or intestinal NETs as compared with placebo (CLARINET study). Length of PFS was not obtained in the lanreotide group but was shown to be at least 24 months and is estimated to be 32.8 months during open label data collection.[11]

IMAGE-GUIDED LIVER-DIRECTED THERAPIES

Advances in image-guided liver-directed therapies have led to improved outcomes for patients with liver metastases (Fig. 1). Improvements in catheters, embolic agents, chemotherapy drugs, and delivery systems have been linked to further technical breakthroughs sparking interest in combination approaches with systemic therapies. Median overall survival for patients with NET with liver metastases is less than 5 years.[4] Image-guided tumor

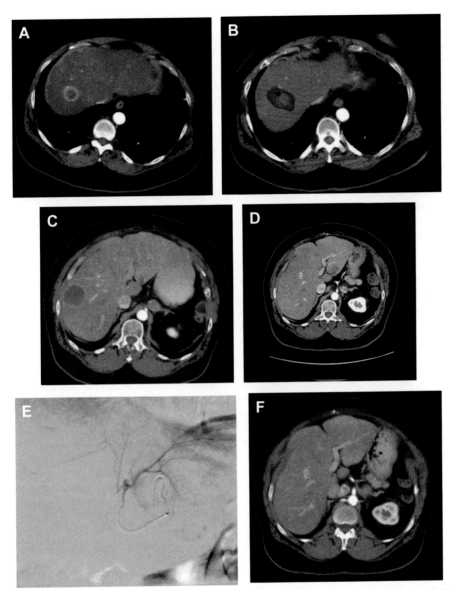

Fig. 1. Long-term (>5 years) disease control by using a combination of different image-guided local therapies. A 65-year-old woman with intermediate-grade pancreatic neuroendocrine tumor metastatic to the liver referred to interventional radiology after disease progression on lanreotide, everolimus, and sunitinib. After successfully undergoing RFA for initial dominant lesion in right liver, transcatheter arterial embolization was used to treat remaining liver lesions resulting in durable complete response. (*A*) Axial contrast-enhanced computed tomography shows a ring-enhancing metastatic lesion in right liver. (*B*) Axial contrast-enhanced computed tomography shows optimal post ablation defect with complete coverage of target lesion. (*C*) Axial contrast-enhanced CT shows a separate metastatic lesion in the right liver considered too large for RFA and referred for transcatheter arterial hepatic embolization. (*D*) Axial contrast-enhanced CT shows separate enlarging lesion in left liver. (*E*) Digital subtraction angiography of left hepatic artery during left liver lesion embolization. (*F*) Axial contrast-enhanced CT shows complete resolution of both right and left liver lesions after TAE.

ablation is considered a potential first-line treatment in many patients with single and/or small liver tumors, and it can be accomplished using chemical agents or thermal energy. Chemical ablation can be achieved by direct intratumoral percutaneous ethanol injection and, less commonly, ablation using acetic acid or chemotherapeutic agents that induce tumor cell death. Thermal ablation modalities include high-energy radiofrequency ablation (RFA) and microwave ablation (MWA); these procedures can be performed under imaging guidance by interventional radiologists or by surgeons in the operating suite. A systematic review of studies evaluating the use of ablative techniques for neuroendocrine liver metastases combining both percutaneous (26%) and surgical (74%) approaches for a total 595 patients showed local recurrence rates of approximately 20% on contrast-enhanced computed tomography (CT) of the thorax, abdomen, and pelvis within 2 years.[12–14] Transarterial embolization, chemo-embolization, and radioembolization consist of transcatheter intra-arterial delivery of a single or combination of embolic agents, chemotherapy drugs, or radioactive microspheres into a liver tumor. These treatments are based on the fact that blood flow to liver neoplasms is supplied virtually entirely through the hepatic artery, whereas supply to the normal liver parenchyma occurs predominantly through the portal vein. Moreover, tumor ischemia caused by embolization of the dominant arterial supply has a synergistic effect with the chemotherapeutic drugs. Only retrospective data are available comparing the different modalities in metastatic NET context with expected imaging response rates ranging between 60% to 95%. A retrospective multicenter study assessing 155 patients with NET with liver metastases undergoing conventional transarterial chemoembolization (TACE) (n = 50), transarterial radioembolization (TARE) (n = 64), and transarterial embolization (n = 41) demonstrated equivalency between the different modalities without significant differences. Radioembolization showed a higher hazard ratio for overall survival than chemoembolization (hazard ratio 1.8, P = .11). A more recent retrospective study of 248 patients from 2 academic medical institutions comparing TACE (79%) and TARE (21%) showed no difference in median overall survival, but disease control rate was greater for TACE on first posttreatment imaging. There was also no difference in PFS between TARE versus TACE (15.9 months vs 19.9 months). Despite their similar objective response outcomes, these different embolization strategies differ importantly on their toxicity with reports of increased risk for biliary injury in patients with NET after chemoembolization using drug-eluting beads transarterial chemoembolization (DEB-TACE).[15,16] Based on these studies, attention should be directed at diagnosing early bile duct dilatation and intrahepatic bilomas throughout DEB-TACE follow-up, since they may require percutaneous drainage.

NEW TARGETED AGENTS

Better understanding of the molecular underpinnings of NET tumor growth has led to increased role for molecular targeted agents in the treatment of these tumors. Everolimus is an mTOR inhibitor that is, used for patients with progressive, metastatic gastrointestinal or bronchopulmonary tumors. In the RADIANT-4 study, 302 patients with progressive nonfunctional gastrointestinal tract or lung NET were randomized to receive either everolimus or placebo. Median PFS for the study was 11 months for patients undergoing treatment with everolimus versus 3.9 months with placebo. Everolimus was associated with a 52% reduction in the estimated risk of progression or death (hazard ratio 0.48, P<.00001) with infrequent grade 3 or 4 adverse events.[17] National Comprehensive Cancer Network (NCCN) NET guidelines recommend everolimus for patients with progressive metastatic gastrointestinal tract NETs. In addition, a recent subgroup analysis of the RADIANT-4 lung patients showed a median PFS improvement of 5.6 months with similar safety profile supporting the use of the agent in patients with advanced nonfunctional lung NET, as well.[18] Vascular endothelial growth factor (VEGF), a key driver of angiogenesis, is also implicated in NET progression with prognostic implications. In addition, NET tissues also exhibit overexpression of platelet-derived growth factor receptors (PDGFRs) and stem-cell factor receptor (c-kit). Sunitinib is a tyrosine kinase inhibitor that exerts its antitumor activity by inhibiting several of these pathways. A randomized, double-blind, placebo-controlled phase 3 trial of sunitinib in patients with advanced, well-differentiated pancreatic neuroendocrine tumors showed improved PFS (11.4 months in treatment group vs 5.5 months in placebo group) and objective response rate of 9.3% in the sunitinib group.[19]

PEPTIDE RECEPTOR RADIONUCLIDE THERAPY

In the past decade, ^{68}Ga-labeled SSTR analog PET/CT has emerged as a more sensitive imaging solution for NETs, due to the increased affinity of these agents for somatostatin receptors subtype 2.[20,21] Thus, the next logical therapeutic step consisted of combining of one of these imaging isotopes with a therapeutic radioactive element, to develop a targeted theranostic agent. PRRT is a synthetic somatostatin analog that is radiolabeled with lutetium 177 (^{177}Lu-DOTATATE).[22,23] PRRT is emerging as the standard of care for patients with inoperable low-grade (1 or 2) NETs expressing somatostatin receptors. Once bound to the SSTR 2 receptors, the radionuclide is internalized, and cell death ensues due to lethal beta radiation. The 2 most common radionuclides used for PRRT are [yttrium-90 DOTA Phe-1-Tyr^3-] Octreotide (^{90}Y-DOTATOC) and [Lutetitium-177 DOTA-phe1-Tyr^3]Octreotate   (^{177}Lu-DOTATATE). In

2018, ^{177}Lu-DOTATATE (Lutathera; Advanced Accelerator Applications, Milburn, NJ) was approved by the US Food and Drug Administration for the treatment of SSTR-positive gastroentero-pancreatic NETs, including foregut, midgut, and hindgut tumors. NCCN guidelines recommend Lu177-DOTATATE for low-grade and intermediate-grade patients with NET who progress on SSAs. A phase III randomized study (NETTER-1) evaluated 229 patients assigned to [177]Lu -DOTATATE or high-dose octreotide. Patients treated with PRRT showed significant improvement in PFS (not reached vs 8.4 months) with objective imaging response observed in 18% of patients.[24] A subsequent study including 610 patients with metastatic gastroenteropancreatic and bronchial NETs showed PFS and overall survival for all patients of 29 months and 63 months.[25]

IMAGING TREATMENT RESPONSE AND FOLLOW-UP

Optimal NET imaging assessment and follow-up require familiarity the entire range of disease sites, morphologic manifestations, as well as the impact of the various therapeutic options on their clinical course. Meticulous evaluation requires both subjective and objective assessments, the latter fundamental in the context of clinical trials and currently dominated by size measurement(s). Changes in lesion attenuation on CT, MR imaging, and PET/CT can also be used as objective criteria of response, but these criteria are not as universally accepted as changes in tumor size defined by RECIST criteria.[26] An accurate assessment of treatment response should rely on changes in lesion size and number; presence and magnitude of contrast enhancement; and finally changes in functional imaging. In addition to cursory measurements of primary and nodal sites, an active search for small peritoneal implants and bone metastases should be systematically carried out when evaluating follow-up scans for neuroendocrine patients. The indolent nature of NETs often translates into several consecutive imaging studies with minimal deviation from baseline scans.[27] Typically, imaging surveillance requires more than a year to allow recognition of any appreciable change. Finally, because most well-differentiated NETs display increased vascular density, a salient feature of NETs is their exuberant enhancement on contrast-enhanced studies. Thus, it is important to recognize that, when subjected to antivascular therapies, objective response rates may not provide the full picture of treatment response; incorporation of both size and magnitude of lesion enhancement is needed to more accurately predict drug efficacy.[28–30]

ANATOMIC IMAGING

Multi-detector CT (MDCT) is a widely available technique, with a high spatial and temporal resolution as well as multi-planar capabilities, which makes it one of the modalities of choice in the anatomic assessment of NETs.[31] NETs are generally imaged using a multiphase imaging protocol that incorporates precontrast scans followed by late arterial phase (25–30 seconds), porto-venous phase and delayed imaging. This technique should be obtained with 100 to 120 mL of iodinated contrast (Omnipaque 350; GE Health Care, Princeton, NJ) injected at 3 to 5 mL/s with slices reconstructed at 2.5 to 5 mm. The requirement of multiple phases of contrast enhancement reflects the variable conspicuity of these tumors, seen in both the primary tumor and liver metastases. In some studies, the tumors are more conspicuous on the arterial phase, and in other studies they are better seen on the porto-venous phase. This is because although these tumors are traditionally viewed as hypervascular, they may have little or no enhancement on the arterial phase and may be optimally identified only on the portal phase.[32] The precontrast series is an underappreciated but essential element of the imaging protocol for NET liver metastasis, as some liver metastases may only be evident on this acquisition.[33] This basic multiphase CT protocol is not only ideal for the diagnosis and follow-up liver metastases but also for the detection and definition of regional extent of pancreatic neuro-endocrine tumors. However, the protocol needs slight modification for the localization of small bowel tumors; this evaluation may be performed with CT enterography using a negative or low attenuating oral contrast agent to distend the bowel.[31]

Regarding liver metastases, MR imaging provides an alternative and reliable imaging modality for NET surveillance (**Fig. 2**). The imaging protocol relies on a similar use of multiphase postcontrast imaging to CT, using a T1-weighted fat-suppressed breath-hold 3-dimensional gradient-recalled echo sequence and includes the acquisition of precontrast, arterial phase, porto-venous, equilibrium and delayed phases, (typical parameters 3 mm, 288 × 155, 1 NEX). In addition, the protocol includes a T2-weighted fast spin echo sequence with fat suppression (5 mm, 128 × 156, 3 NEX), a diffusion-weighted sequence (b values 0, 600, 1000; 5 mm, 128 × 102, 6 NEX) (**Table 1**). The use of diffusion-weighted imaging has shown improved sensitivity in the detection and

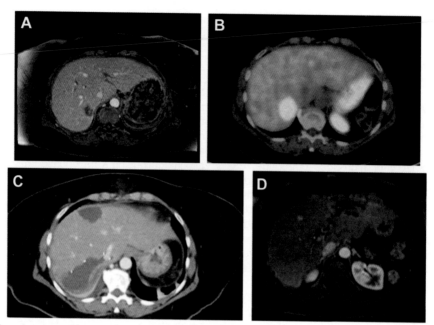

Fig. 2. Early recurrence after curative surgery emphasizes the need for close follow-up. A 62-year-old woman with G2 pancreatic NET metastatic to the liver referred for curative surgery. After successfully undergoing surgical resection of primary and 4 separate lesions, the patient presented with early recurrence and is currently treated with lanreotide. (A) Axial post contrast fat-saturated MR image shows a peripherally enhancing hepatic lesion. (B) Axial 68Ga-DOTATATE PET/CT image showing a segment 7 liver lesion with SUV 32.7, consistent with metastasis. (C) Axial contrast-enhanced CT shows successful surgical resection of target lesions. (D) Axial post contrast fat-saturated MR image obtained 3 months after surgery shows a new enhancing hepatic metastasis, consistent with early recurrence.

characterization of NET liver metastasis.[34] When needed for problem solving, MR imaging can be performed with liver-specific contrast, where the absence of contrast accumulation within the tumor on the images acquired 20 minutes after injection allows for a sharp tumor-to-normal liver interface. One downside to keep in mind when using exclusively MR imaging for follow-up is the greater difficulty to detect small peritoneal implants in comparison to CT.

FUNCTIONAL IMAGING

Diagnostic indium (^{111}In-penteotride) and, more recently, gallium-1,4,7,10-tetraazacyclododecane-N,N′,N″-tetraacetic-somatostatin receptor (^{68}Ga-DOTA-SSTR) tracers can be used to visualize and quantify the increased expression of somatostatin receptors in patients with NET. Whole-body planar imaging without or with single-photon-emission CT (SPECT) [111]In scans have been the cornerstone of NET functional imaging since 1994. Recently, ^{68}Ga-labeled SSTR analog PET/CT supplanted ^{111}In imaging, due to its increased sensitivity and lower radiation dose. ^{68}Ga-DOTA-SSTR imaging is now indicated for NET initial staging, detection of occult disease,

diagnosis of recurrence, patient selection before PRRT, as well as disease confirmation in sites not amenable to biopsy.[35,36] [68]Ga -DOTA-SSTR PET/CT is particularly useful in detection of recurrent NET.[20] Several studies have shown that, when compared with MDCT alone, addition of ^{68}Ga-SSTR scans, improved detection of disease recurrence during NET treatment follow-up imaging and, more importantly, resulted in change in patient management. In a series of 143 patients with metastatic pancreatic and small intestine NETs undergoing surveillance with cross-sectional imaging consisting of MDCT every 6 months and ^{68}Ga-DOTA PET/CT yearly, functional imaging affected management in 73.4% of patients, including both octreoscan (32.7%) and DOTA scan (36.9%). Functional imaging detected 75.8% of new lesions, including 29.3% that were missed by MDCT.[5] The optimal timing for [68]Ga -DOTA-SSTR PET/CT imaging remains undetermined with most consensus guidelines recommending routine surveillance with SSTR PET imaging only for patients with disease that is, only seen predominantly on SSTR PET/CT or at the time of clinical or biochemical disease progression.[37] Decreased ^{68}Ga-DOTATATE uptake in tumors after the first cycle of PRRT predicts time

Table 1
MR imaging scan parameters for follow-up imaging

MRI Parameter	ABD Cor T2	ABD Ax Dualecho	Ax T2	+C ABD Ax 3D T1	+C ABD Ax DWI
Pulse sequence	2D Spin Echo	2D SPGR	2D FSE	3D LAVA	2D Spin Echo
Imaging option	NPW, EDR, TRF, Fast, ZIP512, SS, ARC	EDR, Fast, ZIP512, Asset	FC, EDR, TRF, Fast, ZIP512, Nav	EDR, Fast, ZIP512, ZIP2, ARC	EDR, EPI, DIFF, Asset, Nav
TR, ms	590.9	220.0	N/A	3.6	N/A
TE, ms	140	2.1/4.4	85	1.7	67.6
Flip angle, deg	N/A	85	N/A	12	N/A
RBW, Hz	62.50	62.50	41.67	62.50	250.00
FOV, cm	38 × 38	38 × 30.4	38 × 30.4	38 × 30.4	38 × 30.4
Slice thickness, mm	5	5	5	6	5
Spacing, mm	0	0	0	−3	0
Frequency encoding	256	256	256	256	96
Phase encoding	224	192	192	192	128
NEX	1	1	2	1	50: 1 400: 3 800: 6
Number of slices	53	51	53	Locs per Slab: 50	61
Scan time, min:s	0:31	0:57	5:00	0:15	7:45
Acceleration	Phase: 2.5	Phase: 2	Phase: 1	Phase: 1.5 Slice: 1	Phase: 2
B-Value, s/mm² (NEX)	N/A	N/A	N/A	N/A	50, 400, 800

Abbreviations: ABD, abdominal; ARC, autocalibrating reconstruction for cartesian imaging; FOV, field of view; EDR, ECG derived respiration; N/A, not applicable; NPW, no phase wrap; RBW, receiver bandwidth; TE, echo time; TR, repetition time; TRF, tailored radiofrequency; 2D, 2-dimensional.

to progression and clinical improvement in patients with well-differentiated NETs.[27]

RESPONSE ASSESSMENT

RECIST 1.1 criteria are the mainstay for response evaluation and rely on changes in the largest diameters of target lesions before and after treatment.[26] Response is categorized in 1 of 4 groups based on the percentage of decrease or increase in the sum of the largest diameters of the target lesions. While measuring diameters of hepatic tumors with contrast-enhanced CT is objective, the main limitation in the context of NETs is to accurately localize the tumor margins. However, objective measurements used in RECIST 1.1 do not always offer the most accurate evaluation for targeted therapy response, given the slow-growing nature of tumors like NETs.[29] Alternative response criteria using not only lesion attenuation, but also morphology offer promising results and seem better suited to assess response to target agents.[38] These studies, although limited, have established the relevance of such criteria and emphasized the need for more investigation (**Fig. 3**).

Response to hepatic regional therapy performed with bland embolization, chemoembolization, or radioembolization is also based on change in size and attenuation secondary to decrease in enhancement and development of necrosis. Posttreatment

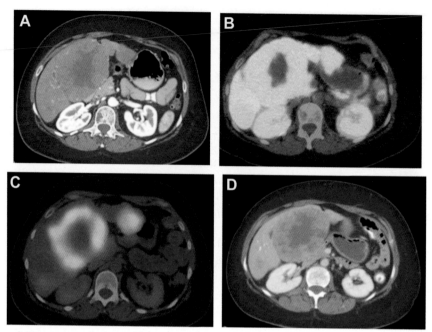

Fig. 3. Successful treatment of advanced metastatic NET with PRRT with follow-up study showing multiple areas of tumor necrosis in the dominant lesion without any appreciable change in the lesion greatest diameter. The findings illustrate the fact that RECIST 1.1. criteria are not always accurate in determining treatment response. A 46-year-old woman with G2 sigmoid NET metastatic to the liver referred for PRRT. (*A*) Axial contrast-enhanced CT shows large centrally-necrotic liver metastasis. (*B*) Axial ^{68}Ga-DOTATATE PET/CT image demonstrates that the mass is somatostatin-avid with SUV 18.95. (*C*) Axial SPECT/CT obtained 24 hours after administration of 210 mCi of ^{177}Lu-DOTA-Octreotate shows expected localization to active liver lesion. (*D*) Axial contrast-enhanced CT obtained 6 weeks after therapy shows multiple new areas of decreased attenuation in the previously enhancing component of the dominant liver metastasis, consistent with treatment response.

imaging is typically performed 6 to 8 weeks after the procedure. It is important to note that TARE patients may exhibit a decrease in target tumor size up to 4 to 6 months after treatment.[39] In cases with a persistent area of enhancement, it is important to monitor the enhancing tissue for growth; the absence of growth is compatible with response and observation is appropriate in this situation. Tumor viability can be predicted by persistent enhancement on scans performed earlier, and the observation of a decrease in the degree of tumor enhancement might also be delayed.[40] Response evaluation after RFA follows the same principles as with other tumor types, and the most important predictor of recurrence is the size of the ablative margin, which can be evaluated by comparing pre and post procedure studies.[41]

SPECIFIC IMAGING CONSIDERATIONS
Functional Imaging Selection of Potential Peptide Receptor Radionuclide Therapy Candidates

[111]In scintigraphy has a well-established semi-quantitative scoring system to determine degree of radiotracer uptake on octreoscan. This scale was conceived for planar imaging and consists of comparing the target uptake to the uptake in the liver or spleen. The relative uptake score ranges from none (0), much lower than liver (1), slightly less than or equal to liver (2), greater than liver (3) and greater than spleen (4).[42] Such standardized criteria are still being developed for PET/CT studies, but growing evidence supports the use of ^{68}Ga-DOTA-SSTR uptake to select optimal candidates for PRRT, as well as a reliable predictor of treatment response. Using the maximum standardized uptake value (SUVmax) of ^{68}Ga-DOTA-Phe-1–Tyr^3—octreotide (DOTA-TOC), Kratochwil and colleagues[43] demonstrated significant differences in values for SSRT2 expressing lesions exhibiting response to PRRT (33.55 $\pm$ 4.62) versus non-responding lesions (18 $\pm$ 3.59) with a proposed cutoff value of 16.4 to select patient for treatment. In a more recent study, 55 patients with metastatic NETs with uncontrolled symptoms or disease progression, baseline, single lesion SUVmax predicted both response and PFS with tumoral SUVmax correlating with SSTR2 expression and a SUVmax

cutoff of 13 yielding high specificity and sensitivity.[44] Important pitfalls of PET SSTR imaging include physiologic distribution in the pituitary, thyroid, and adrenal glands, as well as the head of pancreas, where it can be particularly challenging to distinguish between benign versus malignant uptake. In addition, focal areas of inflammation and infection can lead to false-positives.

Role of Transarterial Radioembolization in the Age of Peptide Receptor Radionuclide Therapy

With the advent of PRRT as treatment of choice for patients with advanced metastatic NET, the role of TARE in the NET treatment algorithm is being revisited, due to potential of increased risk for radiation-induced liver damage with cumulative radiation doses.[45] In a single-institution retrospective analysis including 106 patients undergoing TARE, of whom 54% had a NET diagnosis, chronic hepatotoxicity (occurring at least 6 months after treatment) was observed in 13% of patients. Tumor involvement greater than 50% of liver parenchyma and cirrhosis were the comorbidities most commonly associated with this outcome. A separate study including solely patients with NET treated with TARE revealed that bilobar treatment was associated with increased long-term risk for portal hypertension.[46] Given this theoretic risk, TARE should be used for patients with NET without somatostatin receptor expression and in patients with history of prior biliary tract instrumentation, due to lower risk of hepatobiliary infection, when compared with thermal ablation, TAE, and TACE.[47]

SUMMARY

The management of NETs continues to evolve and effective therapeutic options are increasingly available, even for patients with advanced disease. Management of these complex patients often requires a combination of 2 or more modalities. Modern imaging strategies provide anatomic and functional information to help guide appropriate selection of best treatment approaches. The recent approval of ^{68}Ga-DOTA-SSTR imaging has changed the role of imaging in the initial staging, detection of occult disease, diagnosis of recurrence, patient selection before PRRT, and disease confirmation in sites not amenable to biopsy. PRRT is emerging as the standard of care for patients with inoperable low-grade (1 or 2) NETs expressing somatostatin receptors and advances in image-guided liver-directed therapies have led to improved outcomes for patients with

liver metastases. Imaging of NETs treatment and follow-up after these novel therapies will help determine treatment combinations with best long-term outcomes.

REFERENCES

1. Kaltsas GA, Besser GM, Grossman AB. The diagnosis and medical management of advanced neuroendocrine tumors. Endocr Rev 2004;25(3):458–511.
2. Oronsky B, Ma PC, Morgensztern D, et al. Nothing but NET: a review of neuroendocrine tumors and carcinomas. Neoplasia 2017;19(12):991–1002.
3. Dasari A, Shen C, Halperin D, et al. Trends in the incidence, prevalence, and survival outcomes in patients with neuroendocrine tumors in the United States. JAMA Oncol 2017;3(10):1335–42.
4. Man D, Wu J, Shen Z, et al. Prognosis of patients with neuroendocrine tumor: a SEER database analysis. Cancer Manag Res 2018;10:5629–38.
5. Merola E, Pavel ME, Panzuto F, et al. Functional imaging in the follow-up of enteropancreatic neuroendocrine tumors: clinical usefulness and indications. J Clin Endocrinol Metab 2017;102(5):1486–94.
6. Glazer ES, Tseng JF, Al-Refaie W, et al. Long-term survival after surgical management of neuroendocrine hepatic metastases. HPB (Oxford) 2010; 12(6):427–33.
7. Woltering EA, Voros BA, Beyer DT, et al. Aggressive surgical approach to the management of neuroendocrine tumors: a report of 1,000 surgical cytoreductions by a single institution. Coll Surg 2017; 224(4):434–47.
8. Pavel M, O'Toole D, Costa F, et al. ENETS consensus guidelines update for the management of distant metastatic disease of intestinal, pancreatic, bronchial neuroendocrine neoplasms (NEN) and NEN of unknown primary site. Neuroendocrinology 2016;103(2):172–85.
9. Shah MH, Goldner WS, Halfdanarson TR, et al. NCCN guidelines insights: neuroendocrine and adrenal tumors, version 2.2018. J Natl Compr Canc Netw 2018;16(6):693–702.
10. Rinke A, Muller HH, Schade-Brittinger C, et al. Placebo-controlled, double-blind, prospective, randomized study on the effect of octreotide LAR in the control of tumor growth in patients with metastatic neuroendocrine midgut tumors: a report from the PROMID Study Group. J Clin Oncol 2009;27(28): 4656–63.
11. Caplin ME, Pavel M, Cwikla JB, et al. Anti-tumour effects of lanreotide for pancreatic and intestinal neuroendocrine tumours: the CLARINET open-label extension study. Endocr Relat Cancer 2016;23(3): 191–9.
12. Mohan H, Nicholson P, Winter DC, et al. Radiofrequency ablation for neuroendocrine liver

metastases: a systematic review. J Vasc Interv Radiol 2015;26(7):935–42.

13. Akyildiz HY, Mitchell J, Milas M, et al. Laparoscopic radiofrequency thermal ablation of neuroendocrine hepatic metastases: long-term follow-up. Surgery 2010;148(6):1288–93.

14. Amersi FF, McElrath-Garza A, Ahmad A, et al. Long-term survival after radiofrequency ablation of complex unresectable liver tumors. Arch Surg 2006; 141(6):581–7.

15. Bhagat N, Reyes Dk, Lin M, et al. Phase II study of chemoembolization with drug-eluting beads in patients with hepatic neuroendocrine metastases: high incidence of biliary injury. Cardiovasc Intervent Radiol 2013;36(2):449–59.

16. Monier A, Guiu B, Duran R, et al. Liver and biliary damages following transarterial chemoembolization of hepatocellular carcinoma: comparison between drug-eluting beads and lipiodol emulsion. Eur Radiol 2017;27(4):1431–9.

17. Yao JC, Fazio N, Singh S, et al. Everolimus for the treatment of advanced, non-functional neuroendocrine tumours of the lung or gastrointestinal tract (RADIANT-4): a randomised, placebo-controlled, phase 3 study. Lancet 2016;387(10022):968–77.

18. Fazio N, Buzzoni R, Fave GD, et al. Everolimus in advanced, progressive, well-differentiated, non-functional neuroendocrine tumors: RADIANT-4 lung subgroup analysis. Cancer Sci 2018;109(1):174–81.

19. Raymond E, Dahan L, Raoul JL, et al. Sunitinib malate for the treatment of pancreatic neuroendocrine tumors. N Engl J Med 2011;364(6):501–13.

20. Treglia G, Castaldi P, Rindi G, et al. Diagnostic performance of Gallium-68 somatostatin receptor PET and PET/CT in patients with thoracic and gastroenteropancreatic neuroendocrine tumours: a meta-analysis. Endocrine 2012;42(1):80–7.

21. Sadowski SM, Neychev V, Millo C, et al. Prospective study of 68Ga-DOTATATE positron emission tomography/computed tomography for detecting gastro-entero-pancreatic neuroendocrine tumors and unknown primary sites. J Clin Oncol 2016;34(6): 588–96.

22. Pool SE, Krenning EP, Koning GA, et al. Preclinical and clinical studies of peptide receptor radionuclide therapy. Semin Nucl Med 2010;40(3):209–18.

23. Essen MV, Krenning EP, Kam BLR, et al. Peptide-receptor radionuclide therapy for endocrine tumors. Nat Rev Endocrinol 2009;5(7):382–93.

24. Strosberg J, El-Haddad G, Wolin E, et al. Phase 3 trial of 177 Lu-dotatate for midgut neuroendocrine tumors. N Engl J Med 2017;376(2):125–35.

25. Brabander T, Zwan WA, Teunissen JJM, et al. Long-term efficacy, survival, and safety of [177 Lu-DOTA 0,Tyr 3] octreotate in patients with gastroentero-pancreatic and bronchial neuroendocrine tumors. Clin Cancer Res 2017;23(16):4617–24.

26. Eisenhauer EA, Therasse P, Bogaerts J, et al. New response evaluation criteria in solid tumours: revised RECIST guideline (version 1.1). Eur J Cancer 2009; 45(2):228–47.

27. Haug AR, Auernhammer CJ, Wangler B, et al. 68Ga-DOTATATE PET/CT for the early prediction of response to somatostatin receptor-mediated radionuclide therapy in patients with well-differentiated neuroendocrine tumors. J Nucl Med 2010;51(9): 1349–56.

28. Choi H. Response evaluation of gastrointestinal stromal tumors. Oncologist 2008;13(Suppl 2):4–7.

29. Faivre S, Ronot M, Dreyer C, et al. Imaging response in neuroendocrine tumors treated with targeted therapies: the experience of sunitinib. Target Oncol 2012;7(2):127–33.

30. Luo G, Javed A, Strosberg JR, et al. Modified staging classification for pancreatic neuroendocrine tumors on the basis of the American Joint Committee on Cancer and European Neuroendocrine Tumor Society Systems. J Clin Oncol 2017;35(3):274–80.

31. Sahani DV, Bonaffini PA, Castillo CFD, et al. Gastroenteropancreatic neuroendocrine tumors: role of imaging in diagnosis and management. Radiology 2013;266(1):38–61.

32. Kaur H, Hindman NM, Al-Refaie WB, et al. ACR appropriateness criteria ® suspected liver metastases. J Am Coll Radiol 2017;14(5S):S314–25.

33. Oliver JH 3rd, Baron RL, Federle MP, et al. Hypervascular liver metastases: do unenhanced and hepatic arterial phase CT images affect tumor detection? Radiology 1997;205(3):709–15.

34. d'Assignies G, Fina P, Bruno O, et al. High sensitivity of diffusion-weighted MR imaging for the detection of liver metastases from neuroendocrine tumors: comparison with T2-weighted and dynamic gadolinium-enhanced MR imaging. Radiology 2013;268(2):390–9.

35. Virgolini I, Ambrosini V, Bomanji JB, et al. Procedure guidelines for PET/CT tumour imaging with 68Ga-DOTA-conjugated peptides: 68Ga-DOTA-TOC, 68Ga-DOTA-NOC, 68Ga-DOTA-TATE. Eur J Nucl Med Mol Imaging 2010;37(10):2004–10.

36. Yang J, Kan Y, Ge BH, et al. Diagnostic role of Gallium-68 DOTATOC and Gallium-68 DOTATATE PET in patients with neuroendocrine tumors: a meta-analysis. Acta Radiol 2014;55(4):389–98.

37. Hope TA, Bergsland EK, Bozkurt MF, et al. Appropriate use criteria for somatostatin receptor PET imaging in neuroendocrine tumors. J Nucl Med 2018; 59(1):66–74.

38. Smith AD, Shah SN, Rini BI, et al. Morphology, Attenuation, Size, and Structure (MASS) criteria: assessing response and predicting clinical outcome in metastatic renal cell carcinoma on antiangiogenic targeted therapy. AJR Am J Roentgenol 2010; 194(6):1470–8.

39. Memon K, Lewandowski RJ, Mulcahy MF, et al. Radioembolization for neuroendocrine liver metastases: safety, imaging, and long-term outcomes. Int J Radiat Oncol Biol Phys 2012;83(3):887–94.

40. Atassi B, Bangash AK, Bahrani A, et al. Multimodality imaging following 90Y radioembolization: a comprehensive review and pictorial essay. Radiographics 2008;28(1):81–99.

41. Yeduuri S, Terpenning S, Gupta S, et al. Radiofrequency ablation of hepatic tumor: subjective assessment of the perilesional vascular network on contrast-enhanced computed tomography before and after ablation can reliably predict the risk of local recurrence. J Comput Assist Tomogr 2017;41(4):607–13.

42. Kwekkeboom DJ, Krenning EP. Somatostatin receptor imaging. Semin Nucl Med 2002;32(2):84–91.

43. Kratochwil C, Mavriopoulou MSE, Holland-Letz T, et al. SUV of [68Ga]DOTATOC-PET/CT predicts response probability of PRRT in neuroendocrine tumors. Mol Imaging Biol 2015;17(3):313–8.

44. Sharma R, Wang WM, Yusuf S, et al. 68 Ga-DOTATATE PET/CT parameters predict response to peptide receptor radionuclide therapy in neuroendocrine tumours. Radiother Oncol 2019;141: 108–15.

45. Strosberg JR, Halfdanarson TR, Bellizzi AM, et al. The North American Neuroendocrine Tumor Society consensus guidelines for surveillance and medical management of midgut neuroendocrine tumors. Pancreas 2017;46(6):707–14.

46. Tomozawa Y, Jahangiri Y, Pathak P, et al. Long-term toxicity after transarterial radioembolization with yttrium-90 using resin microspheres for neuroendocrine tumor liver metastases. J Vasc Interv Radiol 2018;29(6):858–65.

47. Devulapalli KK, Fidelman N, Soulen MC, et al. 90 Y radioembolization for hepatic malignancy in patients with previous biliary intervention: multicenter analysis of hepatobiliary infections. Radiology 2018; 288(3):774–81.

UNITED STATES POSTAL SERVICE®

Statement of Ownership, Management, and Circulation
(All Periodicals Publications Except Requester Publications)

1. Publication Title	2. Publication Number		3. Filing Date
RADIOLOGIC CLINICS OF NORTH AMERICA	596 – 510		9/18/2020

4. Issue Frequency	5. Number of Issues Published Annually	6. Annual Subscription Price
JAN, MAR, MAY, JUL, SEP, NOV	6	$513.00

7. Complete Mailing Address of Known Office of Publication (Not printer) (Street, city, county, state, and ZIP+4®)

ELSEVIER INC.
230 Park Avenue, Suite 800
New York, NY 10169

Contact Person
Malathi Samayan

Telephone (Include area code)
91-44-4299-4507

8. Complete Mailing Address of Headquarters or General Business Office of Publisher (Not printer)

ELSEVIER INC.
230 Park Avenue, Suite 800
New York, NY 10169

9. Full Names and Complete Mailing Addresses of Publisher, Editor, and Managing Editor (Do not leave blank)

Publisher (Name and complete mailing address)

DOLORES MELONI, ELSEVIER INC.
1600 JOHN F KENNEDY BLVD. SUITE 1800
PHILADELPHIA, PA 19103-2899

Editor (Name and complete mailing address)

JOHN VASSALLO, ELSEVIER INC.
1600 JOHN F KENNEDY BLVD. SUITE 1800
PHILADELPHIA, PA 19103-2899

Managing Editor (Name and complete mailing address)

PATRICK MANLEY, ELSEVIER INC.
1600 JOHN F KENNEDY BLVD. SUITE 1800
PHILADELPHIA, PA 19103-2899

10. Owner (Do not leave blank. If the publication is owned by a corporation, give the name and address of the corporation immediately followed by the names and addresses of all stockholders owning or holding 1 percent or more of the total amount of stock. If not owned by a corporation, give the names and addresses of the individual owners. If owned by a partnership or other unincorporated firm, give its name and address as well as those of each individual owner. If the publication is published by a nonprofit organization, give its name and address.)

Full Name	Complete Mailing Address
WHOLLY OWNED SUBSIDIARY OF REED/ELSEVIER, US HOLDINGS	1600 JOHN F KENNEDY BLVD. SUITE 1800 PHILADELPHIA, PA 19103-2899

11. Known Bondholders, Mortgagees, and Other Security Holders Owning or Holding 1 Percent or More of Total Amount of Bonds, Mortgages, or Other Securities. If none, check box ▶ ☐ None

Full Name	Complete Mailing Address
N/A	

12. Tax Status (For completion by nonprofit organizations authorized to mail at nonprofit rates) (Check one)
The purpose, function, and nonprofit status of this organization and the exempt status for federal income tax purposes:
☒ Has Not Changed During Preceding 12 Months
☐ Has Changed During Preceding 12 Months (Publisher must submit explanation of change with this statement)

PS Form **3526**, July 2014 [Page 1 of 4 (see instructions page 4)]   PSN: 7530-01-000-9931   PRIVACY NOTICE: See our privacy policy on www.usps.com

---

13. Publication Title	14. Issue Date for Circulation Data Below
RADIOLOGIC CLINICS OF NORTH AMERICA	JULY 2020

15. Extent and Nature of Circulation			Average No. Copies Each Issue During Preceding 12 Months	No. Copies of Single Issue Published Nearest to Filing Date
a. Total Number of Copies (Net press run)			847	766
b. Paid Circulation (By Mail and Outside the Mail)	(1)	Mailed Outside-County Paid Subscriptions Stated on PS Form 3541 (Include paid distribution above nominal rate, advertiser's proof copies, and exchange copies)	592	548
	(2)	Mailed In-County Paid Subscriptions Stated on PS Form 3541 (Include paid distribution above nominal rate, advertiser's proof copies, and exchange copies)	0	0
	(3)	Paid Distribution Outside the Mails Including Sales Through Dealers and Carriers, Street Vendors, Counter Sales, and Other Paid Distribution Outside USPS®	198	179
	(4)	Paid Distribution by Other Classes of Mail Through the USPS (e.g., First-Class Mail®)	0	0
c. Total Paid Distribution (Sum of 15b (1), (2), (3), and (4))		▶	790	727
d. Free or Nominal Rate Distribution (By Mail and Outside the Mail)	(1)	Free or Nominal Rate Outside-County Copies included on PS Form 3541	40	25
	(2)	Free or Nominal Rate In-County Copies Included on PS Form 3541	0	0
	(3)	Free or Nominal Rate Copies Mailed at Other Classes Through the USPS (e.g., First-Class Mail)	0	0
	(4)	Free or Nominal Rate Distribution Outside the Mail (Carriers or other means)	40	25
e. Total Free or Nominal Rate Distribution (Sum of 15d (1), (2), (3) and (4))		▶	830	752
f. Total Distribution (Sum of 15c and 15e)		▶	17	14
g. Copies not Distributed (See Instructions to Publishers #4 (page #3))		▶	847	766
h. Total (Sum of 15f and g)			95.18%	96.67%
i. Percent Paid (15c divided by 15f times 100)		▶		

* If you are claiming electronic copies, go to line 16 on page 3. If you are not claiming electronic copies, skip to line 17 on page 3.

16. Electronic Copy Circulation		Average No. Copies Each Issue During Preceding 12 Months	No. Copies of Single Issue Published Nearest to Filing Date
a. Paid Electronic Copies	▶		
b. Total Paid Print Copies (Line 15c) + Paid Electronic Copies (Line 16a)	▶		
c. Total Print Distribution (Line 15f) + Paid Electronic Copies (Line 16a)	▶		
d. Percent Paid (Both Print & Electronic Copies) (16b divided by 16c × 100)	▶		

☒ I certify that 50% of all my distributed copies (electronic and print) are paid above a nominal price.

17. Publication of Statement of Ownership

☒ If the publication is a general publication, publication of this statement is required. Will be printed in the NOVEMBER 2020 issue of this publication.   ☐ Publication not required.

18. Signature and Title of Editor, Publisher, Business Manager, or Owner

Malathi Samayan   Date 9/18/2020

Malathi Samayan - Distribution Controller

I certify that all information furnished on this form is true and complete. I understand that anyone who furnishes false or misleading information on this form or who omits material or information requested on the form may be subject to criminal sanctions (including fines and imprisonment) and/or civil sanctions (including civil penalties).

PS Form **3526**, July 2014 (Page 3 of 4)   PRIVACY NOTICE: See our privacy policy on www.usps.com

Moving?

Make sure your subscription moves with you!

To notify us of your new address, find your **Clinics Account Number** (located on your mailing label above your name), and contact customer service at:

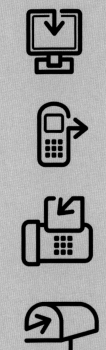

Email: **journalscustomerservice-usa@elsevier.com**

800-654-2452 (subscribers in the U.S. & Canada)
314-447-8871 (subscribers outside of the U.S. & Canada)

Fax number: **314-447-8029**

Elsevier Health Sciences Division
Subscription Customer Service
3251 Riverport Lane
Maryland Heights, MO 63043

*To ensure uninterrupted delivery of your subscription, please notify us at least 4 weeks in advance of move.

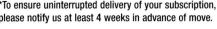